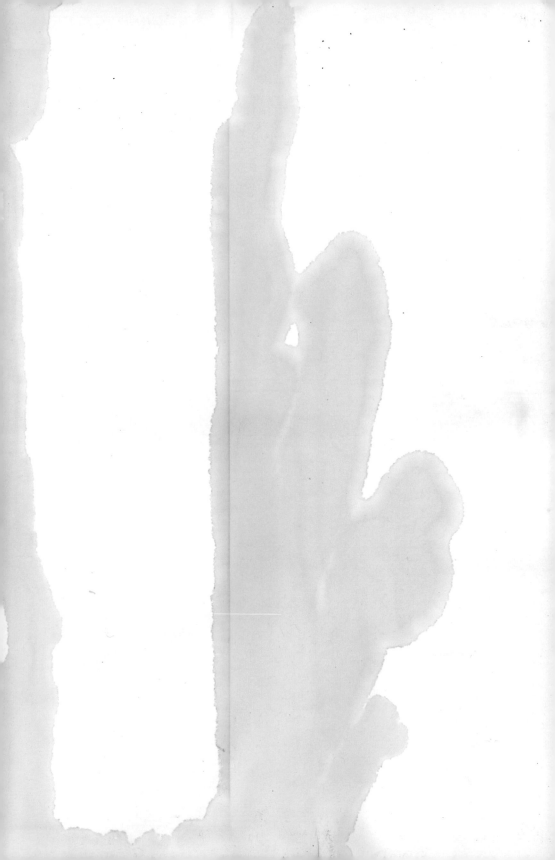

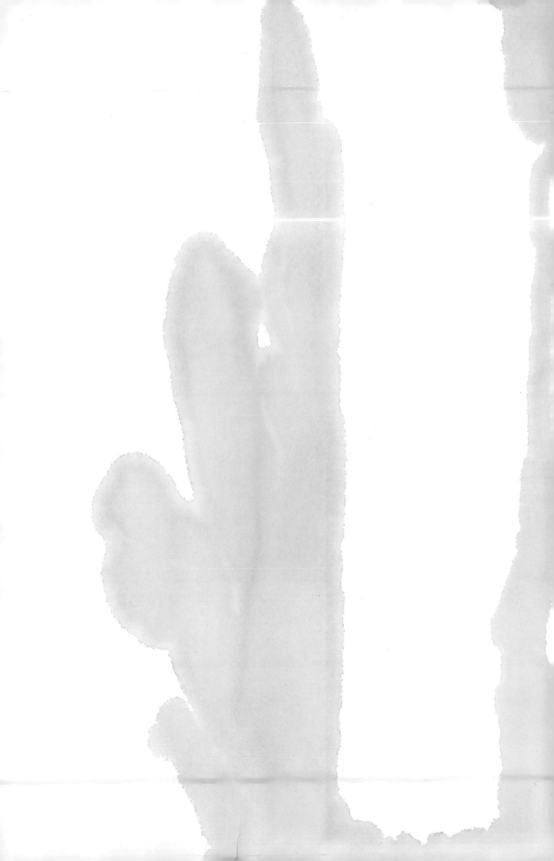

ATTACHMENT IN PSYCHOTHERAPY

Attachment in Psychotherapy

DAVID J. WALLIN

THE GUILFORD PRESS
New York   London

Library of Congress Cataloging-in-Publication Data

Wallin, David J.
  Attachment in psychotherapy / David J. Wallin.
     p. ; cm.
  Includes bibliographical references and index.
  ISBN-13: 978-1-59385-456-0 (hardcover : alk. paper)
  ISBN-10: 1-59385-456-0 (hardcover : alk. paper)
  1. Attachment behavior. 2. Object relations (Psychoanalysis) 3. Psychotherapy. I. Title.
  [DNLM: 1. Object Attachment. 2. Psychoanalytic Therapy—methods.
WM 460.5.O2 W211a 2007]
  RC455.4.A84W3557 2007
  616.89'17—dc22

                                               2007001234

For Gina, Anya, and Gabriel

Only connect! That was the whole of her sermon. Only connect the prose and the passion, and both will be exalted, and human love will be seen at its height. Live in fragments no longer. Only connect, and the beast and the monk, robbed of the isolation that is life to either, will die.
　　　　　　　　　　　　—E. M. FORSTER (1910/1999)

The being who is the object of his own reflection, in consequence of that very doubling back upon himself, becomes in a flash able to raise himself into a new sphere. In reality, another world is born.
　　　　　　　—PIERRE TEILHARD DE CHARDIN (1959)

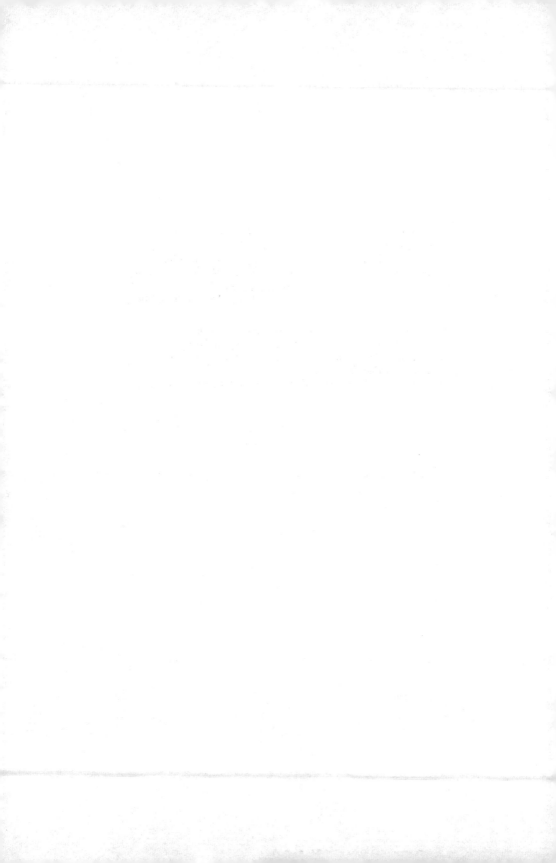

About the Author

David J. Wallin, PhD, is a clinical psychologist in private practice in Mill Valley and Albany, California. A graduate of Harvard College who received his doctorate from the Wright Institute in Berkeley, California, he has been practicing, teaching, and writing about psychotherapy for nearly three decades. Dr. Wallin is the coauthor (with Stephen Goldbart) of *Mapping the Terrain of the Heart: Passion, Tenderness, and the Capacity to Love.*

Preface

A single question launched the odyssey that produced this book: *How does psychotherapy enable people to change?*

This question has inspired my deepest curiosity for more than three decades, no doubt for personal as well as professional reasons. As a graduate student seeking a dissertation topic, I considered trying to solve the mystery by observing what master clinicians actually *did* with their patients. Years later I learned that attachment researchers had taken a related tack by observing what sensitively responsive parents actually did with their children.

Because "what good therapists do with their patients is analogous to what successful parents do with their children" (Holmes, 2001, p. xi), studies of developmentally facilitative relationships in childhood should teach us a great deal about the kinds of therapeutic relationships that most effectively foster change. Similarly, attachment research into the consequences of development gone awry should offer a scientifically grounded basis for understanding the suffering and vulnerabilities that bring our patients to therapy in the first place.

But exactly what *are* the clinical implications of the research and how can they make our work as therapists more effective?

That these questions have been so long in the answering is partially due to an accident of history. With the deepening of Bowlby's conviction that it is the *real* relationships of early childhood—not our internally driven fantasies about them—that fundamentally shape us, the man who would become the father of attachment theory found himself increasingly at odds with his psychoanalytic peers. For locating attachment (rather than the sexual or aggressive drives) at the heart of human development, he was effec-

tively marginalized by the analytic establishment of his day. The result was that attachment theory became the intellectual property primarily of academic researchers rather than psychotherapists. Hence, the irony that while Bowlby spent most of his own time treating patients, his theories—initially formulated to augment the effectiveness of treatment—were tested and elaborated by investigators, the majority of whom were not practicing clinicians.

These researchers brought empirical rigor to the study of the most intimate human bonds, generating the wealth of knowledge about parent–child relationships, the internal world, and psychopathology that has made attachment theory the dominant paradigm in contemporary developmental psychology. No other research-based framework tells us more about how we become who we are. Yet until quite recently therapists were largely left to draw their own inferences about how the theory is to be applied. Thus the clinical promise of attachment theory has remained unfulfilled.

This book represents my contribution to realizing that promise. Drawing on neurobiology, cognitive science, trauma studies, and Buddhist psychology as well as attachment theory and relational psychoanalysis, I aim to convey how therapists can make practical use of three key findings of attachment research. Accordingly, I focus on the therapeutic relationship as a developmental crucible, the centrality of the nonverbal dimension, and the transformative influence of reflection and mindfulness.

As originally conceived three years ago, the writing was to have been quickly completed. I'd been teaching about attachment and psychotherapy since the mid-1990s, and expected to be able to turn a transcript of that teaching into a book in no more than six to nine months. But the project of transposition became a process of discovery both far lengthier and more rewarding than I could have anticipated. I hope the following chapters record the outcome of that process in such a way that, as a reader, you may be able to share my experiences of discovery.

Acknowledgments

With the writing finally done, it's enormously gratifying to be able to thank all those who helped make it possible.

There from the inception were Nancy Kaplan, who really introduced me to attachment theory; Owen Renik, who inspired me to take risks in making bridges from attachment theory to clinical practice; and Karlen Lyons-Ruth, who encouraged my synthesis of developmental research and relational psychotherapy. Phillip Shaver proved extraordinarily generous with his insight and experience. Upon hearing he'd made a presentation on attachment to the Dalai Lama, I immediately called Phil and found that he, too, was intrigued by the therapeutic promise of partnering attachment with mindfulness. I'm also grateful to Erik Hesse and Mary Main for making themselves accessible to me in Berkeley, and for their thoughtful suggestions and support. On the other side of the Atlantic, Peter Fonagy has been unfailingly responsive. Talking with him about his ideas and mine has been a tremendous pleasure and help.

To Cindy Hyden I offer heartfelt thanks for her invaluable editorial input, wise counsel, and expert handholding. From book proposal to project's end she provided me with a secure base. To Jim Nageotte at The Guilford Press, I owe a special debt of gratitude. From the start, he recognized the book's potential and, all along the way, made important contributions to its substance and form.

Among the many friends, family members, and colleagues who read sections of the book, discussed its content, and/or extended their support to its author, I am grateful to Stephen Seligman, Richard Tarnas, Michael Blumlein, Lloyd and Catherine Kamins, Stephen Goldbart, Freda Wallin,

Michael Wallin, Laurie Cohen, David Shaddock, Michael Guy Thompson, Diana Fosha, Judy Pickles, Lynnette Beall, Barbara Holifield, Jules Burstein, Johanne Busch, Ava Charney-Danysh, Sara Fisher, Michael Gray, Linda Hendricks, and Horacio Miller. Thanks also to Bob Cassidy for his help in getting my ideas into the world and for inadvertently nudging the book into being. And thanks especially to Linda Graham for conversations over lunch that were always informative and often inspiring.

To my patients, and in particular to those who permitted me to use our shared experience in the book, I owe a very great deal. As they've let me into their lives, hearts, and minds, I've not only learned about how to be more helpful as a therapist, I've also learned about myself.

For her uniquely valuable contributions to my personal, professional, and creative life, I thank Alice Jones.

Finally, and foremost, I want to thank—but can't ever thank enough— my wife, Gina, and my children, Anya and Gabriel, whose love, (nearly) inexhaustible patience, and, yes, sacrifice made the writing possible. Beyond these gifts, Gina's intelligence, sensitivity, and clinical acumen have made her a remarkably insightful partner—and a valued collaborator—in shaping the ideas that became this book.

Contents

xv

CHAPTER 1

Attachment and Change

. . . the therapist's role is analogous to that of a mother who provides her child with a secure base from which to explore the world.

—JOHN BOWLBY (1988, p. 140)

In the world according to Bowlby, our lives, from the cradle to the grave, revolve around intimate attachments. Although our stance toward such attachments is shaped most influentially by our first relationships, we are also malleable. If our early involvements have been problematic, then subsequent relationships can offer second chances, perhaps affording us the potential to love, feel, and reflect with the freedom that flows from secure attachment. Psychotherapy, at its best, provides just such a healing relationship.

Precisely how as psychotherapists we can enable our patients to grow beyond the limits imposed by their history is a question that attachment theory does not directly address. Yet the ongoing research inspired by Bowlby's original insights has enormous clinical value, offering us a progressively clearer view of the development of the self in a specifically relational context.

In attempting to harness the power of this research, I have identified three findings that appear to have the most profound and fertile implications for psychotherapy: first, that co-created *relationships of attachment* are the key context for development; second, that *preverbal experience* makes up the core of the developing self; and third, that the *stance of the self toward experience* predicts attachment security better than the facts of personal history themselves.

1

In drawing out the clinical implications of these three core conclusions, I reach into the attachment literature, of course. But I also reach beyond it, not only to intersubjective and relational theory but also to affective neuroscience—which Allan Schore (2004) calls the "neurobiology of attachment"—as well as cognitive science, trauma studies, and explorations of consciousness. The present chapter plumbs the three core findings regarding the developmental centrality of attachment relationships, preverbal experience, and the reflective function. And it distills their clinical yield in a model of psychotherapy that involves the *transformation of the self through relationship*. My aim here is to convey the orientation to emotional healing—the clinical philosophy derived from reviewing research, theory, and personal experience—that underlies all the various approaches I take in order to be of help to my patients.

As I will explain, the proposed model of psychotherapy as transformation through relationship describes a trajectory that parallels the unfolding story of attachment theory itself. Bowlby (1969/1982) began by recognizing that attachment is a biological imperative rooted in evolutionary necessity: The attachment relationship to the caregiver(s) is critical to the infant's physical and emotional survival and development. Given the requirement to attach, the infant must adapt to the caregiver, defensively excluding whatever behavior threatens the attachment bond. Mary Ainsworth's research (Ainsworth, Blehar, Waters, & Wall, 1978) then clarified that it is the quality of the *nonverbal* communication in the attachment relationship that determines the infant's security or insecurity—and along with it, the infant's approach to his or her own feelings. Mary Main's investigations (Main, Kaplan, & Cassidy, 1985) illuminated the ways in which these early biologically mandated nonverbal interactions register in the infant as mental representations and rules for processing information that influence, in turn, how freely the older child, adolescent, and adult is able to think, feel, remember, and act. Finally, Main (1991) and Peter Fonagy (Fonagy, Steele, & Steele, 1991a) highlighted the crucial importance of the stance of the self in relation to its own experience. They showed that security of attachment, resilience, and the ability to raise secure children all are correlated with the individual's capacity to adopt a reflective stance toward experience. Thus, from Bowlby to Ainsworth, Main, and Fonagy, the evolving narrative of attachment theory has unfolded through a focus on intimate bonds, the nonverbal realm, and the relation of the self to experience.

The same three themes organize the model of therapy as transformation through relationship. In this model, the patient's attachment relationship to the therapist is foundational and primary. It supplies the secure base that is the *sine qua non* for exploration, development, and change. This sense of a secure base arises from the attuned therapist's effectiveness in helping the patient to tolerate, modulate, and communicate difficult feel-

ings. By virtue of the felt security generated through such affect-regulating interactions, the therapeutic relationship can provide a context for accessing disavowed or dissociated experiences within the patient that have not—and perhaps cannot—be put into words. The relationship is also a context within which the therapist and patient, having made room for these experiences, can attempt to make sense of them. Accessing, articulating, and reflecting upon dissociated and unverbalized feelings, thoughts, and impulses strengthen the patient's "narrative competence" (Holmes, 1996) and help to shift in a more reflective direction the patient's stance toward experience. Overall, the *relational/emotional/reflective process* at the heart of an attachment-focused therapy facilitates the integration of disowned experience, thus fostering in the patient a more coherent and secure sense of self.

TRANSFORMATIVE RELATIONSHIPS

Very much as the original attachment relationship(s) allowed the child to develop, it is ultimately the *new* relationship of attachment with the therapist that allows the patient to change. To paraphrase Bowlby (1988), such a relationship provides a secure base that enables the patient to take the risk of feeling what he is not supposed to feel and knowing what he is not supposed to know. The therapist's role here is to help the patient both to deconstruct the attachment patterns of the past and to construct new ones in the present. As we have seen, the patterns played out in our first attachments are reflected subsequently not only in the ways we relate to others, but also in our habits of feeling and thinking. Correspondingly, the patient's relationship with the therapist has the potential to generate fresh patterns of affect regulation and thought, as well as attachment. Put differently, the therapeutic relationship is a developmental crucible within which the patient's relation to his own experience of internal and external reality can be fundamentally transformed.

THE UNTHOUGHT KNOWN

Given the prelinguistic roots of the patient's original attachment patterns, and the disavowals and dissociations they may have demanded, the therapist must tune in to the nonverbal expressions of experience for which the patient has as yet no words. That is, the therapist must find ways to connect with what Christopher Bollas (1987) has called the patient's "unthought known." Grasping the unspoken (or unthinkable) subtext of the therapeutic conversation requires what several writers (Bateson, 1979; Bion, 1959) have referred to as the clinician's "binocular vision" that

tracks the subjectivity of both the patient and the therapist. The underlying assumption here is that the patient who cannot (or will not) articulate his own dissociated or disavowed experience will *evoke* it in others, *enact* it with others, or *embody* it. The clinical implication is that the therapist must pay particular attention to her own subjective experience, to the transference–countertransference enactments jointly created by patient and therapist, and to the nonverbal language of emotion and the body—for all these are routes to accessing and eventually integrating what the patient has had to deny or disown.

THE STANCE TOWARD EXPERIENCE:
REPRESENTATION, REFLECTION, AND MINDFULNESS

Along with its emphasis on the centrality of relational and nonverbal experience, attachment research underscores the salience of the reflective function and metacognition. More broadly, this research reveals the decisive impact of the stance of the self toward its own experience.

Secure attachment is clearly associated with a reflective stance toward experience. In Main's (1991) account, this stance rests on the metacognitive capacity to recognize the "*merely* representational nature" of our own beliefs and feelings (p. 128). With such a stance, we can step back from the immediate "reality" of experience and respond in light of the mental states that might underlie it—to use Fonagy's term, we can "mentalize." With greater freedom to mentalize, we are less likely to be inescapably gripped by emotional reflexes laid down in the course of our first relationships. As research using Main's Adult Attachment Interview has revealed, the reflective stance toward experience is entirely different from that found in insecure individuals who tend either to minimize and deny the impact of their experience (in the dismissing state of mind) or to be overwhelmed by it (in the preoccupied state of mind). As a rule, the more we are able to mobilize a reflective stance the more resilient we will be, and the more capable of raising secure children.

By the same token, to "raise" secure patients, we must cultivate in ourselves this capability for reflection in psychological depth. And, of course, we must nurture it in those who come to us for help. As therapists, our efforts to foster or disinhibit our patients' mentalizing capacities are an essential feature of the help we offer. To the extent that we make it possible for patients to mentalize, we strengthen their ability to regulate their affects, to integrate experiences that have been dissociated, and to feel a more solid, coherent sense of self.

Beyond the capacity for a reflective stance, I would argue that there exists the potential for a stance toward internal and external experience that

is, in some sense, "deeper" and closer to the subjective center of ourselves. I am thinking here about a stance that involves deliberate nonjudgmental attention to experience in the present moment—that is, a stance of *mindfulness* (Germer, Siegel, & Fulton, 2005; Kabat-Zinn, 2005). While mindfulness is not part of the vocabulary of attachment, this construct from Buddhist psychology seems a natural outgrowth of attachment theory and research. In fact, Phillip Shaver, coeditor of the *Handbook of Attachment,* told me that recently, in preparing a scientific presentation for the Dalai Lama, he had occasion to read nearly a dozen books on Buddhism. To his surprise, he found the psychology there to be not only consistent with but in many respects virtually identical to the psychology of attachment theory (Shaver, personal communication, 2005).

To clarify what is meant by a stance of mindfulness, imagine four concentric rings each of which represents an element that contributes to the moment-to-moment experience of being a "mindful self."

The outermost ring stands for external reality. The world of external reality includes not only the events that happen to us and the situations we co-create but also, perhaps most importantly, the people with whom we are involved.

Moving inward there is a second ring that stands for the representational world: that is, the mental models of previous experience that relieve us of the necessity to reinvent the wheel with every new moment. These representational models orient us, shaping our interpretations of past and present, and establishing our expectations for the future.

Within the second ring is a third, standing for that part of ourselves that is capable of a reflective stance toward experience—in shorthand, the "reflective self." Here our representations, including our internal working models, are understood to mediate or filter our experience of external reality. We neither equate the subjective world of representations with the objective world of external reality nor deny the impact of external reality upon our subjective experience. With such a stance we can reflect, consciously and unconsciously, on the meaning of our experience rather than simply take that experience at face value. This affords us a significant measure of internal freedom.

Attachment theory deals explicitly only with the elements represented by these first three rings: external reality, the representational world, and the reflective self. It seems to me, however, that there is a trajectory to the evolving narrative of attachment theory that points like an arrow to a fourth ring inside the other three. This fourth ring represents what I am calling the mindful self.

To put it somewhat cryptically, this self is the answer to the question, Who (or what) is it that actually reflects on experience? For if a reflective stance involves metacognition—thinking about thinking—then it seems

natural to ask *who is it that is thinking the thoughts about thinking.* You might try, as I did, to close your eyes and pose this question to yourself. My own (experientially derived) response to the question took me by surprise. It was: *no one.* Dovetailing with a fundamental tenet of Buddhist psychology, this elusive understanding reflects the paradox that the mindful self can be at once a secure self and no (personal) self at all, but only awareness (see Goldstein & Kornfield, 1987; Kornfield, 1993; Engler, 2003).

Jeremy Holmes (1996), who writes eloquently about attachment, touches on the same paradox when he acknowledges borrowing from Buddhism the term *nonattachment* to describe an "equidistant position" that includes awareness *both* of the depth and breadth of the self's experience *and* of the fact that the self is "ultimately a fiction" (p. 30).

Another angle on this matter of mindfulness: While the reflective stance toward experience entails metacognition, a mindful stance involves *meta-awareness*—that is, awareness of awareness. Put differently, the self that *reflects* on experience attends to the contents of experience while the self that is *mindful* attends to the process of experiencing. Such mindful attention illuminates the process by which experience is constructed (Engler, 2003).

Fonagy alludes to research highlighting the clinical potential of mindfulness meditation as an adjunct to psychotherapy. He notes that "what we would call 'mentalizing' is directly enhanced by meditation practice" (Allen & Fonagy, 2002, p. 35). Fonagy's point is undoubtedly well taken. Yet mindfulness involves more than formal meditation. And meditation supports more than mentalizing.

The regular exercise of mindful awareness seems to promote the same benefits—bodily and affective self-regulation, attuned communication with others, insight, empathy, and the like—that research has found to be associated with childhood histories of secure attachment (Siegel, 2005, 2006). Although there may be other explanations for these parallel outcomes, I would suggest that they arise from the fact that mindfulness and secure attachment alike are capable of generating—though by very different routes—the same invaluable psychological resource, namely, an *internalized* secure base.

Secure attachment relationships in childhood and psychotherapy help develop this reassuring internal presence by providing us with experiences of being recognized, understood, and cared for that can subsequently be internalized. Mindfulness practice can potentially develop a comparably reassuring internal presence by offering us (glimpsed or sustained) experiences of the selfless, or universal, self that is simply awareness. Such experiences are often marked by profound feelings of security, acceptance, and connection, in relation as much to others as to ourselves (Linda Graham, personal communication, 2006).

As therapists, our own capacity to be mindful may be critical to our efforts to be of help to our patients. First, and perhaps most crucially, a mindful stance fosters the experience of being firmly lodged in the present moment. The British psychoanalyst Wilfrid Bion (1970) captures this state of open presence as well as any Buddhist philosopher when he extols the advantages of approaching the patient "without memory, desire, or understanding" (pp. 51–52). Thus rooted in the here and now—rather than the remembered past, the wished-for future, or the abstractions of theory—we are less vulnerable to our own tendencies to be either dismissing or preoccupied. A mindful stance allows us to be more fully present, open, and capable of responding—like the "good enough" attuned parent—to the requirements of the moment as these emerge in our interaction with the patient. Second, a mindful and present-centered stance fosters an experience of being inside, and aware of, the body. The resulting attunement to our own somatic responses amplifies the signals that allow us to tune in to the non-verbal expressions of the patient's internal state. Thus, mindfulness can potentially enhance accurate empathy as well as our ability to connect with the patient's unarticulated, and perhaps dissociated, experience. Third, mindfulness (like a secure state of mind with respect to attachment) fosters an attitude of acceptance—a nondefensive openness and receptivity to experience *as it is* that can help us make room for the full spectrum of the patient's feelings, thoughts, and desires. In this way, mindfulness in the therapist may facilitate a relationship with the patient that fosters the process of integration.

Such integration may be not only a primary goal of psychotherapy but also (as previously suggested) a consequence both of secure attachment and of the practice of mindful awareness. As part of what makes the therapeutic relationship a transformative one, the therapist's mindful stance may have a "contagious" quality—kindling the patient's own experience of mindfulness very much as expressions of the therapist's reflective stance help to kindle the patient's ability to mentalize. With some patients, in addition, it may be helpful for the therapist to encourage the formal practice of meditation.

I trust I have made it clear that, viewed through the lens of attachment theory and research, the healing power of psychotherapy derives primarily from the therapeutic interaction. The new relationship of attachment that the patient forms with the therapist can potentially function as a developmental crucible. In the chapters to follow, I delve more deeply into the three key themes—the relationship, the nonverbal dimension, and the stance of the self toward experience—that orient my work with every patient. The chapters in Part I summarize the story of attachment theory and research, establishing in the process the book's conceptual foundation. Part II de-

scribes the impact of attachment relationships on the developing self. Part III makes the first bridges from attachment theory to the practice of psychotherapy. Part IV explains the clinical implications that follow from identifying the patient's prevailing pattern(s) of attachment. Part V details further the nature of therapeutic work in the nonverbal realm as well as the ways in which we can attempt to both cultivate in ourselves and elicit in our patients a more reflective and mindful stance toward experience.

PART I

BOWLBY AND BEYOND

John Bowlby was, of course, the father of attachment theory. His seminal contributions were empirically tested and eventually elaborated by Mary Ainsworth. Their intellectual relationship was a cross-fertilizing, mutually influential one in which Bowlby's ideas provided the initial impetus for Ainsworth's research, which then reshaped Bowlby's thinking—thus sparking further rounds of research and refinements in theory. Their collaboration gave birth to the fundamental structure of attachment theory and led to the explosion of empirical investigation the theory has triggered.

The conclusions of Bowlby and Ainsworth were extended through the work of Mary Main, who brought the focus of attachment research from infancy to adulthood and from nonverbal behavior to mental representation. In turn, Main's contributions inspired Peter Fonagy and his colleagues, who identified intersubjective attachment relationships as the key context within which the vital human capacities for insight and empathy can develop.

In relating the story of attachment theory research, Part I concentrates on those findings that have the most direct and fertile implications for psychotherapy. As such, it can be seen to supply the conceptual foundation for the clinically focused chapters that come later.

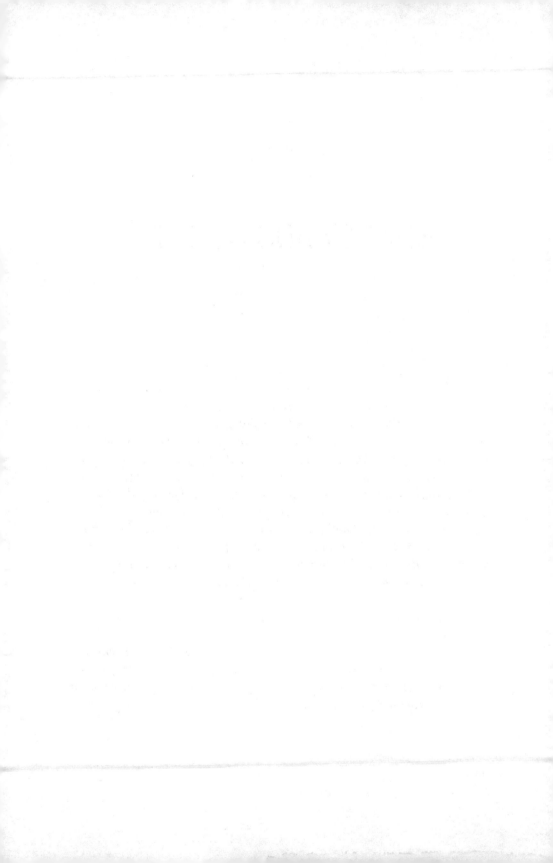

CHAPTER 2

The Foundations
of Attachment Theory

While Bowlby is commonly described as the father of attachment theory, there are those like Inge Bretherton (1995) who assert that the theory is actually the brainchild of *two* parents, the (m)other being Mary Ainsworth. Although Ainsworth is said to have remarked more than once that "Bowlby does the theory" (Karen, 1994, p. 434), I believe that here she was vastly understating her own importance. When I asked Bowlby's son how his father regarded Ainsworth's role, Sir Richard Bowlby replied that from his father's point of view,

> they were the dynamic duo. You couldn't say who did the theory anymore than you could say of a set of stairs, this one's part of the staircase, but the one above isn't. Their relationship was one long conversation. Without Ainsworth my father would have been a shadow . . . [though] without my father Ainsworth would have been nothing. (R. Bowlby, personal communication, 2004).

JOHN BOWLBY: PROXIMITY, PROTECTION, AND SEPARATION

Bowlby's core contribution was to recognize the biologically based evolutionary necessity of the attachment of a child to its caregiver. Bowlby understood that the primal nature of attachment as a motivational system is rooted in the infant's absolute need to maintain physical proximity to the

caregiver, not just to promote emotional security but in fact to ensure the infant's literal survival. In the natural environments to which our human ancestors had to adapt, a host of predators and other mortal threats made it extremely unlikely that an infant separated from protective figures could survive for many minutes, much less hours (Main, Hesse, & Kaplan, 2005). Thus what Bowlby called the *attachment behavioral system* was "designed" by evolution to enhance the probability of survival and reproductive success. As such, the attachment system is no less a component of human genetic programming than are feeding and mating (Bowlby, 1969/ 1982).

This collection of inborn, instinctively guided responses to threat and insecurity is evidenced in three kinds of behavior:

1. *Seeking, monitoring, and attempting to maintain proximity to a protective attachment figure*—or one of a tiny hierarchy of attachment figures—who is usually but not invariably a relative. While it might seem that whomever the child is most involved with (mother, father, or another caregiver) would be at the top of the attachment hierarchy, this place of preference turns out in fact to be regularly occupied by the mother—regardless of the extent of the child's involvement with her.[1] Crying, clinging, calling, and crawling to the attachment figure(s) are all part of the young child's biologically engrained repertoire for establishing the security of proximity.

2. *Using the attachment figure as a "secure base"* (in Ainsworth's phrase) from which to explore unfamiliar settings and experiences (Ainsworth, 1963). Consider, as illustrations of the secure base phenomenon, Margaret Mahler's well-known observations of infants and toddlers who briefly venture away from mother, only to return to her for a few moments in order to "refuel" before once again resuming exploration (Mahler, Pine, & Bergman, 1975). What Bowlby called the *exploratory behavioral system* is intimately related to the attachment system. When a child's attachment figure is available as a secure base to provide protection and support when needed, the child generally feels free to explore. When, on the other hand, the attachment figure is temporarily absent, exploration abruptly ceases.

3. *Fleeing to an attachment figure as a "safe haven" in situations of danger and moments of alarm.* In common with other ground-dwelling primates but unlike many other species, human beings who are threatened seek safety not in a *place* (like a burrow or a den) but rather in the company of a *person* regarded as "stronger and/or wiser" (Bowlby, 1988, p. 121). Internal and external threats to the infant's survival, "natural clues of danger" (e.g., darkness, loud sounds, and unfamiliar settings), and actual, or impending, separation from the mother can all trigger the proximity seeking that is the hallmark of attachment behavior.

If physical proximity per se was the "set goal" of attachment when Bowlby first began to articulate his theory, the vision has since been elaborated and refined. Bowlby himself came to realize that physical proximity, crucial in its own right, is also a symbol signifying the comforting availability of the caregiver. In this light, the goal of attachment behavior is not only protection from present danger but also reassurance of the caregiver's ongoing availability. And given that a caregiver could be at once physically accessible and emotionally absent, Bowlby defined the attachment figure's "availability" as a matter not just of accessibility but of emotional responsiveness as well.

To this broadened understanding he eventually added the specifically internal dimension of attachment, asserting that it was actually the child's *appraisal* of the caregiver's availability that was critical and that this appraisal in the present largely depended on the child's experience of the caregiver's availability in the past (Bowlby, 1973). In much the same vein, Sroufe and Waters (1977a) argued that the set goal of the attachment system is not primarily distance regulation but rather "felt security"—a subjective state that hinges not on the behavior of the caregiver alone but on the child's internal experience as well, including his or her own mood, physical condition, imaginings, and so on.

Keep in mind that while Bowlby originally focused on the behavior of infants and young children, he came to believe that the manifestations of the biologically driven need to attach are significant across the entire lifespan. This belief is suggestively corroborated by statistics and everyday experience. Actuarial data demonstrate that people who are partnered and/or have close friends live longer than those who are isolated, just as the data of nearly universal experience confirm that in times of threat—think of September 11, 2001—we reach out to those with whom we are intimate. The more extreme the threat the stronger is the desire for connection, not infrequently through the literal proximity of skin-to-skin contact. Evidently bodily closeness, essential to the infant's survival, can often be experienced as an emotional necessity among older children and adults.

Throughout our lives we are prone to monitor the physical and emotional whereabouts—the accessibility and responsiveness—of those to whom we are most attached. Thus, especially once felt security is added to proximity as the set goal, attachment must be seen as an ongoing human need rather than a childlike dependency that we outgrow as we grow up. As Bowlby (1980) put it:

> Intimate attachments to other human beings are the hub around which a person's life revolves, not only when he is an infant or a toddler, but throughout his adolescence and his years of maturity as well, and on into old age. (p. 442)

But what makes secure attachments possible in early childhood and, for that matter, across the entire lifespan? Bowlby was profoundly discontent with the psychoanalytic explanations of his day—like those of Melanie Klein that located the origins of healthy and pathological development exclusively in the fantasies of the child, rather than in the actualities of the child's formative relationships. Less than a year before he died in 1989, Bowlby expressed his own vision in an interview with Robert Karen (1994):

> I held the view that real-life events—the way parents treat a child—is of key importance in determining development, and Melanie Klein would have none of it. . . . The notion that internal relationships reflect external relationships was totally missing from her thinking. (p. 46)

Bowlby had been supervised by Klein during his analytic training. Working five days a week with an anxiety-ridden boy, Bowlby was dismayed when Klein forbade him to meet with his young patient's overwhelmingly anxious mother. His dismay turned to horror, however, when three months into the case the mother was hospitalized with agitated depression and Klein's only reaction was annoyance that now there was no one to bring the child to treatment:

> The fact that this poor woman had had a breakdown was of no clinical interest to her whatever. . . . [T]his horrified me, to be quite frank. And from that point onwards my mission in life was to demonstrate that real-life experiences have a very important effect on development. (p. 46)

Bowlby's emphasis on the *realities* of how we are treated by those who matter most to us arose only partly in reaction to the psychoanalytic shibboleths of his day. More important, perhaps, was his exposure to children *in extremis*—specifically children whose relationships with their mothers had been disrupted by deprivation, separation, or loss. Working in the late 1930s as a psychiatrist at London's Child Guidance Center, Bowlby spent nearly three years treating and studying delinquent boys; he detailed the catastrophic impact of protracted separations in early childhood in "Forty-Four Juvenile Thieves: Their Characters and Home-life" (1944). As a result of that work, the World Health Organization (WHO) commissioned Bowlby in 1949 to compose a monograph on the emotional fate of children made homeless in the aftermath of World War II (Bowlby, 1951). Finally, as deputy director of the Tavistock Clinic's children's department, Bowlby witnessed the psychic devastation that resulted when prolonged hospitalization or institutionalization of toddlers separated them from their parents.

The factual realities of separation and loss had an undeniably calamitous impact on the delinquent, homeless, and hospitalized children he had observed. Bowlby (1969/1982) discovered that this impact regularly played out in a sequence of responses that reflected the child's struggle to cope with painful reality. The initial reaction to traumatic separation was protest, followed by despair that, in turn, finally gave way to detachment.

While Bowlby's studies of separation and loss had a profound influence on his approach to understanding human development, it is also true that these kinds of trauma became the primary focus of his investigations in large part because they could be empirically documented and scientifically researched (Bowlby, 1986; Bretherton, 1991). By contrast, in his WHO monograph on children ravaged by the dislocations of war, Bowlby had alluded to the much harder-to-investigate but equally corrosive effects of chronically inadequate parenting. In the same report, he theorized that to make healthy development possible "the infant and young child should experience a warm, intimate, and continuous relationship with his mother (or permanent mother substitute) in which both find satisfaction and enjoyment" (Bowlby, 1951, p. 13). The point is this: Bowlby knew that more universally than the trauma of separation and loss, it was the ongoing, everyday interactions of children and their parents that shaped psychological development—and yet he lacked the empirical tools to study them. In due course, these ordinary, but exceedingly hard-to-research interactions would become the focus of exploration for Bowlby's colleague Mary Ainsworth.

MARY AINSWORTH: ATTACHMENT, COMMUNICATION, AND THE "STRANGE SITUATION"

A developmental psychologist and researcher at the University of Toronto, Ainsworth was also a brilliant diagnostician who eventually coauthored a book with the leading Rorschach expert of the day, Bruno Klopfer. When she married in 1950, Ainsworth relocated with her husband to London, where late in the year she responded to a job advertisement placed by Bowlby in the *Times* seeking a researcher into the psychological impact of early childhood separation from the mother. Thus began a reciprocally influential collaboration that lasted for nearly 40 years during which Ainsworth took on the initial task of empirically testing Bowlby's hypotheses. Her investigations—first in Uganda, then in Baltimore—transformed attachment theory and research.

While her studies clearly confirmed many of Bowlby's ideas, Ainsworth also made independent contributions that proved absolutely critical to the evolution of the attachment concept. Most important, perhaps, she discovered that the inborn, biologically driven attachment system is actually

malleable—and that qualitative differences in the attachment behavior of individuals depend on the differential behavior of caregivers (Grossman, 1995). This discovery led to the classification of attachment styles in infancy and adulthood that is such a central part of what attachment theory brings to psychotherapy.

Ainsworth also identified, in a preliminary way, the kinds of parent–child interactions most likely to produce secure attachment, on the one hand, or the varieties of insecure attachment, on the other. The key to security or insecurity, she realized, was to be found in the *patterns of communication* between infant and caregiver.

In addition, Ainsworth was responsible for the "secure base" concept and had a pivotal role in moving attachment beyond the exclusive focus on proximity, so as to include the influence of the child's *expectations* of the caregiver—expectations that eventually gel in the mental maps or representations that Bowlby dubbed "internal working models." Finally, there is the contribution—bearing her name—that became virtually synonymous with the study of attachment: the Ainsworth Strange Situation. First devised and deployed in Baltimore in 1964, this laboratory procedure for studying infant–parent relationships set off the explosion of research that has made attachment theory the dominant paradigm of contemporary developmental psychology.

Ainsworth in Uganda

The investigative journey that culminated in the Strange Situation began 10 years earlier when Ainsworth again relocated with her husband, this time to Uganda. Like Bowlby, with whom she had been researching the impact of traumatic separation for three and a half years, Ainsworth had become convinced that the study of "development gone awry" was inadequate as a basis for understanding the normal development of attachment (Marvin & Britner, 1999). Therefore, shortly after settling in Kampala, she launched the first ever naturalistic, longitudinal study of infants in interaction with their mothers. For nine months, Ainsworth observed 26 families with infants who had yet to be weaned. Visiting each family for two hours every two weeks, she collected data that began to answer fundamental questions about the ontogeny of attachment: What characterizes the "gestation" of an attachment bond and what signals its "birth"? What promotes secure attachment and what impedes it?

The data (Ainsworth, 1967) suggested that attachment develops through stages in which the infant's initial lack of differentiation of mother from others is replaced by a clear preference for her that—between six and nine months—crystallizes in a powerful bond. The crystallizing of attachment proper was reflected in (among other behaviors) the infants' flight to

mother when distressed or alarmed, their use of her as a secure base for exploration, and their active approach to her upon reunion. Ainsworth's documentation of the infants' shared developmental trajectory offered clear empirical support for Bowlby's theory. Yet it was actually the differences among these infants (rather than the commonalities) that she found most intriguing.

Whereas the majority of infants were unmistakably attached, a minority could not be soothed by their mothers and largely failed to explore, while a smaller minority showed virtually no evidence of attachment at all. Ainsworth theorized that these unexpected variations reflected differences in the nature of the caregiving the infants had experienced. While the infants who received the greatest amount of care and attention from their mothers were generally the most likely to be secure, there were striking exceptions that led Ainsworth to believe that it was not the quantity of care that counted but, rather, the *quality*. On the basis of interviews with the mothers, she tentatively concluded that the mother's sensitivity to her infant's signals was of paramount importance. She also found a positive correlation between the infant's attachment security and the mother's pleasure in breast feeding (Bretherton, 1995; Marvin & Britner, 1999). The latter finding supported Bowlby's early hypothesis (Bowlby, 1951) that healthy development hinges on *both* parties' enjoyment of the attachment relationship. While Ainsworth was ultimately unable to specify which kinds of maternal behavior were conducive to the development of secure attachment and which were not, her identification of the probable link between maternal attunement and attachment hinted at what she would discover eight years later in Baltimore upon replicating, but also very significantly refining, the study she had conducted in Uganda.

The "Strange Situation"

In 1963, Ainsworth enlisted 26 pregnant mothers to participate in a home-based study of early development. Once the babies were born, their interactions with their mothers were meticulously documented over the course of a year. During 18 four-hour visits to each family, Ainsworth and her team collected data demonstrating a near-perfect overlap between the attachment behaviors noted in Baltimore and those originally observed in Uganda. This cross-cultural correlation lent support to Bowlby's assertion that attachment was a universal instinctive need. Yet Ainsworth was also aware of a puzzling and provocative difference between the two groups: While the Ugandan infants at home conspicuously displayed secure base behavior, the Baltimore cohort did not.

For Ainsworth, the secure base phenomenon was central, its presence signifying the security that was reflected in a balanced capacity for explora-

tion and attachment. In Uganda, infant exploration had taken off in the presence of the attachment figure, only to be abruptly terminated by distress at her departure. In Baltimore, by contrast, exploration seemed to go on whether the attachment figure was present or not.[2] To help determine whether secure base behavior was, in fact, a genetic given as Bowlby had theorized, Ainsworth conceived (with Barbara Wittig) an initially controversial procedure that skirted the problem of familiarity by presenting the Baltimore infants with a "strange situation" (Ainsworth, Blehar, Waters, & Wall, 1978).

In this structured laboratory assessment lasting roughly 20 minutes, mothers and their infants—now 12 months old—were introduced to a pleasant, toy-filled room. What followed in a series of three-minute episodes included opportunities for the infant to explore, in the mother's presence, two separations from the mother, two reunions, and the infant's exposure to a stranger (always a trained baby watcher). The expectation was that the disquieting combination of an unfamiliar setting, separation, and a stranger would trigger the predictable, biologically based manifestations of the attachment behavioral system. Ainsworth predicted that using the mother as a secure base, the infants who had been judged secure in the home would play in her presence, experience distress at her departure, and be sufficiently reassured by her return to make continued playful exploration possible. Ainsworth also expected that infants judged insecure in the home would be highly upset during the episodes of separation. As it happened, however, the Strange Situation behavior of some of the infants took Ainsworth completely by surprise.

The majority of the Baltimore babies—who turned out to be those judged "secure" on the basis of a year's worth of observations in the home—did indeed respond as they were predicted to, demonstrating a flexible capacity both to explore freely and to be consoled by connection. What Ainsworth failed to anticipate, and initially could not understand, was the substantial minority of infants who seemed to have sacrificed connection altogether in favor of exploration. Because they not only explored throughout the entire procedure but also avoided mother upon reunion, these infants were described as "avoidant." In contrast, a smaller minority of infants appeared to have given up exploration completely in favor of connection. Because they not only remained continuously preoccupied with mother's whereabouts but also were angrily or passively inconsolable upon reunion, these infants were called "ambivalent" (or, alternatively, "resistant").

Undoubtedly, Ainsworth's greatest contribution to attachment theory was her detection through the Strange Situation of three distinct attachment patterns each of which was associated with a correspondingly different pattern of mother–infant interaction in the home. Because both the

infant classifications and the styles of interaction that seem to produce them are profoundly relevant to clinical work, it is important to summarize them in some detail.

The Attachment Classifications of Infancy

Secure Attachment

Secure babies appear to have equal access to their impulses to explore when they feel safe and to seek solace in connection when they do not. Ainsworth had concluded that it was the infants' responses to reunion, rather than separation, that revealed the most about attachment security or insecurity. Secure infants—however distressed by separation—were almost immediately reassured by reconnecting with their mother and readily resumed play.

This kind of flexibility and resilience seemed to be the legacy of interactions with a sensitive mother who was responsive to her baby's signals and communications. Generally, mothers of secure infants had been quick to pick them up when they cried and had held them with tenderness and care—but only for as long as the infants wished to be held. These mothers seemed to smoothly mesh their own rhythms with those of their babies, rather than imposing their own pace or agenda. In a fashion that was apparently "good enough" (in Winnicott's idiom), the behavior of these mothers tended to reflect sensitivity rather than misattunement, acceptance rather than rejection, cooperation rather than control, and emotional availability rather than remoteness (Ainsworth et al., 1978).

Avoidant Attachment

Avoidant babies can seem to be peculiarly blasé given that the Strange Situation procedure exposes them to an intrinsically alarming environment. Incessantly exploring while remaining conspicuously unmoved by mother's departure or return, their apparent lack of distress can easily be misconstrued as calm. In fact, their heart rates during the separation episodes are as elevated as those of their visibly distressed but secure peers, while the rise in their level of cortisol (the body's principal stress hormone) pre- to postprocedure is significantly greater than that of secure infants (Sroufe & Waters, 1977b; Spangler & Grossmann, 1993).

Ainsworth came to believe that the superficial indifference of the avoidant baby—as well as the virtual absence of attachment behavior— reflected a defensive accommodation akin to the detachment Bowlby had observed in two- and three-year-olds who had suffered protracted separation from their parents. It was as if these avoidant babies, like the older

children traumatized by separation and loss, had concluded that their over-tures for comfort and care would be of no use—and so, in a sense, they had given up.

Perhaps unsurprisingly, Ainsworth discovered that the mothers of ba-bies judged avoidant had actively rebuffed their bids for connection (Ainsworth et al., 1978), while other researchers would later observe moth-ers like these withdrawing when their infants appeared to be sad (Grossmann & Grossmann, 1991). Inhibition of emotional expression, aversion to physical contact and brusqueness when it occurred were all signatures of the mothering that seemed to produce avoidant infants who regularly went limp when held, rather than cuddling or clinging (Main & Weston, 1982).

Ambivalent Attachment

Ainsworth's research identified two kinds of ambivalent infants: those who were angry and those who were passive. Both were too preoccupied with mother's whereabouts to explore freely and both reacted to her departures with overwhelming distress—so much so that the separation episodes fre-quently had to be interrupted. Upon reunion, those infants categorized as angry oscillated between active overtures for connection to mother and ex-pressions of rejection—ranging from leaning away from mother's embrace to full-blown tantrums. By contrast, the infants classified as passive appeared capable only of faint or even implicit bids for solace, as if too over-come by their helplessness and misery to approach mother directly. Un-happily, the reunions seemed neither to ameliorate the ambivalent infants' distress nor to terminate their preoccupation with mother's whereabouts. It was as if—even in her presence—these infants were seeking a mother who wasn't there.

Ainsworth found, in fact, that the ambivalent babies were the off-spring of mothers who were, at best, unpredictably and occasionally avail-able. And while these mothers were neither verbally nor physically rejecting (as the mothers of avoidant infants had been), their responsiveness to their infants' signals was just as insensitive.[3] Finally, the mothers of ambivalent babies seemed, subtly or not so subtly, to discourage their autonomy—perhaps partly explaining the inhibition of exploration that characterized these ba-bies (Ainsworth et al., 1978).

Communication Is Key

In differentiating between security and the varieties of insecurity, Ains-worth discovered that in the attachment relationship it was the *quality of communication* between infant and caregiver that was of paramount im-portance.

In the secure dyads, the infant clearly expressed his need for comfort after separation, his relief at being soothed during reunion, and his consequent readiness to resume play. The mother accurately read his nonverbal cues (his tearful approach with upraised arms, his molding to her body when held, his eventual restlessness) and responded accordingly (picking him up, holding him tenderly, and releasing him to play). This sequence reflected a kind of attuned communication that has been described as *collaborative* and *contingent*: One party signals while the other answers with behavior that says, in effect, I can sense what you're feeling and respond to what you need.

In the insecure dyads, the communication had a very different quality. Upon separation, avoidant infants failed to express the very marked distress that was revealed indirectly though their elevated heart rates and cortisol levels. Similarly, upon reunion, they failed to express their need to be soothed. In short, the avoidant infants inhibited virtually all communication that invited connection: They expressed no desire for proximity and appeared deaf to whatever affectionate overtures the mother might muster.

Almost the reverse was true of ambivalent infants, who appeared to amplify expressions of attachment. Virtually from the start of the Ainsworth procedure, these infants conveyed their disturbing preoccupation with mother's availability. Their distress upon separation was extremely severe and their relief upon reunion was negligible. Communication of the ambivalent infants' attachment needs seemed to persist at a high volume, so to speak, regardless of mother's ministrations (Ainsworth, 1969; Main, 1990, 1995; Slade, 1999).

Ainsworth came to understand the differing patterns of communication in the Strange Situation as reflections of the infants' need to nurture the best possible attachment to parents with particular strengths and vulnerabilities. "Only connect!" wrote Forster, but to connect—to attach—infants must adapt to the character of their caregivers. In the home the mothers of secure infants had been observed to be sensitive and responsive to their signals, their behavior strikingly contingent upon their baby's—a finding that Mary Main would interpret as evidence of "early attunement" (Main, 1995, p. 417). Thus, it made sense that secure infants would communicate their feelings and needs directly—as if assuming that such communication would evoke an attuned response.

The mothers of avoidant infants had been seen in the home to be rejecting of attachment behavior: They were emotionally unavailable and uncomfortable with physical contact, and they tended to withdraw when their infants were sad. Not infrequently the infants reacted to their mothers' rejections with anger. For these avoidant infants it was adaptive, therefore, to inhibit the communication of attachment needs—both to keep from

being rejected and to sidestep the anger that threatened to push mother away when the infant's needs were frustrated.

The mothers of ambivalent infants were observed to have been inconsistently responsive to their signals and emotionally available only unpredictably. This unpredictability seemed to be a result of the mothers' own states of mind intruding unduly on their ability to tune in to their infants (Siegel, 1999). Given such unpredictable responsiveness on the part of their mothers, it was adaptive for the ambivalent infants to communicate their attachment needs in a persistent and unmistakable fashion—as if keeping up the pressure might keep up the care.

Disorganized Attachment

Ainsworth's research—and, no doubt, her strengths as a person and a teacher as well—proved magnetic to a number of extraordinarily talented students who chose to work with her, including Inge Bretherton, Jude Cassidy, Alicia Lieberman, Everett Waters, and, most prominently, Mary Main. Main's contributions to attachment theory and research will be reviewed in Chapter 3; suffice it to say that they are monumental. In the context of the present overview of the original three "organized" attachment categories, what is crucial is Main's discovery nearly 20 years after Ainsworth's pioneering work of a previously undetected pattern: disorganized/disoriented attachment.

Main and her former student Judith Solomon, while meticulously reviewing 200 videotapes of infants whose Strange Situation behavior simply failed to fit the traditional classifications, became aware that 90% of these infants displayed responses in the parent's presence that were inexplicable, contradictory, or bizarre. Upon reunion, for example, they backed toward mother, froze in place, collapsed to the floor, or appeared to fall into a dazed, trance-like state. Sighting mother, one infant covered his mouth with his hand—a gesture Darwin saw in primates and interpreted as a stifled scream (Hesse, 1999). Disorganized attachment probably resisted detection for so long because behaviors like these (often lasting no more than 10 to 30 seconds) only punctuated, so to speak, the flow of the infant's Strange Situation behavior as a whole (Main & Solomon, 1990). For the same reason, each infant classified as disorganized was also given an alternative classification that best described his overall conduct in the Strange Situation as secure, avoidant, or ambivalent.

Main has hypothesized that disorganized attachment results when the attachment figure is simultaneously experienced not only as the safe haven but also as the source of danger, that is, when the child—preprogrammed to turn to the parent in moments of alarm—is caught between contradictory impulses to approach and avoid. It is an untenable position from which the child's dependency on the parent affords no escape. Little won-

der, then, that the result of such a terrifying "biological paradox" is disorganization and/or disorientation.

For example, in one study of infants who were maltreated by their parents, 82% were classified as disorganized, in contrast to 18% of a matched control group (Carlson et al., 1989). Moreover, disorganized infants were disproportionately represented in high-risk samples involving families burdened by the stressors of poverty, psychiatric illness, substance abuse, and the like. Strikingly, however, disorganization was also found among infants who were neither maltreated nor drawn from high-risk samples.

In trying to understand this finding, Main proposed that infant disorganization is the outcome not only of interactions with parents whose anger or abuse is self-evidently *frightening*, but also of interactions in which the child experiences the parent as *frightened*. In particular, disorganization may result when the parent's fear seems to arise in response to the child and when the parent either reacts with physical withdrawal or retreats into a trance-like state. Summing up, Main suggests that disorganized attachment can be understood to emerge from the child's interactions with parents who are frightening, frightened, or dissociated. In contrast to the organized strategies of secure, avoidant, and ambivalent infants, disorganized attachment should be seen to reflect a *collapse* of strategy on the part of an infant who experiences "fright without solution" (Main & Hesse, 1992).

The Long-Term Effects of Infant Attachment Patterns

In the wake of Ainsworth's landmark research (which has since been duplicated many times over), an abundance of follow-up studies has tended to show that the attachment patterns of infancy have long-term effects. Histories of secure, avoidant, ambivalent, and disorganized attachment have been found to be associated, for better or worse, with subsequent outcomes in childhood, adolescence, and adulthood.

Children with a history of secure attachment show substantially greater self-esteem, emotional health and ego resilience, positive affect, initiative, social competence, and concentration in play than do their insecure peers. In school, children secure in infancy are treated warmly and age appropriately by teachers, whereas the avoidant (often seen as sullen, arrogant, or oppositional) tend to elicit angrily controlling responses and the ambivalent (often seen as clingy and immature) tend to be indulged or infantalized. Avoidant children have frequently been shown to victimize others, while ambivalent children are often victimized; secure children are neither victims nor victimizers (Sroufe, 1983; Elicker, Englund, & Sroufe, 1992; Weinfeld, Sroufe, Egeland, & Carlson, 1999).

As for later development, secure attachment seems to confer a measure of resilience on those so favored early in life. In contrast, disorganized at-

tachment in infancy has been shown to be a very significant risk factor for psychopathology from childhood onward. Borderline patients, for example, often seem to have histories of disorganized attachment (Dozier, Chase, Stoval, & Albus, 1999; Schore, 2002; Fonagy et al., 2002). The organized strategies of insecure attachment are also a risk factor, but far less so. Avoidant attachment has been suggestively tied to obsessional, narcissistic, and schizoid problems, while ambivalent attachment has been linked to hysteric or histrionic difficulties (Schore, 2002; Slade, 1999).

How these findings are to be understood remains something of an open question. The impact of first relationships may endure because the original patterns of behavior, communication, and affect regulation are simply maintained and reinforced through the child's ongoing relationship to the same parents who helped shape these patterns in the first place. On the other hand, it also seems probable that the attachment patterns Ainsworth codified through the Strange Situation are internalized as structured patterns in the mind.

What begin, in other words, as biologically driven interactions may register psychologically as mental representations that continue lifelong to shape behavior and subjective experience whether or not the original attachment figures are physically present. Whereas Ainsworth studied attachment behavior in infancy, it remained for her most gifted student, Mary Main, to illuminate the ways in which early experiences of attachment are encoded in the mind and preserved as influences on the future relationships—with self and others—of the older child and the adult.

NOTES

1. According to Bowlby, the fact that infants preferentially seek proximity to their mother derives from the reality that attachment is mainly a function of availability. Interestingly, Mary Main, citing studies conducted in Sweden, points out that even when the mother works outside the home and father is *de facto* the primary parent, the mother is still strongly preferred. Main suggests that this "startling finding" may be explained by prenatal experience (such as the baby's intrauterine exposure to the voice of the mother and an immediate preference for it) that more or less ensures she will become the primary attachment figure even before her infant emerges from the womb (Main, 1999).

2. Ainsworth tentatively explained this difference with the observation that the American babies—in sharp contrast to their Ugandan peers—were all too accustomed to their mothers' comings and goings. But she was reluctant to believe that secure-base behavior—theoretically a biological universal—would be altogether absent in the Baltimore infants, even though it could not be clearly seen in the familiar setting of the home.

3. They were inept in handling their babies in 41% of the pickup episodes that Ainsworth observed while "tender and careful" in only 2% of the episodes—in stark contrast to the mothers of secure infants who were tender and careful 53% of the time and only very occasionally inept (Ainsworth et al., cited in Main, 1995).

CHAPTER 3

Mary Main

Mental Representations, Metacognition, and the Adult Attachment Interview

Shortly after moving to the University of California at Berkeley in the mid-1970s, Mary Main initiated an ambitious longitudinal study of attachment that aimed to follow a group of middle-class families as their infants developed through childhood, adolescence, and beyond. The opening stage of this project involved each infant in two Strange Situation assessments—one with mother, the other with father. Then five years later, Main began to implement the second stage of her study by conducting videotaped evaluations of 40 families (Main, Kaplan, & Cassidy, 1985). This research, prodigiously inventive in its structure, launched what has been described as a "second revolution in attachment studies" (Karen, 1994, p. 216).

The first occurred when the invention of the Strange Situation gave researchers a laboratory procedure that produced in 20 minutes the same assessment of infant security that had originally taken Ainsworth's team 72 hours of observations in the home. Recall that *behavior* had been the target of Ainsworth's landmark research. As Main said, the Strange Situation assessment derived from observations of "the organization of the physical movements of an infant's body with respect to that of the parent" (Main et al., 1985, p. 93).

By contrast, Main's study of six-year-olds and their parents shifted the focus from the external world of interpersonal interaction to the internal

world of *mental representations*. Her research was designed to tap into the internalized object relations (to use the psychoanalytic phrase) that summed up the individual's attachment history in a complex network of memories, emotions, and beliefs that, in turn, shaped present and future attachment behavior.

To put these developments in context, consider that Bowlby made two extraordinary contributions: First, he identified attachment as a distinct, biologically based, and absolutely fundamental behavioral/motivational system; and second, he theorized that individual differences in the functioning of the attachment system are linked inextricably to the individuals' "internal working models" of self and other (Bretherton, 1985). What Ainsworth's research had done for Bowlby's first contribution, Main's research was about to do for the second: Just as the Strange Situation had enabled investigators to conduct empirical explorations of attachment behavior, Main's innovations made empirical study of the internal working model possible. And much as the Strange Situation in 1964 had opened a window on the attachment relationships of infancy, the Adult Attachment Interview—Main's most important methodological contribution—enabled researchers two decades later to begin to explore the inner world of attachment in late adolescence and beyond. But if we are to fully grasp the significance of Main's innovations and the discoveries to which they led, we first need to circle back to Bowlby's pioneering efforts to understand the internal world.

BOWLBY AND THE INTERNAL WORKING MODEL

Bowlby, of course, had been dissatisfied with then-current psychoanalytic theorizing about the inner world of mental representations. In particular, he had recoiled from the Kleinian conception that internalized object relations and "phantasies" sprang from within the child, rather than emerging—as he believed they did—from the child's actual interactions with real people. He was also reluctant to describe the dynamic and evolving representational world with static metaphors such as "images" or "maps." He was drawn instead to the theory of the "internal working model" that had been proposed by Kenneth Craik, an innovator at the cutting edge of what would come to be called artificial intelligence (Bretherton & Munholland, 1999):

> If the organism carries a "small-scale model" of external reality and of its own possible actions within its head, it is able to try out various alternatives, conclude which is the best of them, react to future situations before they arise, utilize the knowledge of past events in dealing with the present

and future, and in every way to react in a much fuller, safer, and more competent manner to the emergencies which face it. (Craik, 1943, p. 61)

Bowlby was also influenced by the cognitive psychologist Jean Piaget who argued that the infant's actions in relation to objects (grasping, sucking on, or swiping at them) result in knowledge about both the physical world and the infant's impact upon it—knowledge that registers internally as "schemata." In much the same way, Bowlby argued, the infant's repeated interactions with caregivers result in knowledge about the interpersonal world that registers internally as a working model:

> In the working model of the world that anyone builds a key feature is his notion of who his attachment figures are, where they may be found, and how they may be expected to respond. Similarly, in the working model of the self that anyone builds a key feature is his notion of how acceptable or unacceptable he himself is in the eyes of his attachment figures. On the structure of these complementary models are based that person's forecasts of how accessible and responsive his attachment figures are likely to be. (Bowlby, 1973, p. 203)

Bowlby theorized that from early infancy the individual's working model of attachment enables him or her to recognize patterns of interaction with the caregiver that have already repeatedly occurred and thus to "know" what the caregiver will do next. Because the working model influences both expectations and the behavior that flows from them, it can *shape* interactions as well as being shaped by them.

The most functional models of attachment are truly "working" models: They have a provisional quality that opens them to modification on the basis of new experience. Perhaps this explains the clinical impression that the "healthiest" patients are also those most capable of using therapy to help them change. Insecure models of attachment, in contrast, tend to be more rigid and so less open, hence constrained to fit new experience to old expectations. For example, an avoidant patient who has come to expect rejection may read the therapist's acceptance as the result of the therapist's being paid.

Bowlby believed, on the one hand, that internal working models have the potential to be "updated" in light of new and altered relationships, or even through heightened awareness. On the other hand, he observed that these models often resist revision—partly because they so frequently function outside conscious awareness and partly on account of self-protective (if self-defeating) defenses.

How stable, in fact, are these models of attachment? What is their structure? How do they actually develop in infancy and beyond? What differenti-

ates secure from insecure models? Provisional answers could be found in his theory, but questions like these had never been addressed empirically—until the research of Mary Main. Her findings would soon crystallize in a major elaboration of Bowlby's theory of the internal working model.

RECONCEPTUALIZING THE INTERNAL WORKING MODEL

Taking as her starting point the truism that "representational processes cannot be witnessed directly" (Main et al., 1985, p. 78), it was part of Main's genius to invent a research methodology that enabled her to "see" what had hitherto been invisible. Just as archeologists are able to envision long gone civilizations on the basis of excavated artifacts, Main was able— on the basis of what she called "representational artifacts"—to envision the inner worlds of the children and parents her longitudinal study was following (Main, 1991, p. 130).

Main's search for these representational artifacts harked back in part to linguistics (which had been her first love [Karen, 1994]) as well as to the projective tests that had given Ainsworth a window on the human psyche some years before she met Bowlby. Reasoning that an individual's working model of attachment would be revealed in characteristic patterns of narrative, discourse, and imagination, as well as behavior, Main structured her research accordingly.

Most influentially for future attachment studies, she devised a "deceptively straightforward" loosely structured protocol—dubbed the Adult Attachment Interview (AAI)—that asked the parents in her study to recollect and reflect upon the history of their relationships with their own parents, including experiences of loss, rejection, and separation (Slade, 2000, p. 1152; George, Kaplan, & Main, 1984, 1985, 1996). Originally designed, in Main's words, to "surprise the unconscious," the AAI can be seen to "prime" the attachment system. As such, this semiclinical interview has proven to be as powerful a tool for assessing attachment in adulthood as the Strange Situation is for assessing attachment in infancy (Main, 1995, pp. 436–437).

Note, however, that the nature of the "attachment" measured by each of these two instruments is somewhat different: The Strange Situation categories capture the quality of attachment specific to a *particular* relationship— with the result that an infant can, and often is, classified as secure with one parent and insecure with the other. The Strange Situation protocol has been said, in fact, to identify a relationship rather than a trait of the infant's personality. By contrast, because the adult classifications are *independent* of any particular relationship, Main (1995) has suggested that the AAI actually assesses the respondent's current overarching "state of mind with respect to attachment." [1] (p. 437).

The AAI consists of a series of questions (and follow-up "probes") that explicitly draw attention to memories related to attachment. After being asked for an overall description of the childhood relationship with both parents, interviewees are invited to choose five adjectives or phrases that best describe their early relationship with each parent and then are asked to support each of these descriptors, one after the other, with recollections: "*Loving,* you used the word loving to describe your relationship with your mother. Could you tell me about some memories or incidents which would illustrate why you chose that adjective?" (Main, 2000, p. 1078) Subsequently, and at a fairly rapid pace, subjects are asked more complex and detailed questions (see Figure 3.1).

While Main's closest collaborator (and husband) Erik Hesse notes that a proper AAI cannot be conducted on the basis of an abbreviated or modi-

---

1. To begin with, could you just help me to get a little bit oriented to your family—for example, who was in your immediate family, and where you lived?
2. Now I'd like you to try to describe your relationship with your parents as a young child, starting as far back as you can remember.
3–4. Could you give me five adjectives or phrases to describe your relationship with your mother/father during childhood? I'll write them down, and when we have all five I'll ask you to tell me what memories or experiences led you to choose each one.
5. To which parent did you feel closer, and why?
6. When you were upset as a child, what did you do, and what would happen? Could you give me some specific incidents when you were upset emotionally? Physically hurt? Ill?
7. Could you describe your first separation from your parents?
8. Did you ever feel rejected as a child? What did you do, and do you think your parents realized they were rejecting you?
9. Were your parents ever threatening toward you—for discipline, or jokingly?
10. How do you think your overall early experiences have affected your adult personality? Are there any aspects you consider a setback to your development?
11. Why do you think your parents behaved as they did during your childhood?
12. Were there other adults who were close to you—like parents—as a child?
13. Did you experience the loss of a parent or other close loved one as a child, or in adulthood?
14. Were there many changes in your relationship with your parents between childhood and adulthood?
15. What is your relationship with your parents like for you currently?

FIGURE 3.1. Brief précis of the Adult Attachment Interview protocol excerpted from George, Kaplan, and Main (1996). The AAI cannot be conducted on the basis of this brief, modified précis of the protocol, which omits several questions as well as the critical follow-up probes. The full protocol, together with extensive directions for administration, can be obtained by writing to Professor Mary Main, Department of Psychology, University of California at Berkeley, Berkeley, CA 94720. From Hesse (1999). Copyright 1999 by The Guilford Press. Reprinted by permission.

fied list of questions like the one in Figure 3.1, I have found that such queries may be enormously helpful in the clinical setting, especially early in treatment. Recently, for example, I met with a new patient whose escalating conflicts with his wife had become a threat to their marriage. After he described his early relationship with mother and father in the most glowing terms, I asked what he would usually do as a child when he was scared or upset. Initially unable to recall ever having felt either, the patient had a disturbing realization as he touched on the recent night terrors of his four-year-old daughter. While she could turn to her mother for comfort, he had somehow always known that his own parents would not be there for him. Having learned when he was young to "get over it," he now had a nearly impossible time acknowledging his vulnerable feelings; it was far easier for him to get angry.

Knowing that language can conceal as much as it reveals—and that internal representations are largely unconscious, hence unverbalizable—Main concentrated her attention on the particular *ways* the parents in her study used words, rather than the particular words they used: That is, she focused more on process and form than on content. It is specifically this approach to understanding the representational world—through attention primarily to *how*, rather than *what*, people communicate—that has made her work with the AAI invaluable to clinicians.

Main's longitudinal investigation[2] yielded two critical discoveries that effectively moved attachment research from the level of behavior to that of representation—thus making this research immediately relevant to clinicians whose concerns center on the emotions and beliefs that underlie their patients' behavior. Both discoveries depended on inferences from representational artifacts (like the six-year-olds' responses to photos depicting childhood separations, or their parents' AAI transcripts) that were presumed to reflect internal representations.

Studying these artifacts, Main detected two striking correlations: First, she found a correlation between the child's Strange Situation behavior with the primary parent at 12 months and the structure of the inner world of that child five years later. Second, she found an *intergenerational* correlation between the child's Strange Situation behavior, on the one hand, and the parent's "state of mind with respect to attachment," on the other. These two findings—showing that infant patterns of nonverbal behavior can predict representational patterns—were central to Main's elaboration of Bowlby's concept of the internal working model.

Infant Behavior and the Six-Year-Olds' Inner World

The structural parallels between the mother–infant communication patterns Main had observed in the Strange Situation and the six-year-olds' rep-

resentational artifacts turned out to be quite extraordinary.[3] Consider, by way of illustration, the following minidialogues that emerged in response to the separation photos. Having shown each youngster an image portraying an imminent two-week separation, the researcher (whose words are presented in italics) then asked, "What would a child do?"

> *Child 1 (Secure in infancy)*: Cry. [Giggles.] *Cry?* [nods yes.] *Why's she gonna cry?* Cause she really loves her mom and dad. *Cause she really loves her mom and dad?* Mm. *What else is she gonna do?* Play a little bit.

> *Child 2 (Avoidant in infancy)*: I don't know. *What could he do?* I don't know! *Any ideas?* Ow. Ow. [High voice through toy horse.] No, I don't. *No?* Wheww. Sit up lion.

> *Child 3 (Ambivalent in infancy)*: Chase them. *Chase who?* Their dad and mom in his new toy car—he's psssshh—run right off. *Then what's gonna happen?* And then he's gonna, then he is gonna . . . toss a bow and arrow and shoot them. *Shoot his mom and dad?* Yeah. If he want to, maybe.

> *Child 4 (Disorganized in infancy)*: Probably gonna hide away. *Gonna hide away?* Yeah. *Then what's gonna happen?* He'll probably get locked up in his closet. [Forced giggle.] *Locked up in his closet?* Yeah, I was locked up in a closet. (Main et al., 1985, pp. 103–104)

Differences in the children's Strange Situation behavior with mother predicted corresponding differences not only in separation "narratives" like those above but also in the six-year-olds' family drawings, their responses to a family snapshot, and their behavior upon reunion after a brief separation from their parents. Taken together these results demonstrated that "different patterns of mother–infant interaction must have led to the development not only of *different behavior,* but also of *different representational processes*" (Main, 2000, p. 1059). In light of this finding, it clearly appears that our original working models of attachment are forged in the crucible of our earliest interactions.

The Parent's Inner World and the Infant's Behavior: The Adult Attachment Interview and the Strange Situation

Main's second discovery strongly suggests that our *parents'* internal working models exert a decisive influence on the quality of these formative interactions that shape, in turn, our own working models. Main found a significant correlation between the security of attachment of the children in her study (as assessed in the Strange Situation five years before) and the "state of mind with respect to attachment" of their parents (as assessed through the AAI).

More specifically, the Strange Situation classifications *predicted* the AAI results (Main et al., 1985). Importantly, the reverse has also been shown to be true: Subsequent research conducted by Main and replicated by numerous investigators around the world has demonstrated that the AAI classification of the parent predicts the Strange Situation classification of the child with 75% accuracy in regard to security versus insecurity. Astonishingly, such predictions can be made just as accurately when the AAI is administered to parents *before their children are born* (van IJzendoorn, 1995).

Recall that the AAI "primes" the attachment system much as the Strange Situation does. In so doing, it has the potential to generate an extremely evocative, if not stressful, experience for the respondent who therefore has ample opportunity to demonstrate (or fail to demonstrate) the capacity for "coherent discourse" that Main identified as the hallmark of a secure state of mind regarding attachment. Coherent discourse was seen in AAI transcripts that were internally consistent, plausible, and collaborative (Main, 1991, 1995).

Main's study revealed striking differences between the AAI transcripts of the parents who had raised securely attached children and the transcripts of those whose children were insecure. The former clearly reflected the parents' capacity to engage cooperatively with the interviewer, as well as their ease of recall, thoughtfulness, and objectivity while exploring their attachment histories. Precisely because of their objectivity about attachment relationships—whose importance and influence these parents readily acknowledged—Main described them as possessing a "secure/autonomous" state of mind regarding attachment.

In sharp contrast, the parents of insecure children revealed in their AAI transcripts a general pattern of difficulty in maintaining coherent, collaborative discourse—while three *particular* patterns of incoherence and failed collaboration turned out to mirror the three corresponding patterns of insecure Strange Situation behavior. The parents of avoidant infants were termed "dismissing" because they tended to minimize the value and influence of attachment, and to insist on their lack of recall for attachment-related experience. The parents of ambivalent infants were described as "preoccupied" because they seemed to experience past attachments as continually intruding on the present. Finally, because they seemed to become intermittently disorganized or disoriented when discussing past traumas, the parents of disorganized infants were characterized as "unresolved/disorganized" (Main et al., 1985; Main, 1991, 1995, 2000; Siegel, 1999). For a summary, see Figure 3.2.

Main's study revealed an undeniable correspondence between the parent's "mode of discourse" on the AAI—that is, the parent's way of talking

Adult state of mind with respect to attachment	Infant strange situation behavior
Secure/autonomous (F)	Secure (B)
Coherent, collaborative discourse. Valuing of attachment, but seems objective regarding any particular event/relationship. Description and evaluation of attachment-related experiences is consistent, whether experiences are favorable or unfavorable. Discourse does not notably violate any of Grice's maxims.	Explores room and toys with interest in preseparation episodes. Shows signs of missing parent during separation, often crying by the second separation. Obvious preference for parent over stranger. Greets parent actively, usually initiating physical contact. Usually some contact maintaining by second reunion, but then settles and returns to play.
Dismissing (Ds)	Avoidant (A)
Not coherent. Dismissing of attachment-related experiences and relationships. Normalizing ("excellent, very normal mother"), with generalized representations of history unsupported or actively contradicted by episodes recounted, thus violating Grice's maxim of quality. Transcripts also tend to be excessively brief, violating the maxim of quantity.	Fails to cry on separation from parent. Actively avoids and ignores parent on reunion (i.e., by moving away, turning away, or leaning out of arms when picked up). Little or no proximity or contact-seeking, no distress, and no anger. Response to parent appears unemotional. Focuses on toys or environment throughout procedure.
Preoccupied (E)	Resistant or ambivalent (C)
Not coherent. Preoccupied with or by past attachment relationships/experiences, speaker appears angry, passive, or fearful. Sentences often long, grammatically entangled, or filled with vague usages ("dadadada," "and that"), thus violating Grice's maxims of manner and relevance. Transcripts often excessively long, violating the maxim of quantity.	May be wary or distressed even prior to separation, with little exploration. Preoccupied with parent throughout procedure; may seem angry or passive. Fails to settle and take comfort in parent on reunion, and usually continues to focus on parent and cry. Fails to return to exploration after reunion.
Unresolved/disorganized (U)	Disorganized/disoriented (D)
During discussions of loss or abuse, individual shows striking lapse in the monitoring of reasoning or discourse. For example, individual may briefly indicate a belief that a dead person is still alive in the physical sense, or that this person was killed by a childhood thought. Individual may lapse into prolonged silence or eulogistic speech. The speaker will ordinarily otherwise fit Ds, E, or F categories.	The infant displays disorganized and/or disoriented behaviors in the parent's presence, suggesting a temporary collapse of behavioral strategy. For example, the infant may freeze with a trance-like expression, hands in air; may rise at parent's entrance, then fall prone and huddled on the floor; or may cling while crying hard and leaning away with gaze averted. Infant will ordinarily otherwise fit A, B, or C categories.

FIGURE 3.2. AAI classifications and corresponding patterns of infant strange situation behavior. Descriptions of the adult attachment classification system are summarized from Main, Kaplan, and Cassidy (1985) and from Main and Goldwyn (1984–1998). Descriptions of infant A, B, and C categories are summarized from Ainsworth, Blehar, Waters, and Wall (1978), and the description of the infant D category is summarized from Main and Solomon (1990). From Hesse (1999). Copyright 1999 by The Guilford Press. Reprinted by permission.

about her own attachment experience—and her infant's attachment behavior in the Strange Situation. We might reasonably infer that the strength of the parent's capacity to reflect coherently on her past will significantly affect her ability to impart security to her child. And, as we will shortly see, the security of our own "state of mind with respect to attachment" may ultimately depend less on the particular facts of personal history—however problematic—than on the success of our efforts to make meaningful sense of that history.

Working Models as "Rules" not "Templates"

Main was impressed by the fairly stunning parallels her study found among (1) the infants' patterns of nonverbal behavior, (2) the six-year-olds' representations of attachment, and (3) the form and content of their parents' discourse during the AAI. She illustrated these parallels with an example:

> The insecure–avoidant infant turns away from, moves away from, and ignores the parent within the Strange Situation and 5 years later turns away from representational reminders of the parent. In discourse with the child, the parent focuses on objects and activities, asks rhetorical questions, and offers (as does the child) little opportunity for turn taking or topic elaboration. Finally, during the Adult Attachment Interview, the parent of the avoidant infant tends to state that she is unable to recall the events of childhood and/or dismisses or devalues those events as likely influences. Selective inattention to potential cues eliciting attachment or reminding of relationship seems to be a rule preserved by both partners. . . . (Main et al., 1985, p. 100)

Main proposed that internal working models are best conceived not as templates—like the internalized self and object images of psychoanalytic theory—but rather as "*structured processes* serving to obtain or limit access to information" (Main et al., 1985, p. 77, emphasis added). Building on Bowlby's original conception, Main reconceived the internal working model as

> a set of conscious and/or unconscious *rules* for the organization of information relevant to attachment. . . . [T]he secure versus the various types of insecure attachment organizations can best be understood as terms referring to particular types of internal working models . . . *that direct not only feelings and behavior but also attention, memory, and cognition* . . . Individual differences in . . . internal working models will be related *not only to individual differences in patterns of nonverbal behavior but also to patterns of language and structures of mind.* (p. 67; emphasis added)

Main hypothesized that the rules we internalize in the course of our first relationships initially arise in infancy from our experience of what "works" in relation to particular attachment figures. These "rules of attachment" are quite literally rules to live by—given that they emerge out of interactions between the biologically channeled, survival-based attachment system and the actualities of the parenting we experience. Previously, Main had theorized that the differing communicative behaviors of avoidant and ambivalent infants could be understood to reflect correspondingly different *adaptive strategies* for optimizing attachment to parents who were predictably unresponsive, on the one hand, or unpredictably responsive, on the other (Main, 1981, 1995). She now added that the rules originally embodied in a "behavioral/communicative" strategy also eventually generate a "representational/attentional" strategy that determines the extent and nature of our access to attachment-related feelings, desires, and memories. Just as Ainsworth had earlier equated secure attachment with a flexible balance of attachment and exploration, Main now identified flexibility of focus, affect, thought, and memory as markers of security—noting that the most secure dyads in her study were also the freest of "predictable, 'rule-like' regularities and patternings" (Main et al., 1985, p. 101; Main, 1995).

Considering infant communication patterns as nascent representational strategies geared to foster (or avoid disrupting) attachment relationships clarifies a great deal about both the inter- and intrapersonal worlds. In the Strange Situation, Ainsworth had observed communication behaviors variously characterized by flexibility (in securely attached infants) and inhibition or amplification (in infants who were insecurely attached). Main's work suggested that these differing patterns of interpersonal communication were mirrored in correspondingly different patterns in the infants' communications with themselves.

Confident of their mothers' responsiveness, secure infants could well afford to be attuned to their own attachment-related feelings and needs: They could be aware of, and could express, them. Avoidant infants, anticipating mother's rejection and their own anger in response, could afford neither to be aware of nor to express their attachment-related feelings and needs: hence, the avoidant strategy of inhibiting or minimizing such internal experiences. Ambivalent infants, responding to their mother's unpredictable availability, apparently developed a strategy for amplifying or maximizing both the awareness and the expression of their attachment-related feelings and needs, as if to ensure continuing care.

Main makes the additional, clinically crucial point that the rules embodied in these organized representational/attentional/behavioral strategies are implemented *actively*. The avoidant infant, for example, is not merely oblivious to mother: He actively snubs or ignores her, restricting his atten-

tion to the toys—as if to distract himself from the anxiety provoked by the
Strange Situation and the distress of wanting from mother the comfort he
has learned not to expect. We can infer that he is hyperactivating his exploratory system so as to inhibit an attachment system whose output has
not been welcomed. Similarly, the ambivalent infant is not merely preoccupied with mother: He actively seeks contact and strictly confines his attention to monitoring her whereabouts; completely ignoring the toys, he seems
to scan the interpersonal environment, vigilant for the slightest cue that
might amplify his distress. We can infer that he is hyperactivating his attachment system to both capture his mother's unpredictable attention and inhibit the autonomous exploration she has tended to discourage (Main,
1995, 1999).

Very much like these infants, our adult patients can be seen to actively
bolster their adherence to the "rules of attachment." For example, patients
in a dismissing state of mind with respect to attachment frequently find
their attention monopolized by the needs of others—thus facilitating their
habitual denial that they have unmet emotional needs of their own. Correspondingly, patients in a preoccupied state of mind may find themselves
consumed with doubts about their romantic partner's commitment—thus
facilitating a familiar inattention to their own autonomous yearnings.

The clinical implication here is that our patients may unconsciously
deploy their attention in ways that shore up and seem subjectively to "justify" their preexisting expectations and current conduct. To generate what
Main has called "secondary felt security," adults like these have had to
adopt a "second-best strategy" for maintaining proximity (but also self-
organization) in relation to predictably unresponsive or unpredictably
responsive parents (Main, 1995, p. 462). We would do well, in this connection, to consider that much of the thinking, feeling, remembering, and
behaving that we observe in our patients (and ourselves) has arisen and persists in order to preserve outdated—but all-too-enduring—internal working
models of attachment.

The "adhesiveness" of these models has long been central to the concerns of clinicians and researchers alike. Freud, of course, drew our attention to the "repetition compulsion" while Bowlby (1980) remarked on the
"self-perpetuating quality" of internal working models. Main's reflections
on the research attributed the stability of these models—particularly, insecure ones—to the survival–critical context of their original emergence, noting that (1) rules that have enabled an individual to survive are unlikely to
be readily relinquished and (2) rules mandated by internal working actually
function over time to preserve those models. Such rules—determining what
individuals allow themselves to notice, feel, recall, and do—are rigorously
implemented because their violation challenges states of mind and ways of
being that have made emotional survival possible. Thus, the particular

models of attachment originally generated in secure, avoidant, ambivalent, or disorganized infants tended, going forward, to be actively perpetuated by corresponding patterns of awareness, affective experience, and behavior—including, eventually, parenting behavior.

THE INTERGENERATIONAL TRANSMISSION
OF ATTACHMENT PATTERNS

Attachment patterns, as previously noted, have a strong propensity to persist across generations. In the aftermath of Main's original investigation, van IJzendoorn (1995) conducted a meta-analysis of the comparable studies then available (involving 18 samples in six countries) and concluded that the parents' AAI classification generally predicted the Strange Situation classification of their infants. Far more often than not, the secure infant became the secure adult who, as a parent, raised secure children. Likewise, the avoidant infant could be expected to become a dismissing adult whose children were likely to be avoidant, and so on. Similarly, the single study to explore the fate of attachment across three generations suggested that the attachment classifications of grandmothers tended to correspond not only to those of their adult daughters but also to those of their daughters' children (Benoit & Parker, cited in Hesse, 1999). How and why this intergenerational transmission of attachment occurs is a crucial question for researchers and clinicians alike. It's also a question whose answer has significant implications for parenting.

Main's research suggested that secure attachment was the outcome of flexibility in the parents begetting flexibility in their offspring. With a wide behavioral and affective repertoire, and little to restrict the deployment of their attention, secure parents appeared well equipped to provide the sensitive responsiveness to their infants' signals that had been demonstrated by Ainsworth and others to play such a central role in generating security.

As for insecurity, Main proposed that in relation to their children, dismissing and preoccupied parents behaved in ways that were unconsciously calculated to preserve their own states of mind with respect to attachment. These states of mind originally arose in response to the parents' absolutely overriding need for proximity to their own parents. Any and all challenges to such states of mind—including aspects of their own infants' behavior—constituted threats from which these parents protected themselves through rules that dictated selective inattention or misattuned responsiveness. Unfortunately, the very restrictions of attention and behavior that protected such insecure parents also undermined their capacity to be consistently sensitive to their infants' signals. In response, these infants adopted rules that mirrored those of their parents. Thus, the avoidant infants minimized

attachment behavior and maximized exploration of the nonhuman environment, while the preoccupied maximized attachment behavior and minimized autonomous exploration.

Unlike secure, avoidant, and preoccupied infants, those who were disorganized were believed to have repeatedly experienced their parents as frightening—often because these parents were frankly abusive, but sometimes because, in relating to their infants, they appeared to be frightened and/or dissociated. Main's AAI research showed that disorganized parents were themselves gripped by unresolved experiences of childhood trauma or loss.

Never having been consciously processed, these overwhelming experiences were preserved in a dissociated state, lying dormant, yet available to be activated by particular emotionally arousing contexts. When confronted by cues that evoked their trauma or loss—including, for example, their children's distress, demands, or anger—these unresolved parents were liable to be flooded by (formerly) dissociated experiences that too often triggered behavior that terrified their children. These children were then caught in a paralyzing contradiction—turning reflexively to their parents for safety while at the same moment their fear of their parents was provoking their desire to flee. Repeated experiences of this kind led to disorganization during infancy and later to controlling, role-inverting behavior with their parents as a means of "solving" the irresolvable contradiction. The legacy of the parents' unresolved loss or trauma was thus a correspondingly encapsulated and hard-to-resolve trauma in their children, as illustrated in the vignette that follows.

Some time ago, I was exploring with a patient of mine his visceral terror of medical procedures of any kind (more than once he had fainted at the prospect of having his blood drawn). I asked him who had taken him to the doctor when he was a child. "My mother," he replied. I had been working with this man for several years but had never before heard the story he then very matter-of-factly related to me—a story that began to make sense of his lifelong fear:

> "My mom was five when her mother went to the hospital for what was supposed to have been a routine surgery. She died there under the knife but my mom was never told that her mother was dead. She was sent to live with relatives after hearing her dad say that her mother was too sick to take care of her. Then when she was eight, he remarried and mom was brought back home. But when she was introduced to her dad's new wife he just said to her, 'This is your mother.' And she believed it. But years later she learned the truth."

To explain how this kind of trauma and insecurity is transmitted from parent to child, Main proposed that the strength of the attachment impera-

tive is such that even when the developmental cost is exorbitant, young children will respond in ways that preserve their parents' psychological status quo. By the same token, parents as their children grow older will usually collude with them to maintain interactive patterns that reinforce states of mind that now have come to be shared.

For example, unresolved parents may welcome the role-inverting behavior of their disorganized offspring, because that behavior dovetails with their own emotional needs. Having learned long ago to respond solicitously or punitively to their own parents, they may now "invite" the same response from their children because it preserves the originally indispensable internal and interpersonal patterns. Thus the parents' (often unconscious) need to perpetuate these rigid patterns of attention and behavior provokes similarly rigid patterns in their children. Main theorized that this was the mechanism for the intergenerational transmission of insecure attachment (Main, 1995).

Yet the issue remained unresolved. In the meta-analysis mentioned earlier, van IJzendoorn (1995) took a highly sophisticated statistical approach to the relevant studies and concluded that attachment researchers confronted what he aptly referred to as a "transmission gap" (p. 387). The nature of the caregiver's sensitive responsiveness—long thought to be the bedrock of attachment, secure or insecure—appeared to explain partly, but by no means completely, how and why the working model(s) of the parents tended to become the working model(s) of their children. Strikingly, it was Mary Main who, in 1991, introduced to the attachment field two vital concepts—*metacognitive knowledge* and *metacognitive monitoring*—that would later be enlisted by Peter Fonagy to help close the so-called transmission gap.

METACOGNITION: THINKING ABOUT THINKING AND REPRESENTING THE REPRESENTATIONAL WORLD

In Main's attempt to map the representational worlds of the infants, six-year-olds, and adults in her study, she had drawn on Bowlby's concept of the internal working model. At a certain point, however, she came to realize that it was only *secure* individuals who could actually be said to have a singular "model" of attachment. Their experience with a consistently sensitive caregiver—who provided a secure base—seemed to have resulted in the relatively stable expectation that others would be responsive to their needs.

Insecure individuals, by contrast, had grown up with parents who provided no such secure base but instead were rejecting, unpredictable, or frightening. To describe the contradictory, incoherent, and dissociated representations of attachment that resulted from unfavorable experiences such

as these, Main used the term "multiple models." Here she was following Bowlby's lead: "[T]he hypothesis of multiple models," he wrote, "one of which is highly influential but relatively or completely unconscious, is no more than a version, in different terms, of Freud's hypothesis of a dynamic unconscious" (Bowlby, cited in Main, 1991, p. 132).

Unlike the "singular" integrated models of secure individuals that foster flexibility and ease of access to attachment-related information, multiple—that is, incompatible or conflicting—models mandate a defensive narrowing of attention in order to deal with the problem, as Bowlby (1988) put it of "knowing what you are not supposed to know and feeling what you are not supposed to feel" (p. 99). As we've already seen, this rigid exclusion of threatening thoughts and feelings hobbles the ability of insecure parents to respond with sensitivity to their infants' signals. Necessarily, it also undermines the ability of these parents to take a step back and reflect on their own experience.

According to Main, the consideration of multiple models led her directly to *metacognition* (Main, 1991). And here Main brings us just as directly to the clinically crucial matter of the self's stance toward experience, including, in particular, mental experience. Previously researched primarily by cognitive psychologists, metacognition is cognition about cognition: thinking about thinking. It involves the ability, paraphrasing Main, to appreciate the "*merely* representational nature" of our own (or others') mental representations.

Main highlighted the distinction between representation ("I'm a forgettable person") and metarepresentation or metacognition ("I'm a person who often feels she's forgettable—I'm not sure why"). With a functioning capacity for metacognition, we may for the moment find ourselves in a particular state of mind; lacking such a capacity, it's as if we simply *are* that state of mind. Main further distinguished between "metacognitive knowledge" and "metacognitive monitoring."

Metacognitive knowledge centrally involves the ability to grasp what cognitive scientists call the appearance-reality distinction, without which it is impossible to realize that our ideas and perceptions may be without validity, or that others may believe things that are not true. To the extent that our patients are unaware of the "fallible nature of knowledge" their desire as well as their ability to reflect on their experience tends to be limited (Main, 1991, p. 134). For example, a patient recently made an unequivocal assertion that to me seemed quite implausible. When I expressed curiosity about his conviction, he said it simply *felt* true. Then he added decisively, as if this should be the last word on the subject, "Aren't feelings the ultimate facts?"

As therapists, our own capacity for metacognitive understanding of *both* partners in the therapeutic couple is crucial in enabling our patients to

change. For it is this kind of understanding that allows us to respond reflectively, rather than reflexively—that is, to be able to consider the complex meanings of feelings, beliefs, and wishes rather than take them, immediately and unquestioningly, at face value.

Beyond the appearance/reality distinction, metacognitive knowledge makes possible an appreciation of *representational change*, (the sense that beliefs and feelings can change over time), and *representational diversity* (the recognition that, in relation to the same circumstance, others may have beliefs and feelings that differ from our own but may be equally valid). Most fundamentally, perhaps, metacognitve knowledge makes possible the awareness that our ongoing experience is profoundly influenced by underlying mental states, including what we have come to believe, feel, and desire.

Such knowledge provides the foundation for what Main called *metacognitive monitoring*. Metacognitive monitoring involves a stance of active self-scrutiny that situates us at once inside and outside our experience. This reflective stance enables us to step back from experience in order to be aware of aspects of our *ideas* about experience that may be contradictory, biased, or implausible. It also tends to prompt efforts to understand or resolve such contradictions or potential "errors." Metacognitive monitoring thus entails observation of, and curiosity about, the habits of mind that shape our experience. In the AAI context, instances of metacognitive monitoring were seen to be markers of secure attachment, while lapses in such monitoring among parents predicted disorganization in their infants (Main, 1995).

Main proposed that strong metacognitive capacities, among children old enough to have acquired them, might have the potential to diminish the destructive impact of unfavorable attachment exprcience, including trauma. The same, of course, may be true for adults. Conversely, she observed that the developmentally determined *lack* of metacognition among younger children heightened their vulnerability to the impact of problematic attachment-related events. And the same may be true for adults in whom metacognition either has yet to develop or has been defensively inhibited. While metacognition certainly seemed to have a role in conferring resilience or vulnerability, the question of its overall *centrality* in relation to attachment appeared to Main to be unresolved.

It was quite clear to her that a functioning capacity for metacognition was *associated* with security, and its lack with insecurity. However, she was unready to declare whether metacognition fostered secure attachment, *or* secure attachment fostered metacognition, simply because the research necessary to resolve the matter had not as yet been undertaken. For similar reasons (and despite the fact that a parent's high AAI scores for metacognitive monitoring were associated with securely attached offspring) Main

was unready to claim a decisive role for the quality of the parents' metacognition in determining whether their children were securely or insecurely attached (Main, 1991). Several years later, however, Peter Fonagy—a psychoanalyst researching attachment on the opposite side of the Atlantic— was indeed able to make exactly that claim. He did so while extending Main's conceptualization of metacognition in light of the psychological capacity for what is known as a "theory of mind" (Fonagy et al., 1995).

NOTES

1. Importantly, this "state" has been shown by Main's research (and that of others) to have such stability over time that it may as accurately be described as a trait—though by no means an immutable one.

2. Recall that, as the second stage of her longitudinal study, Main and her colleagues in 1982 had conducted two-hour-long videotaped assessments of 40 families. Built around separation and reunion, the process for evaluating the six-year-olds and their parents was specifically geared—like the Strange Situation itself—to activate the attachment system. Each family upon arriving at the research site was asked to pose for a Polaroid photograph. Then the whole family was shown a short film that dramatically depicted a two-year-old child's separation from his parents (Robertson & Robertson, 1971). Next came the separation in real time: The six-year-old was led to a playroom, while in separate offices each parents was given the AAI. Meanwhile the six-year-old was participating for 20 minutes in a "warmup" session with a female examiner who then proceeded to show the child a series of six photographs of children about to undergo separation from their parents. After seeing each photograph the child was asked what the children in the picture would *feel* and what they would *do* when their parents left. Then the examiner showed the child the Polaroid that had been taken earlier saying "But here is a photograph of yourself and your family, and you see, you are all together" (Main et al., 1985, p. 89). The child was also asked to draw a picture of the family. Finally, after the child had been engaged in a period of free play in a sandbox, the first parent returned. The reunion lasted three minutes, following which the second parent returned and joined the reunion for as much as three minutes more.

3. Predictions of the six-year-olds' attachment representations from their Strange Situation behavior with mother ranged from 68 to 88%. Interestingly, only reunion behavior and discourse were significantly related to Strange Situation behavior with father (Main, 1995).

CHAPTER 4

Fonagy and Forward

Main has said that she and Fonagy were drawn independently to the research on *theory of mind* (Main, personal communication, 2004). This term refers to the ways in which all of us, to varying degrees, make sense of our own and others' behavior on the basis of underlying mental states—including beliefs, emotions, and desires. The idea here is that, beginning in childhood, we develop a "theory" that enables us to understand and, to some extent, predict what others will do in light of what we think is going on in their mind. Fonagy may have been inspired by the same literature on theory of mind that influenced Main, but his reading of that literature led to a much broader conceptualization than hers.

PETER FONAGY: MENTALIZING, MODES OF EXPERIENCE, AND THE INTERSUBJECTIVE ORIGINS OF THE SELF

As a junior lecturer at University College London more than a quarter of a century ago, Fonagy had been appointed as liaison to organize the seminars and consultations of the visiting Freud Memorial Professor of Psychoanalysis— who turned out in 1980 to be none other than John Bowlby. Sitting in on Bowlby's teaching that year, Fonagy (who now holds the Freud Memorial Professorship himself) says he was extremely taken not only with Bowlby's ideas but also his profound social concerns:

> Bowlby was deeply committed to the welfare of people who were less privileged than he was. I found his vision enormously impressive—of combining science with concern for the individual and individual subjectivity, together

43

with looking at social forces and social pressures. That remains for me the aspect of attachment theory that is most important and most intriguing. (Fonagy, personal communication, 2006)

Several years later, Fonagy in collaboration with Miriam and Howard Steele launched a study on the transgenerational transmission of attachment patterns. Throughout their study, Fonagy and his colleagues received consultation from Bowlby. They also received training in the AAI from Mary Main.

Mentalizing and the "Reflective-Functioning" Scale

Inspired by Main's groundbreaking work, Fonagy initially attempted to operationalize her ideas about individual differences in metacognitive capacities. But whereas Main had concentrated on the adult's *self*-monitoring of thought and recall during the AAI, Fonagy (taking his cue from the theory of mind) widened that focus to take in the adult's attention to mental states generally, including, in particular, the mental states of others (Fonagy, Steele, & Steele, 1991a). Fonagy would later remark that the hallmark of the ability he referred to as *mentalizing*—that is, "the process by which we realize that having a mind mediates our experience of the world"—was not *self*-knowledge, but rather knowledge of minds in general (Fonagy, Gergely, Jurist, & Target, 2002, p. 3). While such knowledge is largely implicit, Fonagy and Target (in press) use the term "mentalization proper" to describe the activity of "thinking explicitly about states of mind" (p. 2). Mentalizing activity (say, a daughter noting that her father's "rejection" of her might have resulted from his depression rather than his hostility) is rooted in what Fonagy called the capacity for *reflective function*.

Reflective function lets us see ourselves and others as beings with psychological depth. It enables us to respond to our experience on the basis not only of observed behavior, but also of the underlying mental states—desires, feelings, beliefs—that make behavior understandable and give it meaning. As such, reflective function is intimately related to our capacities for insight and empathy.

To evaluate the strength of an individual's mentalizing capacity, Fonagy and his colleagues devised the Reflective-Functioning Scale. Designed for research purposes, this scale can also be used informally to enhance clinical judgments about the kinds of interventions our patients may be able to benefit from. A strong mentalizing capacity—and perhaps in treatment, receptivity to the therapist's interpretations—is likelier to be present when the interviewee (or patient) demonstrates:

- *Awareness of the nature of mental states*—for example, that our understanding of ourselves and others is invariably incomplete; that

people may modify mental states to minimize pain; that people may deliberately disguise internal states; that certain psychological responses are predictable given certain circumstances.

- *Explicit effort to identify mental states underlying behavior*—for example, plausibly accounting for behavior in terms of beliefs, feelings, desires; understanding that our interpretations of others may be influenced by our own mental states; realizing that feelings about a situation may be inconsistent with observable aspects of the situation.
- *Recognition of the "developmental" aspects of mental states*—for example, that what was felt yesterday may be different from what is felt today or tomorrow; that parents' behavior is both shaped by their own parents' behavior and shapes the behavior of their children; that childhood perspectives often need to be revised in light of adult understanding.
- *Awareness of mental states in relation to the interviewer (or therapist)*—for example, that without being told, the therapist cannot know what the patient knows; that the therapist may have her own distinctive emotional responses to the patient's story; that the therapist's history, and consequently, her mental states may well be different from those of the patient (adapted with permission from Fonagy, Target, Steele, & Steele, 1998).

Fonagy makes the point that what we need to listen for here are not enunciations of principles concerning mental states ("One can never know what someone else feels") but rather evidence that such principles are *implicitly* understood ("As a child, I was sure that my mother didn't care for me, but given what I've heard from my father about how *she* felt that I rejected *her*, now I'm not really sure what she felt").

In 1987, Fonagy and the Steeles recruited 100 expectant couples and conducted AAI research using their scale. The study was notable for a number of reasons. First, it documented that the parents' state of mind with respect to attachment—*assessed before the infant's birth*—could predict that infant's Strange Situation classification at 12 months. It also showed that mothers and fathers with a strong reflective capacity were three to four times more likely to have secure children than parents whose capacity for mentalizing was weak. Finally, it demonstrated that a strong reflective capacity could break the "cycle of disadvantage" that ordinarily led parents with adverse attachment histories to raise insecure children.

To test the prediction that an ability to reflect on mental states could function as an "antidote" to the problematic past, the mothers in the study were divided into two groups: the first had experienced severe deprivation (parental mental illness, prolonged separation from parents, and so on); the second had not. It turned out that among the deprived mothers with *strong*

reflective functioning, every single one had secure children. In stark contrast, among those whose reflective functioning was weak, only one in 17 had a secure child. Clearly, the strength of the capacity to mentalize was a protective factor that buffered the impact of difficult early experience and diminished the probability of the intergenerational transmission of insecurity (Fonagy, Steele, Steele, Moran, & Higgitt, 1991b; Fonagy et al., 1995; Fonagy, 2001).

Discoveries such as these led Fonagy to regard mentalizing as absolutely central to attachment. In fact, he has gone so far as to contend that "attachment is not an end in itself; rather it exists in order to produce a representational system that has evolved, we may presume, to aid human survival" (Fonagy et al., 2002, p. 2). This representational system is a *mentalizing* system that offers the enormous evolutionary survival advantage of enabling individuals to understand, interpret, and predict the behavior of others, as well as their own behavior. As such it is a "cornerstone of social intelligence" and critical to work, play, and collaboration of all kinds (Allen & Fonagy, 2002).

Over more than 15 years, Fonagy and his colleagues' extraordinarily active program of research and theory building has made an increasingly powerful case that mentalizing and attachment play critically important, intertwining roles in development, psychopathology, and psychotherapy. In brief, the parent's mentalizing is crucial to promoting secure attachment in the child and secure attachment provides the key context for activating the child's own mentalizing potential. Much of the psychopathology we encounter in our patients can be seen to reflect either an inhibition of mentalizing or a failure to develop it in the first place. Correspondingly, psychotherapy can be understood as an effort to restore or kindle the patient's capacity to mentalize.

Consistent with Main's theorizing about the internal working model, Fonagy has proposed that what is key about the representation of early attachment experience is less the "template" we register than the depth to which our mentalizing ability allows us to probe our experience, especially experience that is emotionally charged. He has offered the term "mentalized affectivity" to describe the capacity to simultaneously feel our feelings and reflect upon their meaning. Fonagy's preeminent collaborator, Mary Target, has put it this way: "Reflective function, at its most developed, involves thinking about feeling and feeling about thinking" (personal communication, 2005).

Modes of Experience

Much of Fonagy's exploration has been aimed at helping us to understand the modes of psychological experience that reflect our sense of the relationship between the internal world and external reality. Fonagy describes three such subjective modes: psychic equivalence, pretense, and mentalizing.

In the *mode of psychic equivalence,* the internal world and external reality are simply equated. There is no differentiating here between beliefs and facts. What we think and feel seems to mirror what occurs to us in the physical world, and vice versa. In this frame of mind, when we are treated badly, for example, we are likely to feel that we *are* bad—and feeling that we're bad, we "know" that we will be treated badly. In such a closed system, the self as psychological agent tends to be submerged: There is no "I" that interprets or creates experience but only a "me" to whom experience happens.

In the *"pretend" mode,* the internal world is decoupled from the external one. Here we are unfettered by actualities: Whatever we imagine is felt to be real and whatever we ignore is rendered immaterial. Dissociation, denial, and extreme narcissistic grandiosity are all examples of the "pretend" mode. In this mode, like the one above, the self as interpreter or creator of experience is constrained, because taking reality into account threatens what has been imagined and opens the door to what has been ignored.

In the *mentalizing (or reflective) mode,* we are able to recognize that the internal world is separate from, but also related to, external reality. Here we can reflect on the ways in which our thoughts, feelings, and fantasies both affect, and are affected by, what actually happens to us. In this mode, our subjective experience is felt to have interpretive depth and thus—because we can grasp the difference between events and our reactions to them—we can enjoy a measure of internal freedom. Mentalizing reveals a world of self and others that is rich, complex, and ambiguous—and one in which we have the potential to revise our mental representations of external reality as our actual realities change.

According to Fonagy, these modes of experience unfold sequentially in the course of development. At first, infants and small children live inescapably in a world of psychic equivalence in which subjective experience is compellingly, and sometimes terrifyingly, real. Then, they find a kind of liberation through the mode of pretense in which subjective experience is decoupled from reality: In play, they can pretend that the constraints of reality simply do not exist. Finally, in normal development, beginning at age four or so, there comes about an integration of these two earlier modes. Now the internal world is neither equated with, nor completely severed from, the external one. With the emergence of the reflective mode comes a growing ability to consider, implicitly and explicitly, the relationship between internal and external reality (Fonagy, 2001; Allen & Fonagy, 2002; Fonagy et al., 2002).

The patients we see in psychotherapy often have trouble extricating themselves from the modes of psychic equivalence and/or pretense. In the first case, they are bullied by feelings and thoughts that demand to be acted on because they are equated with facts. In the second, they are kept aloft by wishful thoughts, but isolated in the process from their feelings and from the people who might matter to them.

For psychotherapists and parents, as well as researchers, the key question must be: What fosters the transition out of the experiential modes of psychic equivalence and pretense into a mentalizing mode? Fonagy's answer—an elaboration on the conclusions of Bowlby, Ainsworth, and Main—is: an intersubjective relationship of attachment that provides first a full measure of affect regulation and then, not unimportantly, a modicum of play in the presence of a reflective other.

Affect Regulation, Intergenerational Transmission, and Intersubjectivity

Fonagy believes that the bridge to a reflective mode of experience is built on a foundation of affect regulation. While the "biological function" of attachment behavior is protection from predators, babies also need the attachment figure to help ensure their *emotional* survival. From the moment they are born, babies are subject to feelings of distress that they are utterly unequipped to manage on their own. To experience the "felt security" that has been described as the set goal of attachment, babies depend on the attachment figure to help them modulate their overwhelming affects.

According to Fonagy, parents who generally succeed in "containing" their infant's distress will usually have a securely attached child with a solid potential for mentalizing. Why should this be so? And what is the tieup between affect regulation, security of attachment, and mentalizing?

Successful Containment and Secure Attachment

The psychoanalyst Wilfrid Bion (1962) proposed that the supportive mother mentally contains emotional experience that the baby cannot manage on his own but manages to evoke in her. Such containment requires the mother to bear within herself, to process, and to re-present to the baby in a tolerable form what was previously the baby's intolerable emotional experience. Drawing on Bion's ideas, Fonagy suggests that parents can contain their infant's distressing affects through communicating affectively and in the language of physical care that (1) they *understand* the cause of the distress and its emotional impact; (2) they can *cope* with the distress and alleviate it; and (3) they can recognize the child's emerging *intentional stance*—by which is meant the child's ability to infer the intentions that underlie behavior, in particular, the behavior of the parent (Dennett, 1987). Strikingly, Fonagy believes that this third element of containment—the parent's recognizing the child as a separate being with a mind of her own, capable potentially of reading her parent's mind as well as her own—"may be the most important in maximizing the likelihood of the child's forming a secure attachment" (Fonagy et al., 1995, p. 248).

Parents who successfully contain their infant's unmanageable emotions

with responses that convey empathy, coping, and appreciation of the child's intentional stance are engaged in a process of interactive affect regulation. Through this process, they are reinforcing their child's confidence in the attachment relationship as a safe haven and secure base. And by acknowledging the child's intentional stance these (mentalizing) parents are providing the building blocks for what will become the child's own mentalizing ability. Note the synergy here of affect regulation, secure attachment, and mentalizing.

MIRRORING THE AFFECTS OF THE CHILD

> *... the precursor of the mirror is the mother's face.*
> —D. W. WINNICOTT (1971a, p. 111)

Fonagy observes that emotionally attuned parents convey their empathy and capacity to cope through affect mirroring that is both "contingent" and "marked." Contingent mirroring is accurate: The parent's facial or vocal displays correspond to the affects of the infant—and thus the parent's affective expressions become the basis for the child's first representations of her own affects. For such contingent displays to be seen as reflections of the *child's* emotional experience, rather than the parent's, the parent must "mark" these displays as pretend or "as if"—for example, by exaggerating the affect that is mirrored or by intermingling the disturbing affect with one that contradicts it (Fonagy et al., 2002). In these ways, the parent's responses are "giving back to the baby the baby's own self" (Winnicott, 1971a, p. 118).

Such emotionally attuned mirroring is absolutely critical, for it is through "resonating with, reflecting on, and expressing the internal state which the infant displays" that the parents allow the child to gradually discover her own emotions as mental states that can be recognized and shared—a discovery that lays the foundation for affect regulation and impulse control (Allen & Fonagy, 2002, p. 11). In addition, by seeing herself in the mirror of her *parents'* image of her as a being with an intentional stance, the child can begin to experience herself as a feeling, believing, desiring, and *mentalizing* individual, who responds to experience not only in terms of physical realities but also in light of mental states (Fonagy et al., 1995). Perhaps most important, it is through the *markedness* of the parents' mirroring that the child develops the awareness that her mind is her own:

> In markedness we deny what we feel while at the same time maintaining our individuality. In effect, we become what the child needs us to be. This is the process at the core of the child's emerging individuality. And if the caregiver is unable to do that—if the caregiver is either too much themselves [noncontingent mirroring] or too much the child [unmarked mirroring]—

the child cannot develop a sense of separateness in the same kind of effective way. (Fonagy, personal communication, 2006)

Broadly speaking, then, this is the process—interactive affect regulation made possible by mentalizing at a high level of contingency in a vital relational context—through which secure attachment is transmitted from one generation to the next. Per Fonagy, it is mentalizing that mediates this process and can potentially enable even parents whose own history of attachment is problematic to raise children who are securely attached.

The Intergenerational Transmission of Insecure Attachment

Fonagy identifies a number of inauspicious scenarios, in all of which the common theme is the inability of the parent to contain the child's unmanageable affects. Preoccupied parents may be able to empathically mirror a child's distress but without being able to deal with it. Dismissing parents may fail to communicate empathy but succeed in conveying a sense of coping and stability. There are also parents whose own vulnerabilities compromise their capacity to respond empathically to the child's intentional stance toward their mental states. Central among these vulnerabilities are the parents' own mentalizing deficits as well as the reverberating anxieties triggered by the child's separateness. For example, an expecting mother told me that she was uncomfortable with babies because she was sure they could "see through her." And what was she afraid they might see? Her scornful intolerance of their crying, their tantrums, their messiness, all the ways they could get in her way.

When parents are chronically unable to contain their child's painful affects, the child tends to behave in ways that reflect an internalization of the parent's characteristic responses to those affects. If a dismissing mother, say, responds to her infant's distress by ignoring or suppressing it, that infant may well develop an avoidant strategy for dealing with her own painful affects—in other words, she will avoid or suppress them. Effectively, the children of insecure parents "borrow" their parents' defenses and, thus, the legacy of parental insecurity is often a parallel insecurity in the child (Fonagy et al., 1995).

PROBLEMATIC MIRRORING

> *If the mother's face is unresponsive, then a mirror is a thing to be looked at but not looked into.*
> —D. W. WINNICOTT (1971a, p. 113)

Fonagy suggests that particular kinds of psychopathology may be associated with particular failures of attunement and mirroring. When the par-

ent's affective mirroring is not "marked" it can lead the child to feel overwhelmed by the contagious nature of his distress—for his upset seems only to provoke an identical emotion in the parent. Repeated exposures to unmarked mirroring are thought to reinforce the psychic equivalence mode because the child's internal experience seems regularly to be matched by his external experience, and there may appear to be no way out. Fonagy theorizes that this may be part of the genesis of borderline pathology.

In contrast, mirroring that is noncontingent can result in a sense of internal emptiness and variations on the false-self theme—because what the child is invited to internalize is an image not of his own emotional self but rather the emotional self of the parent. Because the links here are severed between the child's internal experience and its reflection in the responses of the external world, noncontingent mirroring is thought to reinforce the use of the pretend mode. Thus, according to Fonagy, the child who is regularly exposed to mirroring that is not contingent may be vulnerable to narcissistic pathology in which imagined grandiosity functions as an anodyne for the empty self (Fonagy et al., 2002).

Beyond Containment

If the pathway out of psychic equivalence and pretense begins with containment and affect regulation, it leads to the terrain of reflection in part though the medium of play. When the child is completely absorbed in his or her own play, the worlds of imagination and reality can seem to be entirely separate. But if that play is watched by a parent, an older child, or, for that matter, a therapist, then the pretend world and the real world can start to overlap. With a comment, a look, or an "interpretation" the observer makes links between internal experience and external reality, such that the two can begin to be related—rather than equated or dissociated. Thus, the groundwork is laid for mentalizing and, further, for "metarepresentation"—the ability to reflect on one's own internal experience and that of others in light of the *merely* representational nature of that experience (Fonagy et al., 2002).

Fonagy stresses that such development occurs only in a relational and intersubjective context. The affective mirroring discussed earlier is a core element of the intersubjective process through which we find aspects of ourselves in the minds of others. Whether in the course of childhood development or psychotherapy, it appears that the psychological, emotional, reflective self is discovered (or perhaps created) primarily as it is recognized and understood by others. The optimal setting for such recognition and understanding is, of course, a relationship of attachment.

FROM ATTACHMENT TO INTERSUBJECTIVITY

*The first extended tutorial in intersubjective awareness is
usually conducted with an attachment figure whose presence
and participation are necessary for the child's survival. . . .*
—KARLEN LYONS-RUTH (1999, p. 605)

Intersubjectivity has become a pivotal concept for infancy researchers and
psychoanalytic theorists alike, yet there is no consensus regarding its meaning. Intersubjectivity is variously seen to be a feature of the human condition from birth, a developmental achievement, and/or a theory of therapy.
Given the multiple uses of the word, Beebe, Knoblauch, Rustin, and Sorter
(2003) recommend that we think in terms of "forms of intersubjectivity."
Because intersubjectivity, broadly speaking, describes the interaction between two subjectivities—the interface of two minds—it is clearly central to
the developmental relationships of childhood and psychotherapy that are
the subjects of this book.

Innate Intersubjectivity

Infancy research suggests that rudimentary forms of intersubjectivity are
present virtually from birth. We appear to be preprogrammed—neurologically
"hard-wired"—for intersubjectivity. (The discovery of *mirror neurons* is a
key part of this story that will be taken up in Chapter 5's discussion of the
neurobiology of attachment.) Andrew Meltzoff and Colwyn Trevarthen are
the researchers who first detected evidence among newborns for what
Trevarthen (1979) calls *primary intersubjectivity.*

Meltzoff and his colleagues discovered that at 42 minutes of age, infants intentionally imitate the facial expressions of an adult. While initially
sucking on a "pacifier" and thus unable to imitate, the infants watched the
adult's face—mouth wide open or tongue protruding. Then for the next
two-and-a-half minutes, with the pacifier removed, they were observed
making progressively closer approximations of the expression they had
seen on the adult's face. At six weeks, infants exposed to the facial gestures
of an adult on one day will imitate those gestures on the following day
when confronted with that adult's "neutral" face. Evidently very young infants can detect—and preserve a mental representation of—the correspondence between what they *see* on someone else's face and what they *feel* in
their own face. This deliberate cross-modal matching indicates an extraordinarily early capacity for interconnectedness of self to others—and for the
sense that "I am like you" (Meltzoff, 1985, 1990; Meltzoff & Moore,
1998). Through imitation and the perception of correspondence, infants
discover aspects of themselves in others.

Trevarthen, like Meltzoff, found evidence for innate intersubjectivity in
neonatal imitation. But beyond imitation, Trevarthan observed *mutually reg-*

ulated communication between infant and adult: "Each partner can mirror the motivations and purposes of companions, immediately. Infants and their partners are thus in *immediate sympathetic contact*" (Trevarthen, quoted in Beebe et al., 2003, p. 782). The basis for this contact is the baby's capacity virtually from birth to detect contingent effects—that is, to recognize when the partner's behavior is (or is not) contingent upon the actions of the baby, and vice versa. Babies strongly prefer contingent responsiveness and their ability to recognize such responsiveness makes mutual regulation of joint action possible. According to Trevarthen, it is specifically through "reading" the matches in timing, form, and intensity of each other's communicative behavior that infants and their partners conduct nonverbal "protoconversations." These action dialogues reveal an exquisite mutual intercoordination that seems to reflect a matching not only of behavior but of the corresponding inner states—particularly the motives and intentions—of self and other (Trevarthen, 1998). Fonagy concurs with Trevarthen that human beings are preadapted for intersubjective relatedness: "There *is* primary intersubjectivity. We're born believing that our mind exists in other people. We turn to other people to see what's in our mind and to find out what things mean" (Fonagy, personal communication, 2006).

In much the same vein, Daniel Stern (1985) notes that babies turn to their mothers in order to find out about themselves—but also to find out about others and about the world. At roughly nine to twelve months of age, according to Stern, the infant makes the momentous discovery that he has a mind, that his mother has a mind, and that the subject matter of the mind—inner subjective experience—can be shared. In a classic experiment, for example, a one-year-old is invited to step across a mildly frightening glass surface in order to reach a tempting toy that lies on the other side of the "visual cliff." Confronting this ambiguous situation the baby invariably looks to the mother's face—and the subjective appraisal it conveys—to determine what his *own* subjective experience ought to be: When mother smiles, the baby appears to feel safe enough to boldly venture forth; when she looks frightened, the baby seems upset and he retreats. This kind of "social referencing" involves a form of joint attention in which the child makes up his own mind by looking into the mind of an other.

Such a sharing of the focus of attention is one of the hallmarks of intersubjective relatedness. There are two others: the sharing of intentions and, perhaps most important, the sharing of feeling states. *Affect attunement* is Stern's term for the double process of emotional resonance and communication that allows us both to feel something closely akin to what someone else is feeling and to convey to the other the fact of that shared experience.

Stern observes that in order for the baby to feel that his mother is attuned to his internal state, her imitation of his affects is insufficient because it communicates a response to his behavior rather than his experience. To convey her sharing of the baby's *experience*, the mother must offer a

"cross-modal" response to the baby' emotionally expressive behavior. For example, the mother might vocalize in rhythm with the baby's bodily expressions of excitement or she might convey attunement to the baby's disappointment by making audible sighs that have the same temporal profile as the baby's unhappy cries. The timing, intensity, and form of communicative behaviors (here Stern echoes Trevarthen) are the nonverbal dimensions through which attunement is expressed.

For Stern, it is the *sharing* of intentions, feelings, and focus of attention that define the nature of the child's intersubjective experience and, in due course, the child's experience of him- or herself. Here the crucial developmental question is what can, and cannot, be shared. The answer to this question determines "which experiences are within and which are beyond the pale of mutual consideration and acceptance" (Stern, 1985, p. 208). An intention, feeling, or attentional focus that evokes an attuned response is one that is sharable and thus can be integrated into the child's sense of self, whereas one that fails to evoke such a response can neither be shared nor integrated. From this angle, intersubjective relationships are the crucial context within which subjective experience takes shape. As Stern (2004) puts it, "Two minds create intersubjectivity. But equally, intersubjectivity shapes the two minds. The center of gravity has shifted from the intrapsychic to the intersubjective" (p. 78).

Attachment, Mentalizing, and Intersubjectivity

Stern believes that attachment and intersubjectivity are separate and complementary motivational systems. The attachment system balances our related needs for the security of physical proximity and the learning that exploration makes possible. The intersubjective system is driven by our need to know and be known by others. If attachment exists to foster felt security, intersubjectivity exists to promote the experience of psychic intimacy and belonging. Like attachment, intersubjective experience confers an evolutionary survival advantage. For one thing, it facilitates the formation and effective functioning of groups (including the group of two who fall in love). It also contributes to the formation and maintenance of self-identity. While it is possible to be attached without intersubjective relatedness (think of autism) and intersubjectively related without attachment (think of a chance meeting with a stranger who seems a soulmate), it is generally true that attachment and intersubjectivity are mutually enhancing (think of psychotherapy).

Stern sees mentalizing as a manifestation of intersubjectivity, but also regards the two, I would guess, as quite distinct. *Mentalizing,* as the word's connotations may suggest, is a process that allows us to understand and make meaningful sense of our own experience and that of others. *Intersubjective relatedness*, as the connotations of the phrase may suggest, has less

to do with understanding and meaning than it does with resonance, align-ment, and the "sharing of mental landscapes" between ourselves and others. It is the permeability or "interpenetrability" of personal boundaries that al-lows us to participate in the subjective experience of other people. In this light, the affect attunement that is a signature of intersubjectivity can be seen as a matter not just of communication but also of what Stern calls "in-terpersonal communion"—that is, joining in, being with, or sharing the subjective experience of another person with no attempt to change it (Stern, 1985, 2004).

Intersubjectivity as a Developmental Achievement

Trevarthen and Stern highlight not only the innateness of intersubjectivity and its origins in the perception of correspondence between the experience of self and other, but also the fact that intersubjective experience is mutu-ally regulated. Taking the concept of intersubjectivity a step further, the psychoanalytic theorist Jessica Benjamin proposes that intersubjectivity in the fullest sense depends upon not only correspondence but also difference, not only mutual regulation but also mutual recognition.

Benjamin (1990/1999) asks, "How is the meeting of two subjects dif-ferent from one in which a subject meets object?" (p. 35). In answering the question, she suggests that the capacity for intersubjective relatedness is an evolving and imperfectly acquired one that, at its zenith, makes possible an encounter between two *subjects*—two separate but equivalent centers of initiative and experience. This is a meeting of minds in which, as Benjamin puts it, "you know what I feel, even when I want or feel the opposite of what you want or feel" and "we can share feelings without my fearing that my feelings are simply your feelings" (p. 40). This sort of intersubjective re-latedness exemplifies what Benjamin calls *mutual recognition*—that is, the ability both to recognize and be recognized by another.

Such recognition is fundamental to an "intersubjective" as against an "intrapsychic" experience of others. The first depends on our perceiving the other as a separate subject who primarily exists outside our mental field of operations. The second involves our responding to the other primarily through projection, identification, and other intrapsychic processes—in which case the other is essentially an object in our representational world, to be idealized or devalued, perhaps, but not experienced as a real person. In the terms of Martin Buber's (1923/1970) "interhuman" philosophy of dialogue, intersubjective relatedness makes for an "I–Thou" relationship marked by mutuality, dialogue, and the ability to experience others in their own terms. By contrast, intrapsychic relating confines us to an "I–It" rela-tionship in which mutuality is absent, imposition supersedes negotiation, and preexisting categories dominate our experience of other people.

On the one hand, Benjamin (1990/1999) (rephrasing Freud) asserts in

regard to the aims of psychotherapy, "Where objects were, there subjects must be" (p. 34). On the other hand, she believes (as does Buber) that both kinds of relationship—subject/subject and subject/object—are necessary and that, paradoxically, each makes the other possible.

In clarifying the paradox, Benjamin (1990/1999) traces the development of intersubjectivity from the infant's earliest awareness of correspondence and similarity to the toddler's rapprochement conflicts between separation/individuation and relatedness starting in the middle of the second year:

> We could say that it begins with "we are feeling this feeling," and then moves to "I know that you, who are an other mind, share this same feeling." In rapprochement, however, a crisis occurs as the child begins to confront difference—"You and I don't want or feel the same thing." The initial response to this discovery is a breakdown of recognition between self and other: I insist on my way, I begin to try to coerce you, and therefore I experience your refusal as a reversal: you are coercing me." (p. 40)

Repairing the "breakdown of recognition" is crucial if the child is to begin to acquire the capacity for mutual recognition. Developing this capacity is, of course, not a one-time event, but rather a process that can be initiated early but continues lifelong. It requires that the child become capable first, of asserting her own reality and second, of accepting the opposing reality of the other.

Following Winnicott, Benjamin explains that it is only the child who forcefully expresses her anger and finds that the other "survives destruction"—neither retaliating nor withdrawing—who has the opportunity to learn that the other is, in fact, a separate subject rather than an object. Here is the resolution of the paradox that in being treated as an object, the other may be found as a subject. Through the child's failed attempt to impose his or her will and negate that of the other, the child discovers that differences need not be a barrier to shared experience and that dialogue can obviate the requirement that one must dominate and one submit. This discovery allows the child to take fuller possession of his or her own subjectivity, realizing that a relationship can potentially make room for two—two wills, two views of reality, two subjects.

Note that mutual recognition and mentalizing are conceptual cousins. Without referring to Benjamin's discussion of subjects and objects, Fonagy makes a distinction that parallels hers, suggesting that when we mentalize we respond to others not as *objects* but as *persons*.

Intersubjectivity as a Theory of Psychotherapy

Benjamin gives credit to Robert Stolorow and his colleagues for introducing the term "intersubjectivity" into the arena of clinical theory. Characterizing their own work as an expansion of psychoanalytic self psychology,

they describe intersubjectivity in the analytic context as "the specific psychological field constituted by the intersection of two subjectivities—that of the patient and that of the analyst" (Stolorow, Brandschaft, & Atwood, 1987, p. 1). Similarly, in *A Primer of Clinical Intersubjectivity*, Natterson and Friedman (1995) state, "Intersubjectivity is the over-arching term that refers to the reciprocal influence of the conscious and unconscious subjectivities of two people in a relationship" (p. 1).

While these writers use the word "intersubjectivity" in connection with a specific approach to treatment, I regard it more broadly as the best umbrella term for an invaluable body of clinical research that has taken shape in the last 20 years, that both echoes and extends the clinically fertile insights of attachment theory and infant–parent research. Variously described with the terms "intersubjectivity theory," "relational psychoanalysis," and "social constructivism," these findings from the consulting room have brought about a paradigm shift in the clinical realm that gives us new tools to work with the "unverbalizable" experience attachment research identifies as so central. At the heart of this shift is a rejection of the ideal of the anonymous therapist as objective observer. In its place is recognition of our inevitable involvement in enactments that reflect the interlocking vulnerabilities of patient and therapist—and the challenge of turning these potential obstacles into opportunities for healing.

Attachment and Intersubjectivity in the Healing Relationship

Bowlby's seminal insights as well as the research of Ainsworth, Main, and Fonagy point to the absolute centrality of attachment relationships as the crucibles within which our personalities take shape. By implication, attachment relationships may also be the setting in which—whether in love or psychotherapy—our early emotional injuries are most likely to be healed. The therapist, then, may be a new attachment figure in relation to whom the patient can develop fresh patterns of attachment.

Fonagy, in attempting to make the bridge from attachment research to clinical practice, emphasizes the importance of enabling the patient to find an image of him- or herself in the mind of the therapist as a thinking and feeling being. In this view, psychotherapy "works" by generating a relationship of secure attachment within which the patient's mentalizing and affect regulating capacities can develop. For Fonagy, such a relationship must be an intersubjective one in which the patient comes to know him- or herself in the process of being known by another.

Fonagy is not the only clinician/researcher attempting to bridge the realms of attachment, intersubjectivity, and psychotherapy. In addition, Beebe (2004), Beebe and Lachmann (2002), Beebe et al. (2003), Fosha (2000, 2003), Holmes (1996, 2001), Seligman (2000, 2003), and Slade (1999, 2000), have all made significant contributions to our understanding

of the developmental role of intersubjective attachment relationships. Deserving special note, perhaps, are the contributions that have come from a collaborative effort launched by Daniel Stern in 1995.

At that time, Stern brought together a number of developmental researchers and psychoanalysts (of whom the most prominent were Karlen Lyons-Ruth, Louis Sander, and Edward Tronick) to form what is now referred to as the Change Process Study Group (CPSG) (Stern et al., 1998; Lyons-Ruth & Boston Change Process Study Group, 2001; Boston Change Process Study Group, 1998, 2002, 2005). Leaning on Stern's conclusion that human beings are "hard-wired" for intersubjectivity, the work of this group has emphasized the importance in childhood and psychotherapy of attending to the nuances of interaction in order to understand development. In particular, they have focused on the co-created, implicit, and often unverbalized process through which change occurs in both infant–parent and patient–therapist relationships. From their perspective, the therapeutic relationship as *lived* rather than analyzed is the primary therapeutic intervention. Stern himself, perhaps harking back to his earlier attention to affect attunement as a kind of intersubjective communion, has recently made the case that the pursuit of meaning may short-circuit the deepening of experience—in particular, the experience of intersubjective meeting between patient and clinician that can sometimes produce, in and of itself, the most significant therapeutic change. Without referring directly to mindfulness, Stern highlights in this connection the absolute centrality of a focus on the present moment (Stern, 2004).

Surveying the range of these contributions reveals the outlines of an integrated approach to treatment that fills in the largely missing clinical dimension of attachment theory. As elaborated in the chapters to follow, this approach places the new attachment relationship at the center of therapeutic work. In the context of this co-created intersubjective relationship, implicit and unverbalized communication plays a crucial role in enabling us to recognize, and allowing the patient to revisit, his or her unfinished developmental business. Just as important, we can structure the therapeutic relationship in such a way that it comes to function as an incubator of the patient's more or less undeveloped capacities to freely feel, think, and love. Winnicott (1965) wrote, "The characteristic of the maturational process is the drive towards *integration*" (p. 239). When we can somehow enable that drive in the patient to be reengaged, the new attachment relationship becomes transformative.

PART II

ATTACHMENT RELATIONSHIPS AND THE DEVELOPMENT OF THE SELF

I*t is in the crucible of the child's first relationships that, for better or worse, the self is originally shaped. For patients whose healthy development was derailed by the shortcomings of these formative relationships, psychotherapy may recreate an interactive matrix of attachment in which the self can potentially be healed. In light of the overlap between what is provided by the sensitively responsive parent and the empathically attuned therapist, our work as clinicians can be strengthened to the extent that we understand the change processes of childhood.*

Such understanding requires a somewhat detailed account of the facets of the self—neurobiological as well as psychological—that emerge in the course of development and set the stage for the life experience that will follow. As we are about to see, the trajectory of later development is shaped fundamentally by the ways in which the child first learns (or fails to learn) to manage difficult emotions. Attachment relationships are the school in which this emotional learning originally occurs. In identifying early patterns of interactive affect regulation, both secure and insecure, attachment research enhances our ability as therapists to generate a developmentally

facilitative relationship with our patients in which we are at once reworking old experiences and co-creating new ones.

Chapter 5 describes the multiple dimensions of the self that are first shaped—and can subsequently be reshaped—in an attachment context. Chapter 6 summarizes research that documents the varieties of attachment experience from infancy through adulthood and gives us a uniquely evocative basis for grasping the origin, meaning, and impact of each of the four primary states of mind with respect to attachment. Chapter 7 begins to build bridges between attachment research and clinical practice, with the focus on affect regulation, the co-created attachment relationship, and the qualities of collaborative communication that most effectively foster security in both childhood and psychotherapy.

CHAPTER 5

The Multiple Dimensions
of the Self

In each of us, the ensemble of body proper, brain, and mind interact to generate the relatively stable internal point of reference known as the *self*. This is the part of the human being that *experiences* life—but also shapes it—nonconsciously as well as consciously. The self can also be described in terms of the particular cluster of more or less enduring patterns that determines the character of our unique responsiveness to experience. The present character of the self will vary depending on both our history and current context. The history that is usually most influential here is, of course, the history of the attachment relationships that have formed the self.

THE DOMAINS OF SELF-EXPERIENCE

The impact of attachment relationships registers in the interrelated, indeed overlapping domains of the body, the emotions, and the representational world, shaping the stance of the self toward experience in each. These domains or dimensions of the self are linked and mutually influential to such a degree that distinguishing one from the other can be a difficult matter: Somatic sensations are a component of emotions which shape representations that affect, in turn, the quality of subsequent sensations, emotions, and representations. Yet, despite this kind of loop or overlap, identifying the separate domains of self has considerable clinical value, in part because

it helps illuminate the nature of the integration (or lack of it) that individual patients (and clinicians) bring to the therapeutic relationship.

Largely it is the particulars of attachment history that determine how freely the various dimensions of the self can be accessed and integrated. To what extent can patients experience their bodily sensations, feel their emotions, think their own thoughts? And how effectively can they integrate these domains—for example, by bringing their thoughts to bear on their feelings? Answers to questions like these can help to clarify what our patients may need most from the new attachment relationship we are attempting to provide.

The Somatic Self

> ... the ego is first and foremost a bodily ego.
> —SIGMUND FREUD (1923/1962, p. 20)

The infant's original experiences certainly appear to register in the body: a satisfying fullness after being fed; a comfortable drowsiness that segues to sleep in the mother's arms; the sensation of coldness provoking tears during a diaper change in a chilly room. Daniel Stern (1985) observed in *The Interpersonal World of the Infant* that the "core self" emerges from the baby's early experience of "self-invariants," at the center of which is the baby's own body and its boundaries. The neurobiologist Antonio Damasio (1999) also argues for the "remarkable invariance of the structures and operations of the body" (p. 135) as the source of the stability so pivotal to the experience of self.

Bowlby, of course, grounded attachment theory in evolutionary biology, arguing that the infant's seeking of proximity to the caregiver was originally rooted in the need for bodily protection. Subsequent research shows that ongoing proximity to the attachment figure serves literally to regulate the internal functioning of the infant's body, and evidence suggests that the quality of the attachment relationship—secure or insecure—influences how the infant's developing physiology shapes the bodily self's responsiveness to experience. For example, the secure infants of sensitively responsive mothers have a higher threshold for the activation of physiological stress responses than the insecure offspring of dismissing, preoccupied, and, especially, unresolved mothers (Polan & Hofer, 1999; Lyons-Ruth, 1999).

Thus, the original sense of self is rooted in somatic experience whose nature largely depends on the quality of early attachment relationships. Such experience shapes the self during the first months and years, often with lasting consequences. Potentially, it can allow bodily experience to ground, inform, and enrich the self throughout the lifespan. Alternatively, bodily experience may be denied, dissociated, or distorted—the body itself exploited or attacked for a variety of psychological purposes. Because the

patient's experience of the body is fundamental and because it takes shape in a relational context, an attachment-oriented treatment must include a focus on the somatic self. How to integrate the body in the "talking cure" is a matter I'll take up when exploring the role of nonverbal experience in development and psychotherapy.

The Emotional Self

Feelings of pain or pleasure or some quality in between are the bedrock of our minds.
—ANTONIO DAMASIO (2003, p. 3)

When Sroufe and Waters (1977a) grafted "felt security" onto proximity as the goal of attachment, they explicitly highlighted the centrality of emotion to attachment. Indeed, it is the *feeling of security* that is most fundamental, more even than proximity—for the baby could, of course, be physically close to the attachment figure without feeling secure. Beyond infancy as well, how we *feel* clearly remains central to our sense of who we *are*.

Bowlby (1988) stressed the primacy of emotion[1] when he described the exchange of affects as "the only means of communication we have" in our first years (p. 157). Daniel Stern (1985) echoes Bowlby but goes a step further, observing that "early in life, affects are both the primary medium and the primary subject of communication" (pp. 132–133). Allan Schore (1994) sums up the matter succinctly: "The core of the self lies in patterns of affect regulation" (p. 33).

Emotional responses are fundamental to the developing sense of self for at least three reasons. First, as Bowlby (1969/1982) noted, in the opening volume of his *Attachment* trilogy: "Emotions are . . . the individual's *intuitive appraisals* either of his own organismic states . . . or the succession of environmental situations in which he finds himself" (p. 104; emphasis added).

Second, as suggested in the etymology of the word (from the Latin: *motore,* meaning to move), emotions drive actions—sometimes by triggering inborn behavioral systems, including among others the attachment system. Emotional appraisals had survival value, according to Bowlby, because they facilitated immediate decisions—for example, whether to fight or flee. Built in by evolutionary design, particular emotions automatically spark distinct action tendencies: Anger triggers confrontation or inhibition, fear triggers flight or physical paralysis, helplessness triggers collapse, and so on (van der Kolk, 2006; Damasio, 1999).

Third, emotions are always connected to the body. Bodily sensations are the first form our emotions take, and emotions are regularly expressed through the body. When we feel emotions we are sensing (or imagining) what is going on in the body (Damasio, 2003). As William James (1884)

rather provocatively suggested, our bodies don't run from danger because we're afraid—rather, we're afraid because our bodies run. Grounded in the body, emotions pervade and frequently dominate our subjective experience. When felt intensely, they often trump or preempt rational analysis and decision making.

Emotions, in sum, are the processes by which we *viscerally* appraise the goodness or badness of the experiences we encounter—and it is largely on the basis of such appraisals that we decide (consciously or unconsciously) how we will act. More broadly, our emotions can be seen to provide an internal value system that enables us, throughout our lives, to assign meaning to our experience and make choices about how to proceed (Siegel, 1999).

Fonagy et al. (2002), Schore (2003), and others propose that regulation of emotions is fundamental to the development of the self and that attachment relationships are the primary context within which we learn to regulate our affects—that is, to access, modulate, and use our emotions. The relational patterns that characterize our first attachments are, fundamentally, patterns of affect regulation that subsequently determine a great deal about the nature of our own unique responsiveness to experience— that is, about the nature of the self. Correspondingly, in the new attachment relationship that the therapist is attempting to generate, the patient's emotions are central and their effective regulation—which allows them to be felt, modulated, communicated, and understood—is usually at the very heart of the process that enables the patient to heal and to grow.

The Representational Self

> . . . the idea of a model in the brain is that it constitutes a toy
> that is yet a tool, an imitation world, which we can
> manipulate in the way that will suit us best, and so find out
> how to manipulate the real world, which it is supposed
> to represent.
> —J. Z. YOUNG (1964, quoted in Bowlby, 1969/1982, p. 80)

Bowlby argued that it was an evolutionary necessity to have a representational world that mapped the real one: To function effectively, we needed (and still need) knowledge of the world and of ourselves, and this knowledge must be portable. We derive such knowledge from memories of past experience, and we use this knowledge to make predictions about present and future experience. Hence, the internal working model. But the map, as they say, is not the territory.

The working models of our attachment relationships are selective, more or less representative samplings of lived relational experience. In the framework of Daniel Stern (1985), they are composed of "representations

of interactions that have been generalized" (p. 97). Throughout our lives they continue to provide us with a fundamental orientation, or quality of responsiveness, to experience.

If our early relationships were secure, the result may well be a capacity to respond—that is, to think, sense, feel, and act—with openness and flexibility. In this case, we can modify old representations in light of new experience. Such malleable representations can be used, along with our feelings, as guides in adaptively shaping our conscious choices. If, on the other hand, our formative relationships were marked by avoidance, ambivalence, or disorganization, then our capacity for the "response flexibility" (Siegel, 1999) associated with such alterable representations will be compromised.

Most critical of all, perhaps, is the extent to which our early attachments have (or have not) provided us with the relational experience of a secure base and, thus, the foundation for a mental representation of an *internalized* secure base. This internal representation allows us to restore emotional equilibrium, at times, through obtaining *symbolic* contact with security-enhancing attachment figures, without necessarily seeking actual proximity to them (Mikulincer & Shaver, 2003; Holmes, 2001). When we are able to turn (consciously or otherwise) to such a reassuring internal presence, we gain a degree of resilience—and the resulting confidence to explore our selves and the world—that is missing or diminished when we lack an internalized secure base.

As illuminated by object relations theory, the development of mental representations that "work" entails two fundamental processes: differentiation and integration (Kernberg, 1984). *Differentiation* creates psychological boundaries, particularly between self and other, and between the internal world and external reality. A well-differentiated self-representation allows us to function autonomously without feeling that we are defined by the feelings others have about us. On the problematic side, a lack of differentiation between the inside and outside, between the mental and physical worlds, is exactly what marks the mode of psychic equivalence that undermines many of our insecurely attached patients. *Integration* involves synthesis and connection. Integrated representations of ourselves and of others enable us to bring together emotionally contradictory experiences—so that, for example, we can love someone even when we're angry with them. Integration fosters balance and an awareness of the nuances and complexity of experience. Without integrated representations, we're vulnerable to experiencing our selves and others in extreme and simplistic terms: as all good or all bad, heroes or villains.

Just as the roots of the *emotional self* are found in bodily experience, the *representational self* is fundamentally grounded in emotional experience, often of a highly charged nature. As Bowlby (1969/1982) mentions, experiences of attachment and/or its disruption are prone to evoke the most

intense of feelings. Thus, our representations of ourselves, of others, and of relationships do not merely have a powerful emotional component; they are in most cases actually *dominated*, outside awareness, by the emotions that underpin them.[2]

It is largely the *unconscious* emotional dimension of our inner representations that renders them resistant to revision. If, for example, we learned through our formative interactions that being close to others was risky, then defenses will have been instituted to keep us unaware of our need for closeness; we simply won't be motivated to make the bids for closeness that, if successful, might update our old (avoidant) model of attachment to a more secure one. Likewise, because emotions involve bodily signals to others as well as to our selves, the expectation that our overtures will be rejected may well result in feelings of fear or anger, the unconscious bodily expression of which provokes the very rejection our working model has led us to expect. As both Bowlby and Main emphasize, working models—especially insecure ones—tend to have a self-perpetuating quality. Shaped preverbally in the setting of early attachment relationships, these internal representations inevitably exert a powerful and largely unconscious influence on the nature of the developing self.

It is vital for therapists to be aware that such representations exist in multiple, interacting domains. As Main suggests, internal working models register or encode experience not only in images that can be visualized or beliefs that can be articulated—that is, in symbols—but also in "rules" that determine what we can or cannot attend to, including thoughts, feelings, desires, and memories (Main et al., 1985; Main, 1991). Other attachment researchers have subsequently focused on what Karlen Lyons-Ruth (1999) calls *enactive representations*. These are presymbolic representations of experience that find expression only in action or interaction—that is, in "procedures" or ways of being, especially ways of being with others. For example, although we can't remember our infancy, we might well enact facets of it as a parent with an infant of our own. Finally, from outside the attachment field, investigators of trauma (such as van der Kolk, 1996) and neuroscientists (such as LeDoux, 1996) have discussed *somatic* and *emotional memories* that encode experience in the form of bodily sensations and affective reactions.

Understanding these various forms of representation—bodily, emotional, and enactive as well as symbolic—has enormous clinical value. In therapy, bringing to light representations that have existed in shadow, as invisible imprints of the past, can give patients greater freedom to feel, think, and act in the present. These are matters I'll take up in detail in the chapters on nonverbal experience. For now, suffice it to say that in order to make these implicit representations explicit—and thus potentially subject them to the integrating

influence of conscious reflection—therapists must attune to their patients' bodily, emotional, and enactive as well as linguistic communications.

Of course, what is true here for patients is equally true for their therapists: Only when our representations of experience are illuminated by awareness can we question them. Without the understanding that awareness makes possible, we are no less vulnerable than our patients to believing whatever we might think or feel at any given moment—particularly when the emotional tides of the moment run strong. In such an unreflective state of mind, we are simply embedded or immersed in our subjective experience. Thus deprived of a broader perspective, we fail to grasp the essentially *representational* nature of mental experience and so remain prisoners of (what we take to be) reality.

The Reflective Self and the Mindful Self

While the bodily, emotional, and representational dimensions of the self are inherent in being human, and thus accessible to almost all of us, the domains of the reflective and mindful self are only *potentially* accessible. Yet these potentialities are of critical importance. For in different ways, mentalizing and mindfulness alike are associated with the internalized secure base that makes resilience and exploration possible. Moreover, both are capable of fostering insight and empathy, affect regulation and the sense of personal agency, internal freedom and the capacity to respond with adaptive flexibility to the complex, often difficult, circumstances with which our lives confront us. Thus mentalizing and mindfulness are pathways of psychological liberation.

As discussed earlier, our reflective or mentalizing self generally emerges through a relationship in which experiencing the attachment figure as a secure base makes it safe for us to explore the world, including the internal world. As Diana Fosha (2003) suggests, it is "being understood by and having the sense of existing in the mind and heart of a loving, caring, attuned, and self-possessed other" (p. 228) that gives us the chance to be known as a person rather than an object—that is, a being whose behavior derives meaning from the feelings, intentions, and beliefs that underlie it. Growing up with someone who has our mind in mind equips us as "mental agents" (Fonagy & Target, in press) who can deliberately attempt to make sense of subjective experience, so as to be able to be present for it, rather than feel overwhelmed by or cut off from it. Lacking a childhood relationship that might have supported such mental agency, many of our patients remain swamped by, or estranged from, their internal experience. As therapists, it is largely our mentalizing ability that enables us to provide for these patients the kind of relationship—a new attachment relationship—within which their own capacity for a reflective self can be nurtured.

By a different route, mindfulness (like mentalizing) can allow us to be present for our experience, rather than submerged by or dissociated from it. For if mentalizing promotes internal freedom by enabling us to act as mental agents, mindfulness fosters freedom by enabling us to act as "attentional agents." Exercising voluntary, sustained, and nonjudgmental attention to our here-and-now experience changes that experience—at once deepening and "lightening" it: deepening because we can be more fully present, accepting, and aware, lightening because present-centered awareness is less burdened by the weight of the past and the future, less encumbered by shame and fear. Such awareness can be beneficial in many ways. It contributes to the regulation of difficult emotions. It also tends to deautomatize habitual patterns of response (Engler, 2003; Martin, 1997; Safran & Muran, 2000), enabling us to "wake up" and experience the world afresh—as if with a "beginner's mind" (Suzuki, 1970). Moreover, as I suggested in Chapter 1, the self that is mindful tends to become increasingly identified with awareness itself, rather than the thoughts, feelings, or sensations of which we're aware. This identification with awareness—ultimately an experience of selflessness that lessens the need to protect the (personal) self—can strengthen our sense of an internalized secure base. Finally, mindfulness quiets the mind. Lowering the volume of mental static, it heightens our receptivity to signals from every domain of the self. Experiences of the mindful self are thus not only integrated but also integrating: They foster adaptive connections between different aspects of the self and between the self and others.

Understood in this way, mindfulness can be seen as a vital therapeutic resource that—like mentalizing—both strengthens and is strengthened by the new attachment relationship we are attempting to generate. How to cultivate these complementary capacities in our patients and ourselves is a subject I will address in subsequent chapters on the stance of the self toward experience.

THE NEUROBIOLOGY OF ATTACHMENT

> . . . the evolutionary role of the attachment relationship goes far beyond giving physical protection to the human infant. Attachment ensures that the brain processes that come to subserve social cognition are appropriately organized and prepared to equip the individual for the collaborative and cooperative existence with others for which the brain was designed.
> —PETER FONAGY and MARY TARGET (2006)

Because psychological patterns are also patterns of neural organization, and because the brain as well as the mind develops in the crucible of attach-

ment relationships, a familiarity with the basics of contemporary neuroscience can enrich our understanding of the multiple dimensions of the self. The last 10 years of the 20th century have been called "the Decade of the Brain" because of the explosion of neuroscience research that occurred during this period. Innovative neuroimaging technologies have expanded our knowledge about the structure and functioning of the brain so rapidly that they have begun to make possible the realization of Freud's (1895/1966) dream in the "Project for a Scientific Psychology"—that his theories about the psyche might one day be grounded in the facts of neurophysiology.

Attachment, Experience, and the Brain

The most powerful conceptual links between the brain and the mind—and between neuroscience and psychotherapy—have been forged by Allan Schore (1994, 2002, 2003) and Daniel Siegel (1999, 2001, 2006). Importantly, each writer grounds his understanding of both psychological and brain development on a foundation of attachment theory research. Schore (2002) states unequivocally that healthy *neural* as well as psychological development in early childhood hinges on the attuned responsiveness of attachment figures: "The baby's brain is not only affected by these interactions; its growth literally requires brain/brain interactions and occurs in the context of a positive relationship between mother and infant" (p. 62). When the baby emerges from the mother's womb, his brain—composed of billions of cells called neurons—is the least differentiated of all his bodily organs. The ensuing development of the brain largely depends on how "the genetically programmed maturation of the nervous system" is shaped by interpersonal experience (Siegel, 1999, p. 2). From a neurobiological as well as a psychological standpoint, then, the most vital and influential experience is that which occurs, for better or worse, in the context of attachment relationships.

Siegel explains that what registers in the mind and body as "experience" corresponds at the neural level to patterns in the firing or activation of brain cells. These patterns of neuronal firing establish synaptic connections in the brain that determine the nature of its structure and functioning. Paraphrasing the neuroanatomist Donald Hebb, Siegel (1999) writes, "neurons that fire together wire together" (p. 26). The architecture of the brain is associational: When incoming stimuli (mother's sensitive touch, her soothing voice, her look of calm) trigger activity in the baby's brain, those neurons that fire in synch link up, establishing a "neural network" that associates any or all of these maternal stimuli with a feeling of safety. In this way, experience—especially experience that is repeated—shapes the "circuitry" of the brain. Younger brains are built to learn from older brains, and attachment relationships are the setting in which most of this learning

originally occurs. Thus, relational connections become neural connections that influence, in turn, the responsiveness of the self to new experience. Conversely, the absence of relational connections—say, between the dismissing parent and the distressed infant—can impede the development of neural connections, thus limiting, in turn, the child's ability to feel her emotions. Schore and Siegal make a compelling case—one borne out by my own clinical experience—that a familiarity with basic neuroscience and the impact of early relationships on the brain can help therapists to more effectively help their patients.

The Structure of the Brain

Let's start with the fundamentals. In the crudest of analogies, the brain can be seen as the neural equivalent of a three-story, side-by-side duplex whose structure is divided down the middle (right brain/left brain) and whose three levels (brainstem, limbic system, neocortex) are built one after the other, moving from the bottom up.

The Brainstem

In the course of both individual development and evolution, the brain's "lowest" level or basement—the brainstem—is the first to emerge. Already active in the womb and fully operational at birth, the brainstem owes less to experience and learning than any other region of the brain. Sitting atop the spinal column, the brainstem provides the neural machinery necessary to regulate basic bodily functions (such as heart rate, respiration, digestion) and to activate reflexes, including those that "jump start" the attachment process: "The neonate will orient to the mother's smell, seek the nipple, gaze into her eyes, and grasp her hair. . . . The child's eyes orient to his or her mother's eyes and face. A baby's first smiles are also a reflex controlled by the brainstem to attract caretakers" (Cozolino, 2002, p. 75).

As the neural substrate of the somatic self, the brainstem is significant from a clinical perspective because it modulates arousal and regulates the autonomic nervous system (ANS) that Schore (2003) refers to as "the physiological bottom of the mind" (p. 82). High levels of arousal are associated with the activation of the sympathetic side of the ANS that prepares us for fight or flight by quickening respiration, accelerating the heart rate, and moving blood to the limbs. Low levels of arousal are linked to activation of the parasympathetic system that leads, at the extreme, to tonic immobility or "freezing."

Originating in the brainstem is a double-branched cranial nerve called the vagus that shapes our distinct responses in situations we experience as safe, dangerous, or life threatening. When we feel safe, the more mature

branch, the *myelinated ventral vagus*, puts on the "vagal brake" that downregulates the sympathetic nervous system (calming the body and slowing the heart) so that social engagement becomes possible. When we feel endangered the vagal brake is released, disinhibiting the sympathetic nervous system and mobilizing us for fight or flight. When we feel in mortal danger, the more primitive *unmyelinated dorsal vagus* triggers parasympathetic shutdown and immobilization. Helpless in the face of life-threatening trauma, we "play dead." Dissociation is usually the psychological complement of this physical reaction (Porges, 2006; Schore, 2006).

Importantly, the ventral vagal system has primary control not only of visceral organs like the heart but also of the musculature of the face and head, without which effective social communication (eye contact, vocalizing with an appealing inflection, contingent facial expressions) is impossible. When the ventral vagus is knocked offline by danger or life threat, the resulting sympathetic mobilization or parasympathetic immobilization may well be adaptive. But when past trauma has eroded the efficiency of the brainstem's vagal brake, the resulting propensity to fight, flight, or freezing is almost always maladaptive. Witness the hair-trigger reactivity and/or the expressionless faces and inflectionless voices of the trauma survivors we see in psychotherapy (van der Kolk, 2006; Porges, 2006).

One clinical implication here is that treatment must take into account our patients' brainstem-based patterns of over- and underarousal. The success of therapy, especially with patients who have been traumatized, hinges on our ability to accurately read and effectively modulate their levels of physiological arousal as well as their needs for (and fears of) relational engagement. This requires a focus on the body, nonverbal experience, and the nuances of the therapeutic interaction.

The Limbic System

If, per Paul MacLean's (1990) model of the "triune brain," the brainstem is analogous to the reptilian brain, the limbic system compares roughly to the paleomammalian brain we share with other mammals. Sometimes called the "emotional brain" the limbic system is where we process feelings. Such processing is critical, because emotion provides not only the fundamental means by which we viscerally appraise our experience, but also the nonverbal language that makes effective social interaction possible. The limbic system is also essential for memory, learning, and motivation—including the motivations associated with attachment.

Like the ground floor of a duplex that has easy commerce with the street, the limbic system is where the internal and external worlds meet. Here, at an emotional level, we work out the relationship between our selves and the exigent realities that exist outside our bodies. And on the ba-

sis of our lived experience, we learn what to expect. Literally with mother's first touch we begin to decide whether or not we can safely turn to her for comfort. Whether our cries evoke her reassuring presence or whether our distress provokes her irritation or indifference, these experiences register in emotional memory and guide our ensuing appraisals of security or risk in subsequent attachment-related situations. Clearly, the limbic system is the neural substrate of the emotional self. It houses two key structures.

The *amygdala*, which is well developed at birth, can be been described as the sensory gateway to the limbic system. Along with the brainstem's vagus nerve that brings the visceral sensation of the internal world (heart, lungs, intestines) to awareness, the amygdala is responsible for our "gut" reactions to experience (Schore, 2003). Central to our ability to "read the mind in the eyes," it directs preferential attention to facial cues, and gives us an intuitive "feel" for other people (Baron-Cohen, 1999). The amygdala might also be described as "survival central" (Rothschild, 2000) because of its role in triggering reactions of fight or flight. Within a fraction of a second, the amygdala can appraise sensory input (an angry face, the growl of a dog), especially as this input bears on safety or threat.

By signaling the brainstem to activate the sympathetic nervous system, the amygdala translates near-instantaneous appraisals of danger into physical reactions that prime the body to fight or flee. While a few of these appraisals are grounded in biological universals (human beings instinctively fear snakes, for example), the rest are conditioned by the particulars of personal history.

As much an organ of memory as of appraisal, the amygdala registers experience in the form of nonconscious presymbolic "emotional memories" (LeDoux, 1996). Entirely outside awareness, these linguistically inaccessible traces of the past (particularly the traumatic past) bias our appraisals of experience in the present. Thus, a veteran scarred by the trauma of battle might hear the backfire of a car on a city street and reflexively drop to the ground in a cold sweat. Similarly, patients with a history of traumatic attachment may be automatically prone to read as clues to danger social signals that are ambiguous, nonthreatening, or even positive.

The *hippocampus* modulates the amygdala's bias toward indiscriminate, uncontrolled, hair-trigger reactions. Specialized to organize information according to sequence and context, it enables us to respond very differently to a rattlesnake coiled before us on the trail and a rattlesnake curled up behind glass in a vivarium. If the amygdala, which has no such powers of differentiation, is the accelerator that primes the sympathetic nervous system, the hippocampus is the brake that engages the parasympathetic nervous system, enabling us to settle down (with respiration and heart rate slowed) when the emergency is appraised as a false alarm (Siegel, 1999).

Clinically, it is important to realize that the hippocampus begins to come online only during the second to third year of life, with the conse-

quence that, in the first years of life, experience and learning register in the amygdala as unconscious emotional memories that tend to be global, overgeneralized, and, thus, disproportionately influential. In therapy, such memories may be accessible only through the patient's sensations, feelings, or impulses that, in turn, reflect the bodily, emotional, or enactive representations of early experience.

By contrast, memories that register with the help of the hippocampus—whose connections to the higher brain centers of the cortex continue to mature through late adolescence—are explicit, linguistically retrievable, and contextualized according to time, place, and person. While secure relationships allow the child's developing hippocampus to balance the reactivity of the amygdala, acute and relational trauma can shut down the hippocampus temporarily or inhibit its development, leaving more or less unmodulated the reactivity of the overvigilant amygdala.

It may be that, to paraphrase LeDoux (1996), the amygdala's emotional memories are forever. Yet the fear response is a conditioned one, a product of associational learning. Past attachment trauma may well have created an association between closeness and danger (neurons that fire together wire together). But the patient in psychotherapy who revisits old trauma in the setting of a new attachment relationship can forge fresh associations in the brain and mind. Recalling and reexperiencing childhood fears and hurts in a context of safety can gradually transform the patient's remembered past, and dampen in the process the automatic amygdala-based reactions it has long evoked.

The Neocortex

ANATOMY AND FUNCTION

Layered over the brainstem and limbic system is the cerebral cortex, the upper floor of the neural duplex. Shared with our primate relatives, this "neomammalian brain" makes sense of our experience and organizes our interaction with the world. It is the last part of the brain to emerge, both in evolutionary terms and in the development of the individual, and it matures only gradually with the accretion of experience and new learning, virtually throughout the lifespan. The rear areas of the cortex are dedicated to perception of the physical world through the five senses and the body, while the frontal regions are specialized to process information from other parts of the brain and to guide behavior.

The *frontal cortex* can be seen as the "executive brain" (Cozolino, 2002) that makes possible conscious thought, planning, memory, deliberate action, directed attention, and abstract reasoning. It is the "seat" of language and of those ideas and mental representations that can be raised to the level of awareness, where they may be considered and manipulated.

The frontal cortex can be seen to provide the neural substrate for the symbolic/representational, reflective, and mindful dimensions of the self.

The most advanced area of the cortex—and one that has particular relevance for psychotherapy—is the *prefrontal cortex*. This area is divided into two main regions. The first, specialized for cognitive intelligence, is the dorsolateral region that networks with the hippocampus and the linguistically oriented left brain. The second, specialized for emotional intelligence, is a region Siegel (2006) refers to as the "middle prefrontal cortex," which is richly connected to the amygdala and the emotionally oriented right brain.

The *dorsolateral region* has been described as the "rational mind" (van der Kolk, 2006) and key to the "volitional brain" (Libet, Freeman, & Sutherland, 1999). It enables us to *consciously* think about our experience, deliberately directing attention to our perceptions, memories, and/or ideas, and drawing as needed on our mental representations of the past, present, and future. This region seems to be the neural locale for working memory, the "chalkboard of the mind" (Siegel, 1999) where we use our heads to solve problems, deliberate about decisions, and generally try to make sense of things.

The *middle prefrontal cortex* is an integrative region that links the body proper, brainstem, limbic system, and cortex. Schore (1994, 2002) and Siegel (1999, 2006) have both emphasized the centrality of this region as a mediator of attachment behavior, affect regulation, social communication, and mentalization. They highlight, in particular, the cortical area that sits directly behind the eyes—the *orbitofrontal cortex* (or Ofc)—that may be "as much an extension of the limbic system as it is a portion of the cortex" (Cozolino, 2002, p. 180).

This area appears to be responsible for the decoding of emotional signals through the ability it gives us to "read" nonverbal cues such as facial expression, gestures, and tone of voice. As the "thinking part of the emotional brain" (Goleman, 1995), the Ofc plays a key role in affect regulation, which has been seen as both the purpose for, and the outcome of, relationships of secure attachment. In part, such regulation occurs as the Ofc modulates the amygdala's rapid responses to the perception of threat. While the Ofc responds to threatening facial expressions (as does the amygdala), it also contextualizes the threat and determines its degree (as the amygdala does not). This kind of discrimination facilitates both self-regulation and social relatedness. Conversely, orbitofrontal damage or deficit is associated with difficulty in managing one's emotions, gauging one's impact on others, and responding appropriately to their social signals and states of mind. Uniquely well-connected to every other region of the brain, the Ofc can be seen as a convergence zone and an organ of integration that synthesizes the flow of information conveyed through bodily, emotional, and cognitive channels. This synthesizing capacity is critical to our abilities to update our internal models and get effectively in

synch with other people—both of which, in the face of difficult developmental circumstances, may be essential if we are to become securely attached and capable of imparting security to our children. Of course, these abilities are no less essential to therapists who aim to impart security to their patients.

While the Ofc has been dubbed the "senior executive of the social-emotional brain" (Schore 2002, p. 42), a region above and behind it—the *anterior cingulate*—also plays a critical role in attachment, affect regulation, and mentalizing. It has been suggested that the anterior cingulate may provide the neural foundation for maternal behavior, for the implicit and explicit senses of self, and for the conscious experience of emotion. It may also be the source of the most integrated view of the state of the body. Finally, it appears to be responsible for the moment-by-moment direction of attention and motor responses as these are guided by emotion (Damasio, 1999; Cozolino, 2002; Allen & Fonagy, 2002).

Along with the Ofc and the anterior cingulate, a third region of the middle prefrontal cortex—the *insula*—has special salience for psychotherapy. The insula is vital for "interoception"—that is, attention to, and awareness of, our own bodily states, particularly visceral states. Because somatic sensation underpins emotion, interoception in which "the insula is involved perhaps more significantly than any other structure" (Damasio, 2003, p. 105) may be the primary way in which we know how we feel. In addition, the insula may be key to our ability to feel the emotions of *other*s because it relays from the cortex to the amygdala our sensorimotor impressions—the sight, sound, and "feel"—of *their* affective behavior (Iacoboni, 2005). This is the terrain of empathy and *mirror neurons* to which we will shortly turn.

HOW IT WORKS

Hawkins (2005) has proposed a model of cortical functioning that has important clinical implications. In this model, the neocortex is above all an organ of memory and prediction. Taking in experience through the senses and the body, the cortex registers repeated experiential patterns as memories that shape predictions about what we can expect in the immediate and distal future. Stored as patterns of synaptic connections between neurons, these cortical memories have three defining characteristics: They are *autoassociative*, involve *invariant representations*, and have a *hierarchical structure*.

Visual memory provides the clearest examples. Playing hide-and-seek, I see my daughter's feet peeking out from under the drapes and immediately visualize her whole body. The fact that cortical memory is "autoassociative" means that the part triggers the whole: We may see only a visual fragment but our memory completes the image. As another example, in a dark theater my attention briefly settles on a dimly perceived profile several rows down the aisle; moments later, the vaguely familiar profile becomes suddenly recogniz-

able as—unbidden—the mental image of a friend's face springs into focus. How does this translation from the part to the whole occur?

What Hawkins (2005) calls "invariant representations" are neuronal patterns in the cortex that store experience as *forms independent of variations in detail* (p. 69). When these invariant memorial forms are activated by fragmentary (or distorted) visual inputs, they predict—and, in this way, actually determine in large part—what it is that we will see. Thus, according to Hawkins (2005), "Most of what you perceive is not coming through your senses; it is generated by your internal memory model" (p. 202). Without invariant representations, the world we experience would remain, like that of the infant, a "blooming, buzzing confusion" (James, 1890/1950, p. 488).

Every region of the cortex has six layers of neurons. In the "cortical hierarchy" that Hawkins describes, this six-layered structure generates our subjective experience by combining here-and-now sensory inputs from the three levels "below" with memory-based predictions from the three levels "above." The influence of memory on perception is what cognitive scientists call "top-down" processing, while the buildup of perceptions from sensory inputs is called "bottom-up" processing (LeDoux, 1996). Such a structure is advantageous because it allows us to automatically apply our knowledge of previous experience to that in the present—for example, to recognize a bearded friend's face (invariant representation) even when, for the first time, we're seeing him clean-shaven (real-time visual input). The disadvantage of such a structure in which "observed patterns flow up the hierarchy and predictions flow down" (LeDoux, 1996, p. 159) is that memory-driven expectations often trump new experience—with the result that, for example, our friend's unexpectedly absent beard may go unnoticed. Often what we expect to see is the *only* thing we see.

What is true of the functioning of the visual cortex may be true across the board—not only in other sensory modalities but in all the ways that we take in and process experience. Among the implications here is that what we regard as our perceptions are always (more or less) matters of interpretation. And, of course, these interpretations are rooted in the past. As Hawkins (2005) writes, "Much of psychology is based on the consequences of early life experience, attachment, and nurturance, because that is when the brain first lays down its model of the world" (p. 203).

The Mirror Neuron System

> . . . *an archaic kind of sociality, one that does not distinguish self from other, is woven deeply into the primate brain.*
> —LESLIE BROTHERS (1997, p. 78)

In the mid-1990s the Italian neuroscientist Rizzolati made a momentous discovery. He found in the premotor cortex of macaque monkeys a class of neurons that fired not just during self-initiated movements, but also during

the observation of corresponding movements in other monkeys. Subsequent research has confirmed that human beings, like our primate ancestors, have a "mirror neuron" system that duplicates or simulates in our own brains the actions of others.

But note: It is only *intentional* actions that trigger the firing of mirror neurons. Evidently it is not our perception of action per se that triggers a resonant response but, rather, the perception of action that appears to have an intention behind it. It looks as though our mirror neurons fire as much in response to underlying mental states as to the actions to which they give rise. Underscoring this point is research that demonstrates that it is not only the perceived intentional states of others but also their emotions and bodily sensations that can cause our mirror neurons to fire—for example, when we observe an expression of feeling in someone else or see them receiving a pinprick. As mentioned earlier, it has been theorized (Iocoboni, 2005) that the insula transmits our impressions of others' affects from the cortex that perceives to the amygdala that triggers bodily based feelings.

Mirror neurons thus appear to simulate in our selves both the observed behavior and the inferred mental states (e.g., feelings) of others. As such, the mirror neuron system has been seen as the neural substrate for empathy, affect attunement, mentalizing, and intersubjectivity. It may even be the foundation for our experiences of the "oneness" we share with other living beings (Allen & Fonagy, 2002; Gallese, 2001; Siegel, Siegel, & Amiel, 2006).

Laterality: Two Brains in One

Each hemisphere of the brain is specialized to process and represent experience in a different way. The *right* hemisphere, which Ornstein (1997) calls the "right mind," is specialized to respond emotionally, holistically, nonverbally, intuitively, relationally, and receptively. It has dense neural connections to the limbic system and the body—including, in particular, the amygdala and the ANS—so it can respond to experience viscerally, from the inside out, so to speak. This hemisphere is said to process information "analogically"—taking in and representing experience as an integrated whole. Lacking the kind of "digital" analysis that samples and deconstructs reality in order to make sense of it, the right brain responds directly to what is—the gestalt, the whole context, the parts in relationship to one another rather than in isolation. Because it allows for the awareness of context and multiple perspectives on experience, and because it is attuned to decode nonverbal communication, the right brain can be seen as the neural substrate for the reflective or mentalizing self. The right brain is also thought to be the seat of the unconscious and of Freud's primary process.

The *left* hemisphere is designed to respond in an entirely different register. The wellspring of conscious thought—Freud's secondary process—it

represents experience linguistically, according to a logic that is linear. Its primary unit of information is the word. If we examine our own conscious thinking, we usually find that it consists primarily of a stream of words; while the content of our internal monologue may be informed by the right brain, its verbal expression is mainly the product of the left. If we rely exclusively on the left brain, which is specialized for a focus on detail, we tend to miss the forest for the trees.

There also appears to be a division of emotional labor between the brain's two hemispheres. The left seems to be activated by the experience of moderate and positive emotions, the right by emotions that are very intense and/or negatively tinged. Correspondingly, the left hemisphere appears to mediate approach while the right seems to mediate withdrawal.

Access to both hemispheres is essential to the flexibility that makes effective adaptation possible. Thus, unless they fail to communicate with each other, "two brains are better than one." Fortunately the brain is built to foster such communication across hemispheres: The *corpus callosum*, a band of neural fibers that connects the two halves of the brain, allows us both to capitalize on the special strengths of each and to reap the benefits of their harmonious integration—for example, the integration of right-brain emotional responsiveness and left-brain analysis (Schore, 2003; Siegel, 1999; Cozolino, 2002).

Integration and the Brain

Healthy relationships of attachment, especially in the first years of life, are necessary for the development and integration of right- and left-brain functions—and of limbic and cortical functions as well. Such integration ensures that the various capacities of the brain—sensory, motor, emotional, analytical, and so on—can be functionally linked to make possible the most coordinated and adaptive use of all of the brain's potential resources.

Keep in mind that these varieties of brain integration (right/left, and bottom/up) are the neural corollary of the psychological integration that is not only the reward of secure attachment but also the goal of psychotherapy. This kind of psychological integration—that links differing states of mind as well as mind and body, thought and feeling, self-definition and relatedness—ensures that we can have access to the depth and breadth of the whole of our experience. Such integration allows us to develop and harmonize the multiple dimensions of the self rather than feel the necessity to deny or disown parts of ourselves.

As clinicians, we can be encouraged by research showing that the brain of the adult, like that of the developing child, can be reshaped by current experience that not only establishes new neural connections but also alters

the actual physical structure of the brain. This finding of *neural plasticity* strongly suggests that re-creating an attachment matrix of the kind in which the body, brain, and mind originally develop may be crucial if we are to effectively foster therapeutic change.

BRINGING IT ALL TOGETHER:
ATTACHMENT, THE EMBODIED MIND, AND THE MINDFUL BODY

> *. . . the brain is the body's captive audience.*
> —ANTONIO DAMASIO (1994, p. 158)

In *Descartes' Error,* Damasio (1994) marshals neurobiological evidence to argue for the inseparability of mind and body, asserting that feelings are essentially the mind's readings of bodily states and that reason—to be truly rational—must be anchored in the emotional signals that issue from the body. Yet if the "embodied mind" (Varela, Thompson, & Rosch, 1992; Lakoff & Johnson, 1999) has come to be acknowledged by many scientists and philosophers as a fact of the human condition, its reality is anything but a "given" for those of us—patients and therapists alike—who too often seem to live as if inhabiting a disembodied mind or a mindless body.

Integrating the various dimensions of the self (somatic, emotional, representational, reflective, mindful) and establishing interconnectivity between the separate domains of the brain (left and right, cortical and subcortical) are two sides of the same coin. As the outcome of a secure attachment history and the goal of an attachment-oriented psychotherapy, these kinds of integration may foster the subjective experience of both an embodied mind and a mindful body.

With a mind that is embodied, we feel grounded, our actions directed from within. We have useful, psychologically enriching access to our somatic sensations and our emotions. The felt sense here is that the ways in which we think as well as feel "arise from, are shaped by, and are given meaning through living human bodies" (Lakoff & Johnson, 1999, p. 6).

Patients who might be described in attachment terms as avoidant or dismissing are usually (more or less) "disembodied." As one such patient put it, "I hover over my experience rather than land in my body." For these patients, how the body functions, or looks from the outside, may be important, but what it feels like, or senses, on the inside almost never is. Operating with a left-brain bias, they can appear to live as if uninformed by the emotionally oriented right brain. Yet they are gripped by powerful, subcortical "reflexes" that constrain their actions and divert attention from their feelings and sensations. Being of therapeutic use to such patients usually involves helping them to reclaim the feeling, sensing body as an inherent and essential part of the self.

In sharp contrast to patients who appear to inhabit a disembodied mind are those who seem lodged in a body that is "mindless"—a body that rules the self because its expressions cannot be questioned by the mind. These patients, often preoccupied or unresolved with respect to trauma, can feel tyrannized by the body that seems to betray them. Frequently they are "somatizers" whose emotions and memories mainly find expression in the language of the body. When these emotions or memories have become intolerable, the body that sequesters them is abandoned psychically: Leaving the body—dissociation—provides "escape when there is no escape" (Putnam, 1992, p. 104). Such patients are unable to access the resources of a body that is mindful—a body suffused with awareness so that it can not only be sensed and known but can also sense and know.

As Siegel (2005, 2006) points out, the heart and intestines (whose surrounding cellular structures mimic those of the brain) function as organs not only of circulation and digestion, respectively, but also of perception—hence, the literalness of the expressions "heartfelt feelings" and "gut reactions." When capable of "minding the body" (Damasio, 1994), we have access to a depth of self-awareness *and* awareness of others that is otherwise unavailable. Most important, perhaps, having a body inhabited by the mind and a mind informed and enlivened by the body helps us to be more fully present—a vital point to which I'll return momentarily.

As therapists, we can foster such integration in our patients in much the same way that effective parents foster integration in their securely attached children—that is, by recognizing, and responding in an attuned fashion, to the whole range of their communications, implicit and explicit, whether conveyed through their bodies, their emotions, or their words. This kind of "full spectrum" receptivity and responsiveness can help our patients to develop capacities and integrate experiences—most broadly, those of the body and the mind—for which their original attachments made insufficient room.

Back to the Brain

To further our patients' integration of mind and body—thought and feeling, awareness and experience—we would do well to take seriously the clinical implications of some recent neuroscience findings, including several already touched on above.

The first of these findings (Damasio, 2003; Siegel et al., 2006) are those suggesting that in both evolution and individual development "higher" (cortical/left hemisphere) structures in the brain are built upon—and often dominated by—"lower" (subcortical/right hemisphere) ones. In keeping with this pattern of influence, neural "traffic" is much heavier from the bottom up—from the amygdala (fear response) to the cortex (fear man-

agement)—than from the top down (LeDoux, 1996). These facts argue for a correspondingly bottom-up approach in psychotherapy that consistently grounds clinical work in the bodily sensations and emotions that underpin behavior and thought. They also argue for including a focus on the nonverbal, primarily right-brain-dominated dimension of the therapeutic relationship that is expressed through what is sensed, felt, and done, rather than said (van der Kolk, 2006; Ogden, Pain, Minton, & Fisher, 2005; Schore, 2005).

Second, the neural influence that *does* flow from cortex to amygdala issues mainly from the *middle prefrontal*, rather than the *dorsolateral,* region of the cortex. The former, as you will recall, is an affect-regulating integrator of inputs from throughout the brain, while the latter (the "rational mind") is specialized for conscious, largely verbal information processing. The clinical implication of this (largely) missing linkage between dorsolateral and limbic regions is that simply thinking aloud about difficult emotions with our patients—particularly, traumatized patients—may be useful (see below) but insufficient.

We need, in addition, to activate the middle prefrontal cortex by helping these patients attend to their internal experience, especially bodily experience including in particular, perhaps, the breath. Bringing the mind's attention to bear on the body may go against the grain for these patients. Yet such a focus can be a potent resource for strengthening their capacities for affect- and self-regulation (van der Kolk, 2006). This interoceptive attention is a form of mindfulness that helps ground patients in the present moment, potentially modulating the distress associated with the traumatic past and feared future. Asking our patients to label what they feel in their bodies enlists cortical capacities in the processing of painful subcortical (i.e., somatic/affective) experience. It invites them to *observe* that experience rather than simply identify with it, and feel overwhelmed. Enhanced bodily awareness and the growing sense that feelings can be painful without being intolerable sets the stage for the conscious processing and integration of previously dissociated experience (Ogden, 2006).

Third, recall the theory of the functioning of the layered cortex: The lower three layers process current input from the senses and the body. The upper three layers make predictions about upcoming experience on the basis of memories stored as "invariant representations" that may misrepresent current reality (Hawkins, 2005). One clinical implication here is that in order to loosen the grip of such invariant *mis*representations (e.g., outdated internal working models) we need to cultivate our patients' mindful attention to here-and-now experience. In helping them quite literally to "come to their senses" (Kabat-Zinn, 2005) we diminish the likelihood that the data of present experience flowing up the cortical hierarchy will be swamped by the memories and predictions flowing down.

Finally, there are neuroscience findings that bear directly on mentalizing and mindfulness. With regard to the first, studies show that mentalizing activates not only the prefrontal cortex but also the amygdala (Allen & Fonagy, 2002; Lieberman, in press). The implication here is that in order to actually exercise their capacity to mentalize, our patients need to address their distressing feelings *while they are actually feeling them*—otherwise there is only "pseudo-mentalizing" (Fonagy, personal communication, 2006). Studies show further that bringing language to bear on distressing experience—an essential feature of explicit mentalizing—can reduce its neural impact: Subjects shown upsetting images and instructed to describe them showed much less activation of the amygdala than subjects who were exposed to the images but without the instruction to verbalize (Hariri, Bookheimer, & Mazziotta, 2000; Hariri, Mattay, Tessitore, Fera, & Weinberger, 2003). Similarly, there is evidence that the "reappraisal" or "reframing" of difficult emotional experience can modulate reactivity in the amygdala (see Ochsner & Gross, 2005). Studies like these argue for an integrated—top-down as well as bottom-up—approach to treatment. For it appears that emotion regulation can indeed be strengthened when left-brain/cortical resources (language, interpretation) are enlisted in the real-time processing of right-brain/subcortical experience (bodily based feelings).

Brain research also indicates that emotion regulation may be promoted through a mindful focus on the breathing body. Austin (1999), noting that longer exhalations are produced by meditative attention to the breath, cites findings that suggest that *breathing out reduces firing in the amygdala*, thus "quieting the brain" (p. 94) and calming the body. Lazar et al. (2005) observe that meditators whose practice is anchored in a focus on the breath show cortical thickening, particularly in the insula which links the cortex to the limbic system, integrating thoughts with bodily based feelings. Referencing an earlier study in which people learning to juggle showed thickening in the visual motion areas of the cortex, the authors propose that attending to the breath and other internal sensations is a practice of interoception that could be predicted to "build up" the insula—perhaps facilitating, in the process, access to our own emotions and empathy for those of others.

Broadly, it appears that bringing conscious awareness to bear on particular facets of our experience triggers neural firing in areas of the brain associated with those experiences. When awareness is *repeatedly* focused on such experiences, new synaptic connections are generated, eventually resulting in "cortical remodeling" (Lazar et al., 2005, p. 1895). The clinical implication here is that by repeatedly focusing on, and *linking*, different aspects of the patient's experience—somatic, emotional, representational, and so on—we can establish new connections in the patient's brain. Such connectivity is the neural equivalent of the psychological integration we hope

to facilitate for the patient through a relationship that is more inclusive and collaborative than those that originally shaped him.

To help the patient make the best possible use of the new attachment relationship we are attempting to provide, it is essential to understand the various patterns of early attachment, both secure and insecure. Understanding how caregivers make secure attachment possible can help us tailor our responses to our patients in ways that promote integration and security. Understanding the varieties of insecure attachment can help us to identify those experiences for which our patients' first attachments made no room—and to offer the kind of responsiveness to such experiences that can make their eventual integration possible.

NOTES

1. Note that while some authors employ the terms "emotion," "affect," and "feeling" interchangeably, I prefer to use the word "emotion" in referring to the overarching category of psychophysiological arousal and responsiveness to experience, while reserving "affect" to describe how emotion looks on the outside of the body and "feeling" to describe how emotion feels on the inside of the body (see Rothschild, 2000; Nathanson, 1992; Siegel, 1999; Damasio, 2003).

2. In this connection, Bucci (2003) discusses the "affective core" of our internal representations or working models for which—in light of what drives them—Bucci prefers the term "emotion schemas."

CHAPTER 6

The Varieties
of Attachment Experience

Our first relationships of attachment provide the original blueprint of the mind. The patterns of interpersonal communication in these relationships are internalized as the collection of structured patterns known as the self. At the level of implicit enactive representations—i.e., internal working models—the medium is the message. The structure of our developmental dialogues with those upon whom our survival depends becomes the initial structure of our inner world (Lyons-Ruth, 1999; Main & Goldwyn, 1984–1998; van IJzendoorn, 1995).

At the simplest level, whatever in the infant's nonverbal communication evokes an attuned response from the parent is ruled in, so to speak, while whatever evokes an aversive response (or goes unrecognized) is ruled out. As Main's research reveals, the rules infants derive from these earliest exchanges govern not only how they behave but also what they will allow themselves to feel, want, think, and remember. These rules are encoded in children's internal working models that preserve knowledge of their attachment histories, and shape their current and future relationships to others and to themselves (Main et al., 1985).

But exactly how stable are the attachment patterns of infancy? Summarizing the results of the major longitudinal studies, Fonagy states that secure versus insecure Strange Situation classifications at 12 months accorded with AAI classifications in adulthood 68–75% of the time: "This is an unparalleled level of consistency between behavior observed in infancy and outcomes in adulthood" (Fonagy et al., 2002, p. 40). The current findings

of Mary Main's original study demonstrate a level of consistency from infancy to 19 years that is well over 80%—but only so long as participants with intervening trauma were removed from the analysis. Trauma (for these participants, not abuse but other forms of trauma such as the death of a parent) can apparently change everything, and usually not for the better (Main et al., 2005). On the other hand, there are adults with histories that predict insecurity, but coherent AAI narratives that reflect the achievement of what is called "earned secure" attachment. Promisingly for psychotherapy, evidence like this, as well as a study showing that marriage can transform insecure into securely attached adults, suggests that the individual's working model(s) of attachment can be favorably affected by changes in the nature of the individual's attachment relationships (Hesse, 1999; Crowell, Treboux, & Waters, 2002).

For patients who are insecurely attached, the new attachment relationship with the therapist may be essential in order to integrate experiences that could not be accommodated in their first relationships. While the attachments of childhood initially structure the self, the patient's attachment to the therapist may later *re*structure it, changing an insecure working model to an earned secure one. For psychotherapy to be transformative in this way, it must simultaneously make room for the dissociated past and offer the patient a fresh model of relationship in the present. Importantly, integrating old experiences and creating new ones can turn out to be two sides of the same coin (Lyons-Ruth, 1999; Amini et al., 1996).

As clinicians attempting to foster change by providing a new attachment relationship, knowledge of the varieties of attachment experience— secure and insecure— can help us to identify and eventually make room for the feelings, thoughts, and ways of being with others that were denied a place in the patient's earliest relationships. Such knowledge can also strengthen our ability to imagine, understand, and empathically resonate with the subjective experience, as well as the childhood histories, of our patients. Moreover, it can cue us with regard to the specific therapeutic stance most likely to be in synch with the particular patient's developmental needs.

ATTACHMENT PATTERNS IN INFANCY AND BEYOND

Mary Main's pioneering longitudinal research began in the mid-1970s and followed a group of families as their infants developed through childhood and adolescence into early adulthood. Five years after the infants were involved in two Strange Situation assessments—one with mother, one with father—Main conducted two-hour videotaped evaluations of their families, structured, like the Strange Situation itself, around separation and reunion.

Attempting to move attachment research beyond the Strange Situation, Main not only focused on attachment behavior beyond infancy but also and more significantly sought to illuminate the mental representations—the internal working models—thought to shape attachment behavior across the entire lifespan. Like an archeologist who gathers excavated artifacts in the effort to envision civilizations that can no longer be seen, Main culled "representational artifacts" from her subjects (e.g., the parent's AAI transcripts and the children's family drawings) in order to make their invisible inner worlds visible.

Her findings (Main et al., 1985) regarding the experience and representation of attachment in infants, six-year-olds, and adults illuminate in evocative detail the development, characteristics, and consequences of each of the four primary states of mind with respect to attachment. It Is the intent of the summary that follows, in recognition of the *pervasive* influence of attachment models/rules, to highlight the structural continuity of representational patterns that emerge in infancy, evolve over time, and find expression in multiple modalities (including nonverbal behavior, language, imagery, etc.). That continuity across the various dimensions of the self is what makes our patients' attachment patterns (and our own) so vital to recognize and understand.

Secure/Autonomous Attachment: Free to Connect, Explore, and Reflect

In the Strange Situation an infant classified as secure typically displayed a flexible balance between seeking comfort in proximity to his mother and exploring the toy-filled room on his own: There appeared to be no demand or expectation from mother that she either would or would not be the object of the infant's attention.

Now notice the continuity: As a six-year-old, the same child generally appeared to be emotionally open. Upon being shown an evocative photo depicting separation, he could comfortably discuss the pictured child's feelings and imagine their origins. Moreover, he could envision a constructive solution to the crisis—paralleling the behavior of the secure infant who, after the "crisis" of separation, approached his mother with pleasure, succeeded in finding comfort there, then resumed exploration and play. Similarly, his behavior upon reunion with his parents was immediately warmly welcoming, while his verbal exchanges with them were judged to be "fluent"—fluid rather than stilted, balanced in terms of conversational turn taking, and markedly unrestricted in focus. The secure six-year-old's family drawing was typically realistic, often portraying parents and children standing close to each other with arms outstretched, as if open to contact. Upon being handed a family Polaroid taken at the start of the evaluation, the six-year-old showed pleasure, smiled, or casually commented,

then handed the snapshot back. Main's colleague, Nancy Kaplan, described children like this one as "secure–resourceful" (Main et al., 1985; Main, 1995, 2000).

What does the research reveal about the parents of such secure children? To begin with, their AAI transcripts were typically placed in the "secure–autonomous" category. The content and form of these transcripts demonstrated the parents' capacity to both freely value and objectively reflect upon their attachment relationships. Main described the "mode of discourse" of these parents as coherent and collaborative; their attention seemed to shift flexibly between the interviewer's questions and probes and their own memories, feelings, and thoughts. Revisiting the highly evocative terrain of their attachment histories, these parents appeared to be fully "present," thoughtful, and open to their emotions without being pushed around by them. Even while recalling very troubling experiences with their own parents, they seemed capable of maintaining a balanced perspective that reflected their efforts to understand their parents and sometimes to forgive.

In this connection, Main later identified a subgroup of secure parents—termed "earned secure"—who described problematic and painful childhood histories of the kind ordinarily associated with insecure attachment, but who nonetheless spoke coherently and collaboratively about their histories (Main & Goldwyn, 1984–1998). Very encouragingly for psychotherapy, these "earned secure" adults often have had emotionally significant relationships with close friends, romantic partners, and/or therapists (Siegel, 1999).

The parents of secure children were also seen to be capable of considering—and reconsidering—their attachment experiences in the very process of recalling them. This crucial capacity both to *have* experience and to *reflect* on it—to stand both inside *and* outside one's experience—is what Main (1991) calls *metacognitive monitoring*. Along with the secure parents' ability to be aware of and to integrate a wide range of attachment-related memories, feelings, and thoughts, their capacity for metacognitive monitoring was seen to reflect secure working models or states of mind regarding attachment.

Main proposed that such models or states of mind—precisely because they were open, flexible, and self-monitoring, rather than restricted by particular attentional rules—were what made possible the sensitive responsiveness that enabled secure parents to raise secure children. With little or no need to censor or edit the internal "news" related to attachment, these parents could afford to be receptive to the full spectrum of their child's interpersonal communications and signals. The inclusiveness of the developmental dialogue here provides the relational substrate for the psychological integration—the balance between attachment and exploration, relatedness

and self-definition—that may be the welcome legacy of the child's secure attachment history.

As we are about to see, the offspring of insecure parents appear not to have been so fortunate.

Avoidant/Dismissing Attachment: Not-So-Splendid Isolation

The avoidant infant typically lacked the flexibility and resourcefulness of his secure counterpart. In the Strange Situation, he engaged in exploration to the virtual exclusion of attachment behavior. At 12 months he could be seen to actively avoid his mother, presumably in response to her consistent rejection of his earlier bids for physical and emotional contact—or her intrusive, controlling, and overarousing parenting, as other researchers have suggested (Sroufe, 1996). As if his entire song were made up of a single note, the avoidant infant's display of emotion was restricted to the interest he showed in objects. Yet while appearing unfazed during separation and ignoring mother upon reunion, the avoidant infant was nonetheless reacting *physiologically* in ways that made his actual distress undeniable (Sroufe & Waters, 1977b). He has learned to suppress the automatic expression of emotions associated with separation and attachment—but that does not mean that he has not felt them.

Again, notice the continuity: At age six, the same child who as an infant had behaved as if hopeless about being comforted by mother was capable of naming the sadness experienced by the children in the separation photos but could imagine no solution whatever to the pictured crisis of separation. And just as the infant had ignored mother in the Strange Situation reunion, the six-year-old ignored her now, only more subtly. Their interaction upon reunion was described as "restricted": Leaving all initiative to the parent, the avoidant child responded only minimally; conversation was halting and the topics discussed were impersonal. The family drawing—described by researchers as "insecure–invulnerable"—typically depicted undifferentiated figures, each with a stereotypical "happy face," distant from one another, often floating in the air, and frequently armless. (Here Main asks us to recall the dismissing mother's aversion to physical contact with her infant.) When presented with the family photograph, the avoidant six-year-old turned away, refused it, or casually dropped it to the floor (Main, 1995, 2000).

Almost invariably the parents of avoidant children were classified as "dismissing"—in part, because they seemed so regularly to minimize the importance and influence of attachment relationships. In the AAI context, where the mode of discourse of these parents was neither coherent nor collaborative, their twin signatures were an insistence on lack of recall for childhood experience and the contradiction between the idealized relation-

ships they claimed to have had and the more problematic ones they seem actually to have lived.[1]

Most striking in the AAI transcripts of dismissing parents was the discrepancy between the glowing descriptors they initially chose in characterizing their relationship with their own parents—at worst, "normal," mostly between "very good" and "excellent"—and the often dispiriting recollections they later offered in explaining their choices. Their idealizing or normalizing descriptions were either unsupported ("I don't remember") or actually belied by experience alluded to later in the interview.

Main illustrates such inconsistency with the example of a parent who characterized her mother as "caring, loving . . . and supportive":

> One time I broke my arm playing around in the yard. Things like that would make my mother angry, she hated episodes like that. It hurt a long time but I never told her, she found out from some neighbor, must have been the way I was holding my arm. . . . She didn't like cry-babies. I always tried not to cry because she was a really strong person. (Main, 2000, pp. 1084–1085)

As a child, the parent Main describes had apparently learned to inhibit her attachment-related feelings, impulses, and behavior. As an adult, she avoids such feelings and impulses through idealizing her "caring, loving, supportive" mother. When painful recollection threatens that idealization, she bolsters it through reframing her mother's shortcomings as strength: "I always tried not to cry because she was a really strong person." In this way, dismissing adults frequently "justify" the emotional isolation of their childhoods, explaining that their parents' rejection, neglect, or anger, made for a hard school—but a good one—that fostered self-sufficiency and determination.

The parents of the avoidant children in Main's research appeared actively, if unconsciously, to maintain this emotional isolation. They minimized the evocative potential of past attachment-related experiences through idealization (or devaluation), selective inattention, and insistence on lack of recall. In the here and now of the interview relationship they preserved emotional distance through a stance that bore traces both of their rejecting parents and of their own avoidant infants. Appearing more interested in getting the interview over with than in genuinely collaborating, these parents seemed subtly (or not so subtly) to reject the interviewer: "My mother? A nobody. No relationship. Next question?" (Hesse, 1999, p. 403). And like their infants, they experienced—or else felt they could afford to express—no distress, vulnerability, or anger. Yet as subsequent research using physiological measures of distress has shown, the lack of affect in dismissing adults—like that in avoidant infants—is merely apparent (Dozier & Kobak, 1992).[2]

The avoidant children and dismissing parents shared a mode of experience in which attention to attachment-related matters was radically restricted. Both groups seemed to occupy a representational world governed by rules that minimized awareness of feelings in general and of feelings bearing on attachment, in particular. The "news" about this emotionally flattened world, as registered internally and "broadcast" publicly, all tended to be good—as if reflecting exclusively the requirement to feel (or appear to feel) strong, self-sufficient, and independent. Yet Main's research also pointed to features of this internal landscape that were, so to speak, cloaked in shadow. We can see clinical evidence of such shadowy, hard-to-access experience in dismissing patients who appear to project onto (or into) others their own disavowed needs, vulnerability, and anger.

The motivated inattention to such attachment-related experience imposed significant limitations on the dismissing parents and their avoidant children. Turning their focus *away* from attachment, these parents had to distance themselves both from others and from their own deepest yearnings. In the process, they hobbled not only their capacity to reflect on (internal and interpersonal) experience, but also their ability to sensitively respond to the signals of their infants. To preserve the dismissing state of mind that made their own emotional survival possible, dismissing parents had to ignore or suppress their infants' attachment needs. In response, avoidant infants—their needs blocked—learned to live as if they had none.

Foreshadowing later research into the co-constructed nature of attachment relationships, Main theorized that this kind of "dyadic cooperation" might explain how the dismissing parents' models and rules come to be adopted by their avoidant offspring (Main et al., 1985). Essentially, she was suggesting that what is enacted in relationship with the parents is internalized by the child. Dismissing parents generate developmental dialogues that exclude the expression of needs for physical and emotional contact. In turn, their children internalize these dialogues in the form of unintegrated working models that make no room for the desire, much less the attempt, to satisfy such needs.

Yet the need for comfort and connection in the face of threat or pain is built in by evolutionary design. It cannot be extinguished but only defended against. This is the purpose of avoidant/dismissing strategies that aim to minimize awareness of internal or external attachment-related cues in order to deactivate the attachment behavioral system (Main, 1995).

These "minimizing" or "deactivating" strategies are woven through the contradictory working models—conscious and unconscious—that shape the inner and interpersonal experience of avoidant/dismissing individuals. One model is consciously embraced and involves a sense that the self is good, strong, and complete, while others are untrustworthy, needy, and inadequate. The second model, which is unconscious and feared, entails a

disturbing sense that the self is flawed, dependent, and helpless, while others are likely in response to be rejecting, controlling, and punitive. Deactivating strategies support the first model as a defense against the second (Mikulincer & Shaver, 2003). More specifically, these strategies promote distance, control, and self-reliance (the essence of the conscious model) while inhibiting emotional experience that might activate the attachment system (as it is dispiritingly represented in the unconscious model).

As therapists, we often see clinical evidence of these contradictory models in dismissing patients who seem to "relocate" their own apparent vulnerability and need in others, whom they then experience as weak, burdensome, and undesirable. More generally, the inflated self-esteem of these patients appears to be secured at the considerable cost of finding fault with those they might otherwise depend upon and love.

Ambivalent/Preoccupied Attachment: No Room for a Mind of One's Own

The counterpart of the deactivating strategy Main observed in the avoidant infant is the "hyperactivating" strategy she found in the ambivalent infant. While avoidance was marked by an overregulation of affect, ambivalence involved underregulation. And whereas, in the Strange Situation, the avoidant infant focused exclusively on the toys, the ambivalent infant could focus only on his mother.

Alternately clinging and angrily resistant, on the one hand, or reduced to helpless passivity on the other, the ambivalent infant was extremely hard to soothe. Chronically anxious about mother's whereabouts, he seemed too overwhelmed to explore. This pattern of amplified affect—as expressed in ambivalence and/or helplessness—was seen as the infant's predictable response to a mother who was unpredictably responsive. To the extent that such a response helped secure his mother's erratic attention and curbed the autonomous exploration she seemed to discourage, it could be seen as a necessary and adaptive compromise.

Now consider the typical ambivalent six-year-old in Main's study who—like his infant counterpart—alternated between intense expressions of need and anger. In response to the separation photos, for example, one said the pictured child would buy flowers for his parents but then hide their clothes. Similarly, the ambivalent reunions were characterized by behavior that communicated mixed messages: One child sat obligingly on mother's lap only to wriggle away, while a second ostentatiously expressed affection for the parent, then abruptly broke contact. The ambivalent children's family drawings—described as "vulnerable"—were peopled by very large or very small figures, always placed very close together, and often prominently featuring vulnerable or intimate parts of the body. When handed the family

Polaroid, the ambivalent six-year-olds appeared to become disturbed: One stared at it uneasily, then began to pick at her skin. Unlike the prototypically secure infants who seemed to enjoy the snapshot or the avoidant who turned away from it, the ambivalent infants appeared to be singularly absorbed by the photographic image of attachment—but also troubled by it (Main, 1995, 2000).

The parents of ambivalent children were deeply absorbed in their own troubling concerns about attachment. And like their infants whose worry about mother's whereabouts had undermined their Strange Situation exploration, these parents appeared to labor under the burden of an "excessive, confused, and either angry or passive preoccupation with attachment figures" that compromised exploration of their own attachment histories (Main, 1995, p. 441). The observation that such parents tend to discourage their child's autonomy may be explained by the fears of abandonment and helplessness that seem to underlie their anxiety. Categorized as "preoccupied" and coded "E" (as in enmeshed or entangled), these parents responded in the AAI as if the emotions of the past were swamping their capacity in the present for coherent recall and reflection.

For example, when asked for early memories, a preoccupied adult like those in Main's study might segue from angrily describing a long ago episode with his father to complaining bitterly about an all-too-current grievance against him—while lapsing in this narrative into "unmarked" quotations from father ("So why couldn't you ever listen to your mother?") or directly addressing him now as though his father were actually present ("Don't *ever* talk to me that way again!"). The pervasively disturbing influence of the past was also evidenced in childlike language ("Mommy was mad cause that doggie bit me"); vague usages ("Daddy sat me in his lap, and that"); nonsense words ("dadadada"); grammatically entangled run-on sentences; and/or sentences that are not completed (Main, 1995; Hesse, 1999).

The intense anger, fear, or passivity evoked by past as well as current attachments undercut the preoccupied parents' capacity not only for coherence but also for collaborative discourse. These parents communicated in confused and confusing ways, generating narratives that were hard to follow, tangential to the point of irrelevance, and overly lengthy. In relation to the interviewer, they could be overwhelming, misattuned to ordinary conversational cues, and discouraging of autonomy—just the sort of parental qualities thought likely to produce the "hyperactivating" strategy of ambivalent infants. Recall that in order to secure the parent's unreliable attention, such infants had learned to amplify their expressions of distress. Similarly, the preoccupied parents appeared vulnerable to feelings of distress that they seemed unable (or unwilling) to manage (Main, 1995, 2000).

These parents and their ambivalent children were understood to in-

habit a representational world shaped by multiple, unintegrated working models. These models were thought to be the outcome of contradictory experiences with unpredictable attachment figures. Relatively responsive in one encounter, intrusive or unavailable in the next, such attachment figures evoked in their offspring an abiding preoccupation with the promise of closeness on the one hand and the likelihood of its loss on the other. Presumably, closeness was associated with favorable experience that generated the model of a distressed self in interaction with a sometimes responsive other—while abandonment was linked to problematic experience that resulted in a model of an autonomous self in interaction with an unresponsive other (Mikulincer & Shaver, 2003).

The emotional static created by such conflicting models compromised the capacity of these parents to accurately perceive their infant's signals and respond consistently to their needs. It also interfered with their metacognitive capacity to freely and usefully reflect upon their own experience. For the rules of attachment—amplify distress, inhibit autonomy—that originated in the behavioral strategy of the ambivalent infant continued to impede competent and independent exploration, including self-exploration.

Main concluded that these same rules of attachment were responsible both for the confusing, emotionally overwhelmed AAI responses of the parents and for their inconsistent sensitivity to their infant's nonverbal cues. These parents were simply too distressed by past and present conflicts to effectively process attachment-related information whether it arose from within (memory) or without (their infant's signals). Main's research—as well as clinical experience—suggests that this kind of distress is so welded to the "*false* but *felt* security" it produced in infancy that it remains in adulthood a burden that is hard to lay down (Main et al., 2005, p. 292). As a result, the hyperactivating strategy of preoccupied parents (like the deactivating strategy of dismissing parents) tends to be enacted with—and adopted by—their children.

Disorganized/Unresolved Attachment: Scars of Trauma and Loss

The disorganized/disoriented infant sporadically exhibited behavior with mother in the Strange Situation that appeared inexplicable, bizarre, overtly conflicted, or dissociated. Thought to arise in response to a parent who was frightening to the infant—or whose frightened or dissociated response evoked the infant's fear—such behaviors were understood to reflect the breakdown of an organized attachment strategy when the infant, feeling endangered, faced the irresolvable paradox that his biologically channeled haven of safety was simultaneously the source of his alarm.

Here once again, Main found continuity: The very features of behavior that originally marked the infant as disorganized characterized the "repre-

sentational artifacts" of the typical six-year-old, who appeared "inexplicably afraid and unable to do anything about it" (Kaplan, 1987, p. 109). Upon being shown the separation photos, for example, such children fell silent, too disturbed to respond; or imagined catastrophic outcomes; or else displayed disorganization in language or behavior. Similarly, their family drawings often included disturbing and/or bizarre elements (such as dismembered body parts, skeletons, or figures simply scratched out). When presented with the family snapshot, these six-year-olds became wordless, irrational, or distressed (one child, previously cheerful, bent silently and unhappily over the photograph for a full 12 seconds) (Main et al., 1985; Main, 1995).

Strikingly, however, the children assessed as disorganized in infancy now seemed during the reunions to be making use of a fresh behavioral strategy. Whereas their Strange Situation response had revealed an apparent collapse of strategy, their behavior five years later appeared to reflect a systematic effort *to control* their parents either through reversing roles and taking care of them ("Are you tired, Mommy? Would you like to sit down and I'll bring you some [pretend] tea?") or through being aggressively directive and punitive ("Sit down and shut up, and keep your eyes closed! I said, keep them closed") (Hesse & Main, 2000, p. 1107). In either case, it was as though these children were taking on a parental role in order to maintain proximity to their parents while also dealing with the threat they posed. This controlling/role-inverting strategy was very much in evidence during the reunion discourse in which the "dysfluent" conversations (marked by stammering and false starts) were dominated by six-year-olds who either punitively dismissed or solicitously "scaffolded" their parents' communication (Main et al., 1985; Main, 1995).

Main's study showed that parents of disorganized children had experienced trauma and/or losses that were unresolved. Critically, what appeared to be decisive here was not problematic life experience per se, but how that experience had (or had not) come to be integrated and understood. That is, it was not the parents' history of loss or trauma that bore a statistical relationship to their children's attachment status; it was specifically the parents' *lack of resolution* in relation to such history that predicted disorganized attachment in their offspring (see also Ainsworth & Eichberg, 1991). In the AAI context, this lack of resolution was discernible in disruptions in the parents' capacity to recall and reflect upon potentially traumatic events, such as the death of a close family member or episodes of sexual or physical abuse. When parents revealed "lapses in the monitoring of reasoning or discourse" while attempting to discuss such events, they were classified as *unresolved/disorganized*.[3]

Lapses in the monitoring of *reasoning* were noted when a parent made statements that either reflected incompatible views of the same reality (sug-

gesting, for example, that someone was both dead and alive) or violated consensual assumptions about causality or space/time relations (asserting, for example, that a death resulted from a thought). In response to probes inviting discussion of loss or abuse, the unresolved parents appeared to have been temporarily flooded by the intrusion, into a predominant state of mind, of trauma-related memories or beliefs that were normally confined to a separate, dissociated state of mind.

Lapses in the monitoring of *discourse* were noted when an interviewee suddenly shifted the "discourse register"—for example, switching abruptly from a straightforward description of traumatic experience to an exhaustively detailed one; from a focused account to a prolonged silence, without subsequent recall of what was previously said; or from one "narrative voice" to another (say, from that of someone bereaved to that of someone delivering funeral oratory). Main suggested that during such shifts, an altered state of consciousness had been triggered in which the interviewee was possessed, so to speak, by a particular traumatic experience that had never before been subjected to conscious processing.

These lapses of reasoning and discourse were often brief—punctuating the flow of the interview with an unresolved parent much as the inexplicable or contradictory behavior of disorganized infants had briefly interrupted their usual patterns of interaction in the Strange Situation. Main proposed that the very intrusions of traumatic memory that produced such lapses in the AAI context were responsible at home for the frightening behavior of unresolved parents that produced disorganized attachment in their infants (Main, 1995, 2000; Hesse & Main, 2000).

The parents' lack of resolution of past trauma or loss leads to radically discontinuous states of mind that necessitate the rigid denial of disturbing experience. When emotionally evocative AAI queries or childrearing contexts resembling those of the traumatic past disrupt this denial, unresolved adults can find themselves suddenly falling into states of mind that are overwhelming, chaotic, or trance-like.

Unresolved parents in the grip of such states—triggered, for example, by the cries or tantrums of inconsolable or angry infants—can all too easily behave in ways that terrify their children. And the parental rage that erupts in physical or emotional abuse is doubly devastating because it plays havoc with children's biologically driven responses to fear. Children can neither turn toward nor away from, an attachment figure who is at once the source of perceived danger and the sole haven of safety. Hence, the anomalous behaviors of disorganized infants' that reflect the "contradiction or inhibition of action as it is undertaken, or freezing as though there is no alternative solution" (Ainsworth & Eichberg, 1991, p. 162; Main, 1995; Hesse & Main, 2000).

Importantly, however, it is not only the parents' overwhelming affects

and frightening maltreatment that elicit disorganization. Unresolved trauma can also be expressed in signs of fear—such as physical retreat from their infants or dissociation—that are themselves alarming because the secure base is then felt to be anything but secure. And, because infants are incapable of interpreting the motivations that may underlie their parents' behavior, they are vulnerable to the belief that they are somehow to blame for their parents' fear, withdrawal, or dissociation.

Such experiences of feeling endangered by—or dangerous to—an attachment figure on whom one's survival depends are simply too overwhelming to be integrated. They must be kept at bay, therefore, by disorganized infants and unresolved adults alike. Yet these disowned experiences remain a more or less disturbing presence, lurking on the periphery of conscious awareness and erupting periodically onto center stage.

Clinicians know the exorbitant cost of their unresolved patients' efforts to "exile" past trauma or loss. Such patients feel perpetually threatened from within and without, burdened by an ongoing vulnerability to dissociation, overwhelming emotion, and an external world made dangerous by the projection outwards of unbearable internal experience. In addition, their capacity for metacognitive monitoring is profoundly limited—because looking deeply into themselves or others risks bringing to light what must, of emotional necessity, remain hidden. And finally, as Main's account confirms, the dissociated and dangerous working models of unresolved parents—and the associated foreclosure of self-reflection—place their children at severe risk for disorganized attachment as well as the psychopathologies with which it is all too often linked.

CAVEATS AND A NOTE ON TERMINOLOGY

While I find it extremely helpful to consider patients in light of their prevailing state of mind toward attachment, the fact is that their complexity as whole people can never be adequately captured by a single descriptor—secure, dismissing, preoccupied, or unresolved. For this reason, among others, there has been an ongoing debate concerning the issue of attachment categories (see Brennan, Clark, & Shaver, 1998).

Indeed, social psychologists have argued that it is less meaningful to think about attachment patterns as categories or "types" than as regions in a two-dimensional space, with one dimension corresponding to *avoidance* (of closeness and dependency) and the other to *anxiety* (about abandonment). Note that the term "anxiety" here corresponds to Ainsworth's "ambivalence" and Main's "preoccupation."[4] In this alternative framework, the individual's attachment pattern is defined by the *relative* prominence of avoidance and anxiety (Mikulincer & Shaver, 2003).

More often than not, patients over time reveal multiple states of mind that are, to some extent, context dependent—meaning that a particular state of mind is more likely to emerge in some contexts than in others. In the context of feeling rejected, for example, a patient of mine who ordinarily appeared to be in a dismissing state of mind came to seem preoccupied. That most people have a multiplicity or "layering" of states of mind partly explains the paradox that as therapy moves along and we presumably know the patient better, we often feel less clear about exactly who the patient is—or, at any rate, that clarity is no longer reducible to a single classification.

Moreover, while a patient's attachment classification(s) may suggest a host of clinically valuable implications, it is always the *particulars* of the patient's life and history that are most telling. So, for example, the yearnings for connection that an apparently dismissing patient has needed to disown will have everything to do with the specifics of his experience with his particular attachment figures.

All the caveats notwithstanding, when I've taken a backward look and reviewed summaries of my initial session or two with new patients, I've been struck by the power of first impressions. Particularly in the opening hours of treatment, it is usually possible to develop a clinically useful sense of the patient's *predominant* state of mind with respect to attachment.

Finally, a note on language. Starting with Main, researchers using the AAI have referred to the individual's "state of mind with respect to attachment"—an assessment reflecting the coherence of an adult's discussion of attachment experience and predicting the attachment behavior of that adult's child. Meanwhile, social psychologists have preferred to describe the adults they study in terms of their "attachment style"—an assessment derived from self-reports discussing their experiences in forming romantic or other close relationships. Despite these differences, both "attachment states of mind" and "attachment styles" are tied to internal working models, attachment strategies, and the histories that produce them. For this reason I use the terms interchangeably in the chapters that follow.

NOTES

1. There is a comparatively rare subcategory of Dismissings—Ds2—marked not by idealization but rather derogation of attachment figures (Hesse, 1999).
2. Dismissing adults show a spike in galvanic skin response specifically in response to AAI queries about separation, rejection, and/or experiences of feeling threatened by their parents (Dozier & Koback, 1992).
3. Recently developed, a fifth AAI category—"cannot classify"—also appears to predict infant disorganization. Hesse (1996) proposes that whereas unresolved adults exhibit "brief and circumscribed bouts of disorganization in speech or reasoning," those who cannot be

classified reveal a "global disorganization or collapse of a singular or consistent discourse strategy that runs throughout the interview" (Main et al., 2005, p. 285). Research has shown that the cannot classify category is associated with adult lives marked by psychiatric disturbance, violence, and sexual abuse (Hesse, 1999).

4. Secure attachment is represented by the upper-left-hand quadrant as securely attached individuals are neither avoidant in their behavior nor anxious about abandonment. Ambivalent/preoccupied attachment is represented by the upper-right-hand quadrant because individuals with this pattern are anxious about abandonment yet seek closeness rather than avoiding it. Avoidant/dismissing attachment is represented by the lower-left-hand quadrant: Adults with this pattern appear to be without anxiety about abandonment, yet their behavior is avoidant. The lower-right-hand quadrant, finally, represents what social psychologists call fearful–avoidant attachment: Overlapping with Main's disorganized and unresolved classifications, the pattern of fearful avoidance involves both avoidant behavior *and* abandonment anxiety.

CHAPTER 7

How Attachment Relationships Shape the Self

... one's experiences of relations with others becomes a feature of one's relations with oneself.
—PETER HOBSON (2002, p. 180)

The human infant is an extraordinarily vulnerable and dependent creature. Infants are unequipped with the advanced neural gear necessary to manage on their own the bodily, emotional, and environmental challenges of life outside the womb. To survive, they require the protection of what Bowlby (1988) called "stronger and/or wiser" others (p. 121). Beyond physical survival, infants need attachment figures to help them in forming and maintaining that stable point of reference known as the self.

The infant's utter dependence means that adapting to attachment figures—with their idiosyncratic strengths and vulnerabilities—is mandatory. And because the infant *must* adapt, the infant *will* adapt. (Of course, good-enough attachment figures tend to return the favor, by adapting to their infants: hence, the empirical finding that relationships of attachment are co-created.) Ainsworth's research is essentially a documentation of the variety of adaptive strategies infants develop in order to gain the protection that flows from proximity to their attachment figures.

The infant's automatic adaptations to attachment figures clearly have roots in survival imperatives and instincts. (Recall that the newborn is preequipped at birth with brainstem-based reflexes that jump-start the attachment process.) Yet attachment is driven every bit as much by the need

99

for felt security. Because infants are incapable of manufacturing their own felt security, they need attachment figures to help them manage their difficult emotions.

This emotional management is called *affect regulation*. The psychological fate of the infant (in attachment terms, her security or the lack of it) depends largely on the relative success or failure with which first relationships regulate the infant's affects. From this angle, adaptive attachment strategies can also be seen as strategies of affect regulation that will shape the self in fundamental and pervasive ways.

The self of the developing child emerges as a function of these adaptive strategies and the specific feelings, thoughts, and actions for which the child's first relationships of attachment can effectively make room. The expressions of the child's self that evoke the attachment figure's attuned responsiveness can be integrated, while those that evoke dismissing, unpredictable, or frightening responses (or no responses at all) will be defensively excluded or distorted. What is integrated can then enjoy a healthy maturational trajectory; what is not tends to remain undeveloped.

Attachment relationships are crucial to the process of integration.[1] The difficulties that bring patients to treatment usually involve unintegrated and undeveloped capacities to feel, think, and relate to others (and to themselves) in ways that "work." With this in mind, Bowlby (1985) characterized the psychotherapist's task as follows: "Our role is in sanctioning the patient to think thoughts that his parents have discouraged or forbidden him to think, to experience feelings his parents have discouraged or forbidden him to experience, and to consider actions his parents have forbidden him to contemplate" (p. 198). The role of the clinician is, in short, to facilitate integration and, thus, the resumption of healthy development, starting usually with emotional development.

AFFECT REGULATION AND ATTACHMENT STRATEGIES

The quality of the caregiver's response to the infant's affects is vitally important in determining the nature of the predominant attachment strategy—secure or insecure—that the infant adopts. In the case of secure attachment, the responses of the caregiver help both to alleviate the infant's distress and to amplify her positive emotions. As a consequence, the infant experiences the attachment relationship as a context within which affects can be effectively regulated. What registers internally, then, will be a visceral sense that connection to others can be a source of relief, comfort, and pleasure. What also registers is a sense that the self—in expressing its full range of bodily and emotional experiences and needs—is good, loved, accepted, and competent.

The process of affect regulation here is one in which the infant, through a kind of "social biofeedback," comes to associate the initially involuntary expressions of her emotions with the responses of the caregiver. That is, the infant comes to "know" that her affects are responsible for evoking the caregiver's affect-mirroring responses. Thus, in the most desirable scenario, the infant is learning a number of very useful things: (1) that expressing her feelings can bring about positive outcomes—which generates positive feelings about the self and others; (2) that she can have impact on others—which generates a dawning sense of agency or self-initiative; and (3) gradually, that *particular* affects elicit particular reactions—which helps her begin to differentiate and eventually name her feelings (Fonagy et al., 2002). A relationship of secure attachment can thus be seen as a school in which we learn to effectively regulate affects not only in early childhood but throughout our lives.

The secure pattern I've just sketched reflects what Main calls the *primary attachment strategy*. A biologically preprogrammed product of evolution, it mandates the seeking of proximity to an attachment figure whose affective attunement enables the infant to experience her both as a safe haven at moments of alarm and as a secure base whose availability makes autonomous exploration possible. When, however, the infant's emotional signals evoke misattuned responses from the caregiver that discourage either proximity seeking or autonomy, then this primary attachment strategy will be rejected. More accurately, it will be modified to adapt to the particular vulnerabilities of the (insecure) caregiver: The infant will develop a *secondary attachment strategy* that reflects either a *deactivation* or *a hyperactivation* of the attachment behavioral system. These strategies of infancy can also be seen as the forerunners of psychological defenses that originate in the child's necessary, if sometimes failed, efforts to make the best of a bad situation—that is, to adapt to attachment figures whose own defenses have compromised their ability to interactively regulate the child's affects (Main, 1990, 1995; Mikulincer & Shaver, 2003).

Deactivation is seen in infants classified as avoidant and also in adults whose state of mind is described as dismissing. In contrast, hyperactivation is the adaptive strategy of infants who are ambivalent and adults whose state of mind is preoccupied. Disorganized infants as well as unresolved adults may oscillate between strategies of hyperactivation and deactivation.

As a rule, a predominantly deactivating strategy arises when the parents' responses to the child's attachment-related affects are aversive. Here the child's signals of distress and bids for proximity have evoked reactions that are rejecting and/or controlling. In rejecting her bids for proximity, the parents fail to restore the child's emotional equilibrium, while their intrusiveness can leave the child feeling emotionally overaroused (Sroufe, 1996). In neither case has she received help in managing her difficult feelings—

quite the contrary. In order to maintain the best possible attachment relationship under these circumstances, the child learns to overregulate her feelings and their expression, and to distance from her impulse to connect.

You might think here of obsessive, narcissistic, or schizoid patients whose emotional range is narrow, who can appear more or less blind to the affective signals of others, and whose flattened responsiveness can make them seem low on life—a little as if they were playing dead. Siegel (1999) has suggested that in adults, this avoidant, deactivating strategy is reflected in a bias toward left-brain and parasympathetic nervous system activation.[2] What remains unintegrated in patients with such a strategy are all the emotions, desires, and satisfactions associated with intimate relationships. Needless to say, the avoidance of closeness constricts the development of their capacities for deep feeling, sexual expression, healthy dependency, and trust.

By contrast, the hyperactivating strategy of ambivalent infants appears to be organized around the pursuit of closeness. Adapting to parents whose responsiveness to the infant's emotions is unpredictable and/or misattuned, the child learns that amplifying her affects increases the likelihood of engaging her parents' attention. Yet the quality and quantity of attention evoked does not usually match the child's needs. So she learns not only that her bids for support often fail to produce the desired result, but also that to gain comfort she may have to maintain her expressions of distress at a consistently high volume. In short, she learns to keep the attachment system chronically activated.

The hyperactivating strategy of patients we might see as hysteric or borderline may well reflect their preoccupation with the perceived unavailability of attachment figures (past and present) whose help they have sought to gain by maximizing their displays of distress. Unfortunately for such patients, their need to keep the attachment system chronically activated makes them hypervigilant and prone to exaggerate the presence of threats—particularly threats of abandonment. As with the deactivating strategy, the price of protection here is high. Encouraging a sense of personal helplessness, the strategy of hyperactivation precludes the integration of positive feelings about the self or others for at least two reasons. First, such feelings risk *de*activating the attachment system upon which emotional survival has come to depend. And second, overdependency undermines self-esteem and tends to provoke the very abandonment it is unconsciously intended to avert. Hyperactivating defenses also undermine the development of mutuality in relationships, autonomy in thought or action, and, of course, affect regulation. Relatedly, habitual resort to hyperactivation may lower the threshold for triggering the sympathetic nervous system and diminish the capacity to exert cortical control over emotional reactions. The implication is that our preoccupied patients may need us to help them modulate their emotional reactivity and strengthen their capacity to manage their emotions by making sense of them.

Disorganized attachment is generally seen to reflect the breakdown of an adaptive strategy on the part of a frightened infant instinctively driven to seek proximity to a frightening parent. Yet Main (1995) also notes as evidence of disorganization the sequential or simultaneous display of contradictory behavior patterns:

> An example observed in a maltreated infant consisted of a strong display of attachment behavior (running crying to parent with arms outstretched, followed inexplicably by avoidance (infant suddenly stops, turns her back to the parent, silent). (p. 423)

Correspondingly, it has been suggested that unresolved adults have learned to resort to both deactivating *and* hyperactivating strategies. Such adults frequently have a history of trauma in relation to attachment figures that evoked both an avoidance of closeness and a terror of abandonment (Mikulincer & Shaver, 2003). Patients like these are torn by conflicting impulses (to avoid others out of fear of attack, to turn desperately to others out of a fear of being alone) and often experience their feelings as overpowering and chaotic. As therapists, it can be very helpful to realize that the apparently self-destructive behavior of such patients represents their past and present attempts to contend as self-protectively as possible with these contradictory impulses and overwhelming feelings. The integration we are called on to facilitate here has multiple dimensions, including (but not limited to) the integration of traumatic experience and dissociated affects, as well as the mending of splits in these patients' images of self and others. Making this integration possible depends upon our ability to generate an increasingly secure attachment—a haven of safety and secure base—that can itself become the primary source of the patient's ability to tolerate, modulate, and communicate feelings that were previously unbearable.

In summing up the influence of attachment figures on the development of their offspring (and, by extension, the influence of therapists on their patients' development) it may be useful to recall the perspectives of Fonagy and Main. Per Fonagy, the parents' impact is a function of the quality of their affect-mirroring and their ability to "contain" their child's distress through responses that convey empathic understanding, a capacity to cope, and awareness of the child's emerging intentional stance. The mirroring provided by secure parents is both contingent and marked. Noncontingent mirroring may be associated with avoidant attachment and the "pretend" mode of experience; unmarked mirroring may be linked to preoccupied attachment and the mode of psychic equivalence. In general, security begets security, while the defensive strategies adopted by parents tend to be passed on to their children.

From Main's perspective, security develops as a function of the parents' sensitive responsiveness to affective expressions of the child's need

both for proximity, on the one hand, and autonomous exploration, on the other. Insecurity results when dismissing parents discourage their children's attachment behavior or when preoccupied parents discourage their autonomy. The emotional logic of such parenting flows, according to Main, from the insecure parents' unconscious need to preserve their existing state of mind in regard to the childhood experience they had with their own parents. (This need may partly explain the paradox that while many of us are critical of our parents' parenting, we usually duplicate aspects of that parenting, all our conscious intentions notwithstanding.) Dismissing parents, for example, may ignore, reject, or attempt to suppress their baby's tearful bids for contact and connection because they trigger, outside awareness, anxiety-provoking associations to the painful inadequacies of their own parents' responses to them when they were children.

Parents and therapists alike have the potential to foster a mutually reinforcing synergistic relationship between affect regulation and attachment. To the extent that the parent can attune to the child's emotional signals, there is the potential to respond effectively to the child's emotional needs (either by relieving her distress or visibly enjoying her pleasure). In doing so, the parent strengthens the attachment bond. In turn, the parent—experienced increasingly as a safe haven and secure base—becomes more and more capable of helping the child to access, modulate, differentiate, and use her emotional experience. Much the same can be said of the therapist in relation to the patient.

Attachment figures help their "developmentally disadvantaged" partners (children, patients) to evolve patterns of affect regulation that both shape and are shaped by patterns of relationship. If a child gets help with the feelings he expresses, he will tend to become comfortable and skilled at knowing and showing what he feels—which is, in turn, a big part of knowing how to have a secure relationship. Schore's (2003) definition of attachment as "the dyadic regulation of emotion" (p. 256) underscores that healthy development hinges on a relationship that makes room for, and helps makes sense of, the child's emotional experience—or, in psychotherapy, the emotional experience of the patient.

RELATIONAL PROCESSES AND DEVELOPMENTAL DESIDERATA

The word "desideratum" is defined as "something desired that is essential" (Merriam-Webster Dictionary, 2003). Much of the contribution of attachment theory research—to parenting and therapy alike—lies in its identification of the relational desiderata linked to the development of a secure and integrated self. The underlying assumption here is that, early in life, lived patterns of interaction and affect regulation register internally as representations of various sorts that shape our future responses to experience in

more or less persistent ways. In what follows we'll explore how these patterns are internalized and attempt to identify the sorts of experiences that most effectively foster healthy development.

Bowlby hoped his work might help parents to provide the kinds of relationships that would enable their children to become secure and resilient. Initially he emphasized the importance of the parent's accessibility to the child at times of need. Later, in light of Ainsworth's research highlighting the centrality of the parents' sensitive responsiveness to the infant's nonverbal signals, Bowlby stated that parents must be responsive as well as accessible. The question, of course, is what it means to be "sensitively responsive" as a parent or, for that matter, as a therapist.

With regard to infants, Ainsworth's research is particularly informative. Babies whose crying during the first three months evoked the most prompt and frequent responses of soothing from their parents were, at 12 months, the children who cried least and were most secure. (So much, perhaps, for letting our babies cry.) Ainsworth also highlighted the "attachment/exploration" balance and "secure base" behavior that was successfully fostered by parents equally comfortable with the infant's needs for proximity and autonomy (Ainsworth et al., 1978).

As for life beyond infancy, the attachment researcher Karlen Lyons-Ruth (1999) culled the literature, distilling the empirical findings into a framework for what she calls "collaborative communication." Such communication generally enabled children to develop security, flexibility, and coherent internal working models of attachment. Her framework has four elements.

First, the caregiver should be receptive to the whole range of the child's experience (not just her expressions of distress) and should attempt to learn as much as possible about what the child feels, wants, and believes. Clearly, this kind of openness or inclusiveness can foster the integration so central to attachment theory's understanding of healthy development. Second, the caregiver should initiate efforts at repair when the relationship with the child is disrupted. Doing so builds the child's expectation that, through interaction with others, her lost emotional equilibrium is likely to be restored. Third, the caregiver should actively "scaffold" the child's emerging abilities to communicate—initially, say, by attempting to put into words what the preverbal child cannot yet articulate and, later, by asking the child to "use your words." Fourth, the caregiver must be willing to actively engage with the child, to set limits and allow the child to protest, during periods when her sense of herself and others is in developmental flux. This willingness to struggle makes possible for the child the experience of staying connected even while feeling separate.

The fact that collaborative communication depends on "getting to know another's mind" (Lyons-Ruth, 1999, p. 583) recalls Fonagy's observation that the parents of securely attached children appear capable not

only of empathizing and coping with their child's distress, but also of recognizing the "intentional stance" of the child. That is, they can respond to the child's behavior in light of the feelings, beliefs, and desires that seem to underlie it. Even when the behavior in question is at odds with their own wishes, these parents can respond as if aware of the *context* within which the behavior of the child can be seen to make sense. (Note that these are usually parents who can mobilize a well-developed reflective or mentalizing self.)

Many writers stress the importance in developmental relationships of "contingent communication"—that is, communication in which the caregiver's response to the child matches, fits, or resonates with the child's emotional experience. From birth if not before, according to Trevarthen, Fonagy, and others, the human being is a "contingency detector" whose original preference for perfect stimulus–response contingencies shifts at roughly three months of age:

> Whereas infants' initial focus on perfect contingencies enables them to discover their bodily self in the physical world, their subsequent focus on highly but imperfectly contingent social responsiveness enables them to discover their mental self in the social world. (Allen & Fonagy, 2002, p. 9)

When, subjectively speaking, the caregiver actually *shares* in a version of the child's experience, such contingent communication allows the child to "feel felt," in Siegel's (1999) evocative phrase. Stern covers related ground with his notion of *affect attunement* suggesting that a significant part of what enables a child to feel that her subjective states are valid and sharable are parental responses that echo her emotional experiences, but—crucially—in a different sensory register. This cross-modal responsiveness (the child squeals with joy and her mother's body answers with a responsive shimmy) allows the child to feel known—without it, she may only feel imitated.

Communication that is collaborative, contingent, and affectively attuned is the heart of the prescription to parents who would provide for their children the experience of a secure base. Needless to say, the effort to facilitate this quality of communication is no less vital in psychotherapy than in parenting. As Bowlby (1988) wrote, "unless a therapist can enable his patient to feel some measure of security, therapy cannot even begin. Thus we start with the role of the therapist in providing . . . a secure base" (p. 140).

The affectively attuned responses of the parent or therapist that help the child or patient to feel felt may depend upon what Schore (2003) calls "right-brain-to-right-brain communication" (p. 50). His notion is that our receptivity and responsiveness to the affective signals of others are a product of the right brain's capacity (largely through the orbitofrontal cortex) to

process emotion that is expressed nonverbally—that is, through facial expression, tone of voice, posture, gesture and so on. A patient of mine put it this way, "I say something and then you get this look on your face, so I *know* that you know what I feel."

I believe Schore is right when he suggests that a particular frame of mind is called for if the parent or therapist is to be capable of such right-brain communication. In this connection, he alludes both to Freud's recommendation that the analyst function from a stance of "evenly hovering attention" and to Bion's notion that effective clinicians must have access to their own "reverie." Certainly it has been my experience in relation to my patients and children alike that my ability to tune in emotionally hinges on my capacity to be quite fully present—open and in the moment—rather than preoccupied or distant. In the parent or therapist, such receptive states of mind—which I'm tempted to characterize as "mindful"—seem to engender responses that flow naturally from the requirements of the moment including, in particular, the emotional needs of the child or patient.

Repeated experiences of such emotionally attuned responsiveness contribute to positive expectancies that may gel as increasingly secure internal working models. Put differently, such experiences are lessons in how to have a comfortable and effective relationship—with oneself and one's emotions as well as with others.

It's worth emphasizing here that as a parent or therapist, it is not necessary to be always and perfectly attuned: In this connection, good enough will certainly do. As Stern (2002) has facetiously but instructively noted, it is an empirical finding that the very best mothers generally make a mistake with their infants at least once every 19 seconds. Stern's Change Process Study Group (2005), Beebe and Lachmann (2002), and a host of self psychologists agree that what is more important than avoiding the disruptions that are an inevitable feature of relationships is tolerating and repairing them. In fact, such sequences of disruption and repair, misattunement and reattunement, are vital interactions whose internalization specifically encourages confidence that misunderstandings can be resolved—and, more broadly, that distress can be weathered, because it can be relieved.

CO-CREATION, INTEGRATION, AND INTERSUBJECTIVITY

Thus far we've been looking at what the research tells us about the kinds of responsiveness conducive to the development of a secure and integrated self. Clearly, there are valuable insights here with regard to the stance and behavior that parents in relation to their children—and therapists in relation to their patients—might deliberately attempt to adopt. They include contingent, affectively attuned communication (Siegel, 1999; Stern, 1985);

an approach that conveys empathy, an ability to cope, and an appreciation of the child's "intentionality" (Fonagy et al., 1995); a framework of response that embodies *inclusiveness* in relation to the breadth of the child's subjective experience, *scaffolding* of the child's emerging capacities, a *readiness to initiate repair* when there is disruption, and a *willingness to struggle* with the child when necessary (Lyons-Ruth, 1999).

But it is important to note that—as the "collaborative" part of Lyons-Ruth's framework of collaborative communication implies—a developmentally oriented relationship is never the exclusive creation of one partner or the other. Thus, infant–parent relationships have been described as mutually regulated and co-cocreated. The studies of Jaffe, Beeber, Feldstein, Crown, and Jasnow (2001), Tronick (1989), Sander (2002), and others all conclude that mother and infant constitute a dynamic system in which each partner's conduct affects, and is affected by, the conduct of the other. It's probably no accident that the conclusions of infant–parent research dovetail with those of clinical "researchers" in the relational/intersubjective tradition (Mitchell, 1995; Stolorow et al., 1987; Aron, 1996) who identify "mutual reciprocal influence" as a pervasive feature of the interactions between patient and therapist.

Of course, the degree of influence that a parent exerts in a developmental relationship is generally thought to be greater than that exerted by the child. For example, studies have shown that sensitively responsive parenting can transform infants assessed at three months as temperamentally "difficult" (hard to soothe or arouse) into children who were reassessed at 12 months as "easy"; likewise, when parenting is problematic, so-called easy temperaments have been shown to become difficult (Belsky, Fish, & Isabella, 1991). In addition to having greater influence, the parent has, of course, greater responsibility for helpfully shaping the relationship with the child and, ideally, greater flexibility when it comes to doing so.

Granting these differences, each partner nonetheless has a reverberating impact on the other that generates coordinated and mutually regulating patterns of communication in the interaction of the two. Parent and child "track" each other, lead and follow, take turns, and mirror each other (or fail to) in patterns that are distinctive for every dyad. These patterns reflect the affective attunement of the partners and the quality of contingent responsiveness between them—that is, the degree to which the responses of each partner are contingent upon, or a fitting match with, the initiatives of the other.

Research clearly documents such co-constructed patterns in the face-to-face communication between mothers and infants at play. Sequences of match, mismatch, and repair are seen to occur with split-second coordination. Studies using split-screen video (with the baby's face and torso on one side and the mother's on the other) have revealed such an exquisite syn-

chrony of vocal as well as facial expressions that each partner's behavior in the interaction can be predicted, in twelfth of a second increments, from that of the other. Infants at four months were videotaped interacting with their mothers and at 12 months were assessed using the Strange Situation protocol. Of greatest interest is the finding that what differentiates relationships that foster secure attachment from those that do not is the *degree* of bidirectional coordination in the dyad.

Security at one year was predicted when tracking between mother and infant was in the midrange—such that coordination was "present but not obligatory" (Beebe & Lachmann, 2002, p. 104)—while insecure attachment was predicted when tracking was at either a high or low level. High levels of coordination seemed to reflect excessively vigilant monitoring of the partner, while low levels appeared to indicate withdrawal, inhibition, or simply a lack of fit between the partners. Optimally, in other words, the contingent responsiveness in the communication of infants and parents is close but not perfect. This has implications for psychotherapy as well as parenting.

Beebe and Lachmann help to clarify these implications when they discuss this research in terms of the balance between *interactive regulation* and *self-regulation*. In interactive regulation, one partner focuses on and "uses" the responses of the other to manage his or her own internal states of emotion and arousal. (The infant seeking relief from distress, for example, may tune in to the soothing cadences of the mother's voice.) In self-regulation, by contrast, states of emotion and arousal are managed by turning *away* from the partner and *inward* toward the self (as shown, for example, in the infant's gaze aversion, leaning away, oral self-comforting, and rocking). A balance of interactive and self-regulation is reflected in the kind of midrange tracking that predicts secure attachment. High bidirectional tracking reflects a skew toward interactive regulation (a kind of overinvolvement with the partner) and predicts ambivalent or disorganized attachment, while low tracking reflects a bias toward self-regulation (underinvolvement with the partner) and predicts avoidant attachment.

Thinking in terms of these findings regarding interactive and self-regulation can be helpful when it comes to understanding and being of use to our patients. In treatment, those with a strong tilt in the direction of interactive regulation, rather than self-regulation, are the ones who vigilantly track our every response and/or seem utterly reliant upon us to help them manage their difficult feelings. These are usually patients who would be described as preoccupied with the attachment figure's availability (or, more precisely, their fear of its lack). They behave as if they are hopeless, both about relieving their distress on their own and about the possibility of engaging help without making their distress overwhelmingly obvious to others. The problem for these patients (and their therapists) is not their de-

pendency per se. Instead, it is the fact that their wary need for others monopolizes their attention so thoroughly that they have little opportunity to know and make use of their own resources and desires. What needs reintegrating in these patients is their ability to live, as it were, *inside* themselves rather than feeling that their center of gravity lies *outside* themselves, in the minds and reactions of others.

Of course, we also work with many patients whose vulnerability resides in their overdeveloped capacity for self-regulation. Usually seen to operate from a "dismissing state of mind" with respect to attachment, they tend to be ostentatiously self-sufficient. What Bowlby calls their "compulsive self-reliance" often leaves their therapists (and spouses) feeling as if they have little to offer that is needed or valued by these patients. Their deactivating attachment strategy leaves them distant from the awareness of any feelings or impulses that might bring them close to their disavowed needs to connect with others. Usually, in the psychotherapy of such patients, it is precisely their attachment-related feelings, impulses, and needs that must be reintegrated.

The findings of the face-to-face infant–parent research dovetail with those of Ainsworth's Strange Situation studies. The conclusion that midrange tracking is developmentally optimal is consistent with Ainsworth's understanding that secure attachment is reflected in a balance of proximity seeking and exploration, connection and autonomy, relatedness and self-definition. From the face-to-face videotaped exchanges, one must conclude that a secure outcome is associated with a quality of contingent responsiveness between mother and infant that is close but imperfect. Such responsiveness is part of what enables infants to learn that their own internal states are "sharable" and, at the same time, distinct from those of others.[3]

I would suggest that the developmental desirability of midrange tracking—and the fluid balance of self- and interactive regulation it reflects—underscores the importance in parenting and psychotherapy alike of making room for the subjectivities of *both* partners in the relationship. "Primary maternal preoccupation" (Winnicott, 1975) encourages the likelihood that, for a time, the mother will make a greater priority of her baby's subjectivity than her own; and of course, the helping role and ethical responsibility that therapists assume usually encourage a greater focus on the patient's subjectivity than on their own. Yet the perfectly attuned mother (or therapist) who completely suspends or brackets her own subjectivity is probably neither a feasible ideal nor an entirely desirable one.

In the first place, most of us are simply incapable of parking our own needs and limitations outside the door of the baby's room or the consulting room. When we stretch too far beyond ourselves in trying to do so, there are usually unintended and unwelcome consequences that follow. Second, our children and patients grow not only through experiences of "fit" but

also through experiences of separateness and difference. As Benjamin (1990/1999) has clarified, the capacity for mutual recognition—that is, the ability to recognize (and be recognized by) an other as a separate subject, rather than an object—emerges from the discovery that the other, and the relationship itself, can survive anger and conflict. Put differently, episodes of disruption and repair are a vital part of learning to balance the needs for self-definition and relatedness.

Without the give and take of two distinct subjectivities, the child or patient may learn that "there's only room for one": one voice, one will, one whose needs always dominate, one who controls the interaction. When occupying an avoidant–dismissing state of mind, it may feel as if—of necessity—there's only room for the self. For those in an anxious-preoccupied state of mind, it may feel as if there's only room for the other. Secure attachment makes room for both.

The interaction of two distinct subjectivities—in which each is capable of participating psychologically in the experience of the other—is the essence of intersubjectivity. Stern (2004) has said that we're all "hard-wired" for intersubjectivity. (He points out that our brains are structured in such a way that the real question is why we're not constantly captured by the experience of other people.) Apparently the basic mechanisms of such "interexperience"—Stern references the discovery of mirror neurons—are a feature of the human nervous system virtually from birth. Recall in this connection Meltzoff's (1985, 1990) studies showing that as early as 42 minutes outside the womb, infants will imitate the facial gestures of an adult model. Having observed the adult sticking out his tongue, infants will attempt to do the same. Long before they know much about self and other, or about tongues, babies are apparently capable of making a connection between what they *see* on someone else's face and what they *feel* on their own. Such cross-modal matching appears to demonstrate an astoundingly early-developing capacity for interrelatedness of self and other.

This capacity for rudimentary relatedness—a precursor of more evolved forms of intersubjectivity—is probably an outgrowth of the collection of brainstem-based reflexes that prime the attachment and caregiving systems, making of our first close relationships the vital developmental crucibles that they are. Not only in infancy, but throughout our lives, our interaction with intimate others upon whom we depend provides the key context for psychological growth and change. Tronick (1998) has suggested that both infant–parent and patient–therapist relationships make development possible by generating "dyadically expanded states of consciousness" (p. 290). This is a version of the understanding—shared by clinical theorists of intersubjectivity (Bollas, Mitchell, Stolorow) as well as attachment researchers (Fonagy, Lyons-Ruth)—that we need the mind of another in order to know and to "grow" our own mind.

Through the kinds of co-created, mutually regulated, intersubjective interactions from which security or insecurity emerge, children learn both how to have a relationship and how to regulate their emotions. Similarly, it is in the quintessentially intersubjective setting of the therapeutic interaction that our patients can potentially learn how to have a better relationship with others and with their own feelings as well. Key to the developmental outcome in both cases is the quality of the affective communication in the relationship.

To what extent does such communication allow the partners to get in synch so as to experience a sense of mutual recognition and "fittedness"? To which affective signals from the child (or patient) does the parent (or therapist) respond to in an attuned and collaborative fashion? And which affective signals are ignored, misread, or discouraged? More broadly, how big a container for affective communication and experience does the relationship provide? Circling back to Bowlby, Main, and Stern: That which the attachment relationship(s) can accommodate, the individual has the potential to integrate.

NOTES

1. In the process of integration, developmental experiences of relating, feeling, and thinking are intimately linked and mutually influential. For example, "if a person has not been helped with integrating strong feelings, then action may take the place of thinking" (Hobson, 2002, p. 175).

2. Siegel's conceptualization here is helpful because it highlights both the "deficits" of the predominantly avoidant/dismissing patient and the undeveloped capacities that require therapeutic attention if they are ever to be reintegrated. From a neuroscience angle, such patients may need from the therapist an approach that helps them gain access to the input of the emotionally informed, holistically oriented right brain—from which they can appear to be cut off.

3. Interestingly, several studies have shown that an avoidant outcome is correlated with very high tracking of the infant by the mother, while the infant here responds as if in flight from the mother's attention: This pattern of interaction has been described as "chase and dodge" (Beebe & Lachmann, 2002, p. 111). Evidently, infants—like most of us—need some space. Thus, sensitive responsiveness clearly involves an attunement to the child's needs for self-regulation and "open space" (Sander, 1980) as much as for interactive regulation and the connection it fosters.

PART III

FROM ATTACHMENT THEORY TO CLINICAL PRACTICE

As we have seen, relationships of attachment are the primary context for development. Nonverbal, affective experience within an attachment context constitutes the original core of the self. This is the same context that shapes the stance of the self toward experience, which in turn can exert a decisive influence on development, particularly in the face of adverse circumstances. These are the insights of attachment theory research with the most significant implications for psychotherapy.

Because our first relational experiences are mainly lived outside the domain of language, our crucial internalizations of early relationships register as representations, rules, and models that cannot be linguistically retrieved. For these hard-to-reach representations to later be modified—for old working models to be updated—they must be accessed, that is, experientially engaged. In therapy, such representations in the patient often become accessible only as they are communicated through other-than-verbal channels. Thus a focus on the realms of preverbal, nonverbal, and paraverbal experience is indispensable—both to make sense of the original learning that occurred in the patient's first relationships and to facilitate the relearning that can occur in the new relationship with the therapist. This is the subject matter of Chapter 8.

113

While Bowlby emphasized the formidable influence upon the developing self of the realities of early attachment experience, Main and Fonagy showed that the stance of the self toward experience past and present can ultimately be even more influential. To the extent that we are able not only to have our experience but also to reflect upon it, our sense of security, flexibility, and internal freedom will be very much enhanced. Beyond a reflective stance that allows us to make sense of the contents of awareness (feelings, thoughts, and the like) is a mindful stance that can potentially afford us a calm and spacious awareness of awareness. To the extent that we are mindful, we can be more fully present, more capable of living from within the center of ourselves, and less vulnerable to confusing our shifting feelings and thoughts with who we are. Chapter 9 explores the power in psychotherapy and everyday life of shifting the stance of the self toward experience in a more reflective and mindful direction.

To be able to access our patients' nonverbal experience and strengthen their capacity to reflect and be mindful we need to enlist resources outside the attachment field, because attachment theory is not an explicitly clinical theory. Central among these resources is the clinical research conducted under the banner of intersubjectivity and relational theory—a treatment approach that goes a long way toward fulfilling the clinical promise of attachment theory, as I'll explain in Chapter 10.

CHAPTER 8

Nonverbal Experience
and the "Unthought Known"

Accessing the Emotional Core of the Self

In his final book on attachment, Bowlby quotes Freud who remarked on the characteristic response of the patient who has become aware of something "forgotten": "As a matter of fact I've always *known* it; only I've never *thought* of it" (Bowlby, 1988, p. 101). Perhaps Christopher Bollas (1987) who coined the evocative phrase "the unthought known" was reading the same passage from Freud.

What we "know" but do not (or cannot) think about is also what we cannot talk about. Enormously influential because it registers outside conscious awareness, unverbalized (or unverbalizable) knowledge plays a crucial role in psychotherapy as well as in childhood.

If it is obvious that the therapeutic conversation is always made up of more than words, the case for attending to the nonverbal realm is still vital to make—first, because its clinical centrality is not universally recognized or well understood, and second, because the spell of spoken language can be so hypnotic. We risk allowing the words we exchange in therapy to monopolize our attention when we don't remind ourselves that beneath the words there is a flow of critically important experience that provides the underlying context for the words. Fundamentally emotional and relational, this initially unarticulated experience is often where we find the greatest leverage for therapeutic change.

Having established the crucial importance of the nonverbal subtext, I'll discuss how we might understand it. Finally, I'll begin to explore the research and theory that give us the clinical tools to work with the nonverbal dimension of experience—especially early experience—that investigators of attachment have identified as so central.

THE RESEARCH BRIEF FOR A FOCUS ON NONVERBAL EXPERIENCE

At least two findings from attachment research invite, or perhaps even mandate, attention to experience that our patients are unwilling or unable to put into words. First, there is the fact, established by a multitude of observational and longitudinal attachment studies (see Main et al., 2005), that we learn many of the most significant and lasting lessons about who we are in relation to others by the time we are 12 months old—or perhaps even earlier, if the split-screen studies of mothers and infants at four months prove as telling as they appear to be (Jaffe et al., 2001; Beebe et al., 2000). Empirical evidence clearly indicates that the foundations of our internal working models—as well as the habitual attachment and emotion-regulating strategies encoded in these models—are all laid in place well before the acquisition of language. [1] These are the data that underlie Schore's (2003) conclusion that "the core of the self is ... nonverbal and unconscious and lies in patterns of affect regulation" (p. 46). Because preverbal experience constitutes the basis of the developing self, making room for the reverberation and elaboration of such experience in psychotherapy is absolutely vital.

Second, the parent–child relationships that most successfully foster secure attachment are *inclusive* (Lyons-Ruth, 1999; Bowlby, 1988), meaning that the parent makes as much space as possible for the full spectrum of the child's subjective experience. To generate a therapeutic relationship that is similarly inclusive—that is, to make room for as much of our patients' experience as we can—we have to attend not just to what patients tell us in words but also to what they show us in other ways. Bowlby's theory that the child will integrate only what her attachment relationship(s) can accommodate implies that the child will exclude from awareness those thoughts, feelings, and behaviors that risk disrupting attachment relationships, with the result that those thoughts, feelings and behaviors will remain not only undeveloped and unintegrated but often impossible to verbalize. Hence the requirement to "listen" to what is communicated nonverbally if we are to engage experiences that the patient's original attachment(s) precluded. To integrate what has been defensively dissociated or excluded, we need to access that in the patient that is as yet unspoken, unthought, and, perhaps, unfelt.

Neuroscience research both confirms and elaborates the conclusion of attachment research that patients may lack the words to describe crucial experiences for reasons that are either *developmental* (the experiences occurred prior to the acquisition of language) or *defensive* (the experiences could not be thought, felt, or talked about without jeopardizing vital relationships). Clearly there are neurophysiological as well as psychodynamic barriers that bar linguistic access to formative (and, especially, traumatic) experience (Fonagy, 2001). Research on neural development has shown that the brain centers that mediate language (left cortex, Broca's area) and autobiographical memory (the hippocampus, in particular) are not effectively "online" until 18 to 36 months of age—hence, the near-universal finding of "infantile amnesia." Moreover, overwhelming emotions of the kind evoked by trauma suppress the functioning of these same brain structures. Evidently we lack verbal access to many of the experiences that shape us most profoundly, either because these experiences occurred before we had the neural equipment to encode them linguistically or because this equipment was temporarily disabled by overwhelmingly intense painful emotion.

Patients with posttraumatic stress disorder (PTSD)—flooded by a chaos of disturbing emotions, somatic sensations, images, and impulses—lack the language to give meaning or context to their fragmented, multisensory experience.[2] Trauma, which shuts down Broca's area and the hippocampus, can be understood to both cause and result from an "emotional hijacking" (Goleman, 1995) in which the amygdala with its links to the affectively oriented right brain overwhelms the hippocampus and its associated abilities to encode, retrieve, and contextualize memories of the trauma.[3]

The fact that trauma's impact registers as it does has implications for our work with many, if not most, of our patients. van der Kolk (1996), arguing that the imprint of trauma is somatic and sensory, advocates using bodily sensations to access experiences that patients lack the words to articulate. While he addresses his very helpful recommendation narrowly to therapists working with PTSD, I would broaden its scope in recognition of the fact that patients with trauma represent anything but a narrow category.

The infant's utter dependence upon the attachment figure means that chronic misattunement, depression, and anger on the part of a caregiver may, in and of themselves, be experienced as traumatic. In this connection, Schore (2002) has referred to "relational trauma" that arises from experiences of disorganized attachment and may eventuate in borderline and possibly psychotic disorders. I would further suggest that many of our patients (and many of us) suffer from what psychoanalyst Phillip Bromberg (1998a) has described as "islands" of trauma—and dissociation—whose impact and meaning are initially impossible to put into words. Therapists must

find ways to engage such experiences of trauma if their destructive effects are ever to be mitigated.

Alongside the attachment, neurobiology, and trauma studies, there are findings from cognitive science that help clarify the necessity for a therapeutic focus on nonverbal experience. Cognitive scientists have discovered that memory is not monolithic, and they have identified two distinct systems of memory—explicit and implicit. Here's the shorthand: Explicit memory is roughly coincident with our usual understanding of the term, "memory." As such, it can be consciously retrieved and reflected upon, it is verbalizable and symbolic, and its content is information and images. Implicit memory by contrast is nonverbal, nonsymbolic, and unconscious in the sense that it is not available for conscious reflection. Its content involves emotional responses, patterns of behavior, and skills. Implicit memory entails "knowing how" rather than "knowing that."

Sometimes called early memory because it's available to us even in the womb[4] and originally known as procedural memory (involving procedures, like how to dance or ride a bike or be in a relationship, that cannot be conveyed in words), implicit memory has as its subjective hallmark *familiarity* rather than *recollection*. (While it's often said that once you've learned to ride a bike you never forget how, the fact is that you never actually "remember": so familiar is the skill that you just do it; this "knowing how" to ride a bike is an example of implicit memory.) The most important implicit memories involve procedures for being with others and being with oneself. Taken together, these remembered procedures make up what has been called *implicit relational knowing* (Lyons-Ruth, 1998; Stern et al., 1998).

Implicit knowing is expressed not so much in what we say but rather in how we behave and feel, in how we carry ourselves, and in what we expect from relationships. This knowing usually exists outside reflective awareness—not because we can't bear to know but because what we know has registered in an implicit form that is hard to retrieve linguistically.[5]

Implicit or procedural knowing constitutes the foundation of the internal working model. It has been documented by attachment researchers to emerge early in life as a function of the quality of our first relationships and to persist into adulthood (barring changes in these relationships). An infant may come to know implicitly that his cries of distress will quickly evoke his mother's soothing presence, for example, and this primal knowing will become the enduring expectation that supportive others will be there when he needs them. For many of our patients, however, early interactions have been problematic, registering implicitly as a dispiriting bred-in-the-bone understanding of self and others that they cannot easily articulate but also cannot keep from enacting, often to their own disadvantage.

Paradoxically, perhaps, when these same self-defeating enactments occur in psychotherapy they can be a valuable resource insofar as they enable us to engage and transform the wordless internal representations that hold

our patients hostage to the past. But reaching patients at these noverbal levels requires of the therapist some ability to grasp the unverbalized subtext of the therapeutic conversation.

UNDERSTANDING THE LANGUAGE OF THE NONVERBAL

The words exchanged in psychotherapy float, so to speak, on the stream of nonverbal communication between patient and therapist. The drift of spoken dialogue—what is and is not addressed, and at what depth—is largely determined by the emotional and relational currents that flow beneath the surface of the therapeutic interaction. These undercurrents shape the experience of patient and therapist very much as the infant and caregiver's experience is shaped by the quality of their (necessarily) nonverbal communication.

There turns out to be a rather extraordinary consistency between the nonverbal behaviors that mark the interactions of infancy and those we can observe in the interactions of adults (Beebe & Lachmann, 2002). Studies of these earliest patterns of preverbal communication and their parallels in later life reveal some of the ways in which—inescapably and usually outside conscious awareness—we affect and are affected by those with whom we interact. It is the quality of these nonverbal interactions that largely determines the impact of attachment relationships on the developing self, whether in childhood or psychotherapy.

Facial expression and tone of voice, posture and gesture, the rhythms and contours of speech and behavior—these are the elements that compose what is essentially a medium of body-to-body communication. Such communication during infancy can be seen as a conversation between the baby's somatic/emotional self and the caregiver's somatic/emotional self— or, from a neuroscience perspective, as a "conversation between limbic systems" (Buck, 1994, quoted by Schore, 2003, p. 49). The subject of this conversation is mainly the infant's internal states—particularly, emotions and intentions. As the conversation unfolds through the bodily expression of internal states, the infant learns about herself and others: What are her own emotions and intentions? Will others recognize and attune to them? Will it "work" for her to take the initiative—independently or with the help of others—to attempt to affect her own internal states?

Consider the following account (Sander, 2002) of a filmed interaction of an eight-day-old baby who, having grown fussy in her mother's arms, has just been handed off to her father:

> One sees the father glance down momentarily at the baby's face. Strangely enough, in the same frames, the infant looks up at the father's face. Then the infant's left arm, which had been hanging down over the father's left arm, begins to move upward. Miraculously, in the same frame, the father's right

arm, which had been hanging down at his side, begins to move upward. Frame by frame by frame, the baby's hand and the father's hand move upward simultaneously. Finally, just as they meet over the baby's tummy, the baby's left hand grasps the little finger of the father's right hand. At that moment, the infant's eyes close and she falls asleep, while the father continues talking, apparently totally unaware of the little miracle of specificity in time, place, and movement that had taken place in his arms. (p. 20)

In this "action dialogue" of facial expressions and bodily movements—accompanied by the "lullaby" of the father's talk—we can see an exquisite relational choreography. The baby's nonverbal communication of her needs for soothing and sleep evoked a series of unconsciously coordinated and attuned responses from her father. We might infer that such an experience of attunement registered as a tiny but formative influence on this newborn's dawning implicit knowledge about herself in relation to others.

There is a comparable nonverbal choreography that influences the experience of the patient in psychotherapy and shapes, ideally for the better, his evolving sense of himself in relation to others. Not long ago, for example, while speaking to a patient with whom I had been meeting for several months—call him Eliot—I noticed that my voice sounded louder than usual and that the pace of my speech was accelerated. I realized that I was trying to stimulate myself in order to avoid succumbing to the sleepiness I was just now becoming aware of. After privately asking myself what might be going on (a self-inquiry doubtless hobbled by my heavy-lidded state of mind), I decided to enlist Eliot's participation.

What emerged as I let him in on my experience was that he too had felt sleepy—but, beyond that, he was "gone" emotionally, had withdrawn from me, had (as he put it) "dissociated." It was, he said, his familiar response to feeling anxious, angry, or despairing, and he revealed that he had felt crowded out by me—my chair was too close to him for comfort, I was leaning too far forward, I was talking too much. Note that these troubling concerns only came to the surface through a focus on my own nonverbal (or, rather, paraverbal) behavior and experience, while in parallel fashion Eliot's initially undisclosed distress with me was rooted in the physical facts of our relationship.

Attending to the nonverbal subtext had a therapeutic yield related to several of the developmental desirables discussed earlier. With regard to inclusiveness, we were able to contain within our relationship what Eliot had previously had to leave out: namely, disturbing feelings in relation to me (as well as others) involving boundary issues, closeness, safety, and self-definition—not to mention his self-protective dissociation. With regard to attunement, learning together how easily Eliot could feel crowded out and intruded upon led me to draw back and tone myself down in ways that permitted him to feel safer, closer to me, and more in charge of his own ther-

apy. Overall, our original interaction and the subsequent adjustments it spawned gave my patient an experience of disruption repaired—of "misalignment and re-alignment" (Schore, 2003)—that both of us found quite moving.

It seems plausible to infer that, like the episode of the infant with her father, this one might register internally. Although unlike the baby, Eliot and I of course had the benefit of words in our effort to get in synch, I suspect it was less the content of our verbal exchange than the relational process that had an impact on my patient. In this process, through an initial focus on my own voice and body, I found a way to access and meaningfully respond to emotions that Eliot had previously been unable to articulate. Rooted in the nonverbal subtext, our shared experience—an experience more inclusive, collaborative, and attuned to the patient's needs than his history would have predicted—may well have contributed to a shift in his "implicit relational knowing."

As I have explained, this kind of implicit knowing is always enormously influential and usually very difficult to put into words. Certainly the preverbal or traumatic origins of such implicit knowledge can be impossible to retrieve linguistically. Yet, what we cannot recall explicitly—and cannot put into words—is almost invariably expressed in other ways.

In this connection, I would propose the following shorthand: *That which we cannot verbalize, we tend to enact with others, to evoke in others, and/or to embody.* Before going into more detail, let me illustrate what I have in mind by returning briefly to my experience with Eliot.

Eliot enacted with me a scenario that was simultaneously all too familiar to him and yet impossible for him to recognize—or object to—as it was unfolding. In this jointly created enactment, I found myself talking fast and loudly, as if to drown out the stupefying silence that seemed to hang in the air between us. Only in disclosing my drowsiness did I begin to realize how frustrated I had felt at my failed attempts to have an impact on him. For his part, Eliot was initially mainly aware of my clumsy intrusions on his physical and mental space. As we spoke, however, Eliot began to connect with his guilty anger as he recognized that my efforts to reach him had been feeling misattuned, insufficiently respectful of his vulnerability, and as having more to do with my need to feel effective than his need to feel understood. His emotional reflex had been to withdraw from me, very much as he had pulled away (or tried to) from his intrusively seductive mother.

Eliot evoked several distinct experiences in me, as a function, I suspect, both of what he was communicating nonverbally and of what I was receptive (or vulnerable) enough to be internally affected by. In retrospect, I read my own drowsiness not only as a bodily echo of his (yawn and the world yawns with you) but as a defensive reaction of mine to the feeling of being frustrated and potentially angry—as if I were about to be told that what I had to offer was not merely ineffectual but hurtful. Unsurprisingly, these

experiences of mine, by virtue of their connections to Eliot's own, enabled me to know him in an emotionally direct way—through identification, as it were, rather than through the information conveyed by his words. It was as if rather than hearing what Eliot felt, I simply felt it. Patients who succeed in evoking such subjective responses offer their therapists the opportunity to know them "from the inside out" (Bromberg, 1998a).

Patients may also embody—or induce their therapists to embody— what they cannot or will not communicate in words. Eliot was unable to tell me that he needed to be "gone"—to dissociate or, in effect, to leave his body; I was unable to recognize that Eliot was becoming distant and sleepy, but my body apparently "knew" what my mind did not.[6] With Eliot, the deactivating, parasympathetic branch of my autonomic nervous system was triggered and I became drowsy—as a response to *his* deactivation and/or as a defense against the feelings our interactions were evoking in me.

Enactment, evocation, and embodiment are the primary means by which patients communicate what they know but have not thought—and, therefore, cannot talk about. As such, these channels for conveying the unthought known are absolutely essential for therapists to understand. While the developmental centrality of nonverbal experience has been empirically documented by Bowlby's heirs, it is necessary to turn to contemporary *clinical* theory—specifically, to intersubjective and relational theory—to fully capitalize on this particular finding of attachment research. In subsequent chapters I explore in more detail how therapists can work with these ways of knowing and being known that are largely unmediated by language. What follows should therefore be considered a first pass at some crucial ideas about psychotherapy that will be elaborated as we go on.

WORKING WITH ENACTMENTS OF THE UNTHOUGHT KNOWN

Lyons-Ruth (1999) coined the term "enactive representations" to describe the presymbolic internalizations of early experience that provide the foundations of our internal working models. The term seems apt precisely because of the intense focus among intersubjective and relational theorists on *enactments*. As illustrated in my work with Eliot, enactments are the jointly created scenarios that reflect the initially unconscious, overlapping vulnerabilities and needs of patient and therapist.

Enactments in psychotherapy can be seen as the here-and-now behavioral manifestation of implicit relational knowings whose first (but not only) roots lie in what we—patients *and* therapists—"enacted" with our attachment figure(s) as infants. When, for example, our earliest overtures for comfort were regularly welcomed, we probably learned the advantages of turning to others to soothe our distress; when such early overtures evoked rejection, we probably learned the necessity of concealing our distress from

others whenever possible. Such primal lessons about self and others are learned—remembered, represented, internalized—as they are enacted. Later, rather than being recognized with a sensation of recollection ("Aha! *Now* I remember what happened!") these hard-to-verbalize representations of formative experience are recognized—generally by third parties, if at all— mainly as they are enacted ("Can't you see you're treating our kids exactly as you complain your mother treated you?"). Usually, however, what is known implicitly remains implicit. Rather than become available for conscious reflection, it is simply enacted, automatically and reflexively.

Freud (1958) was insightful on this point: "The patient does not *remember* anything of what he has forgotten and repressed, but *acts* it out. He reproduces it not as a memory but as an action" (p. 147). Freud's discovery that patients *repeat* the past rather than remember it is the cornerstone of his conception of transference. From the intersubjective perspective, what Freud overlooked was the fact that the therapist is never merely a blank screen onto which the patient projects the past. Instead, the patient's transference arises from selective perceptions of the current actualities of the therapist's character and behavior. From this angle, what is enacted in the therapeutic relationship always reflects a spiral of mutual reciprocal influence in which the therapist's contribution is no less significant than the patient's.

As I later elaborate, contemporary intersubjective and relational theories offer clinicians the most powerful tools available for working effectively with transference–countertransference enactments. These theories require that we consider questions such as the following: What is most emotionally compelling in the immediacy of the here-and-now interaction with the patient? What is the interpersonal pattern that is presently being played out—and, in particular, what is the nature of our participation in it? How can the jointly created enactment be understood? Usually questions like these are answerable only in dialogue with the patient. Such dialogue sometimes demands that the therapist "go first": To make the latent enactment manifest, it may be necessary for us to put our own experience of the interaction into words.

Not long ago, for example, in the setting of a treatment newly begun, I was attempting to convey my empathy to a recently separated female patient who was unhappily recounting the difficulties she was having with her husband. While I felt that I was "tracking" her in quite an attuned way, she seemed to find my carefully chosen expressions of understanding consistently useless.

Responding with irritation, the patient ("Carol") dismissed most of what I had to say with words that sounded entirely reasonable but left me feeling thwarted, impatient, and increasingly frustrated. Finally, I told her that I was beginning to feel quite irritated myself, adding that I usually had the feeling here that the two of us were on the same side, as I suspected she

did, but that somehow our conversation today seemed to have turned adversarial. This caught her attention.

I realized as I was speaking to her that, in keeping with my own psychological makeup, I had been ignoring her implicitly provocative devaluation long enough that my exasperation—when I finally felt it—was experienced and expressed with a surplus of intensity. As happens not infrequently, this kind of inadvertent participation on therapist's part can turn out to be a blessing in disguise.

Before long Carol was engaged in a rather troubling consideration of the ways our interaction mirrored that with her husband, with whom at times she felt irresistibly drawn to pick a fight. Hearing this, I shared my thought that perhaps her contentiousness today might be related to her telling me at the end of the last session that therapy was finally starting to help. And now began an exploration—still ongoing—of her fear of her feelings, her strategy of self-sufficiency, and her terror of dependency and rejection. The emotionally charged interaction in this session marked a turning point in our therapy. I believe it illustrates the fact that making optimal use of enactments often has as much to do with the therapist's authentic responsiveness and deliberate self-disclosure as it has with interpretation.

The understanding that enactments in psychotherapy are co-created is entirely consistent with the research suggesting that early attachment relationships are themselves co-constructed. As I mentioned earlier, among the most significant conceptual bridges between the relationships of infancy and psychotherapy are those that have been generated by Daniel Stern, Karlen Lyons-Ruth, and the Change Process Study Group (CPSG). Though Stern et al. might define enactments more narrowly than I do, they consistently emphasize the essentially *enactive*, rather than verbal, processes that make the most significant psychological development—and therapeutic change—possible. In illuminating the healing impact of changes in the "shared implicit relationship" between patient and therapist, their unique approach makes an invaluable clinical contribution (Stern et al., 1998; Lyons-Ruth, 1999; Lyons-Ruth & Boston Change Process Study Group, 2001).

The shared implicit relationship reflects the relatively stable but nonetheless evolving sense in each partner of who the other is, who each is to the other, and who they are together. While it is the product of the actual ongoing personal engagement of patient and therapist, it is also necessarily influenced by the implicit relational knowing—the internal working model, if you will—of each partner. I suspect it is this intersubjective meeting of the self and the other, the internal and the interpersonal, the anticipated experience and the lived experience, that makes the shared implicit relationship a fulcrum of potential change.

In 1998, the CPSG published a landmark paper whose subtitle—"The 'Something More' than Interpretation"—hints at the nonverbal experiences

in therapy that effect change. Specifically, they observed that changes in implicit relational knowing occur as a function primarily of what is enacted in the *intersubjective field* of patient and therapist. When their relationship is altered, it shifts the patient's sense of who the therapist is, who he or she is to the therapist, and who they are to each other.

Stern and his colleagues note that therapy unfolds through a series of *present moments* ("beats" in the terms of drama), each of which embodies a distinct subjective sense of "what is happening now between us." At times these present moments become charged with intense feeling, pulling patient and therapist irresistibly into the immediacy and emotional heat of the here and now: The CPSG refers to these moments as *now moments.*

When a now moment evokes an authentic personal response from the therapist that resonates deeply with the patient, the therapeutic couple may experience a memorable *moment of meeting* that transforms the shared implicit relationship. A moment of meeting offers the patient a glimpse into new ways of being, beyond the constraints of preexisting transference predispositions or implicit relational knowing. Such a corrective relational experience can open the door to sudden, dramatic change.

After initially spotlighting these transformative encounters, the CPSG shifted focus to the ongoing therapeutic relationship—the larger context for the high-impact moments of meeting. As previously mentioned, development in therapy—just as in childhood—is facilitated by a relationship involving collaborative, attuned, and contingent communication. Such communication depends much more on the implicit, affective, interactive *process* between patient and therapist than on the explicit content of the words they exchange. Lyons-Ruth puts it this way: "Process *leads* content in this conception, so that no particular content needs to be pursued; rather the enlarging of the domain and fluency of the dialogue is primary and will lead to increasingly integrated and complex content" (Lyons-Ruth & Boston Change Process Study Group, 2001, p. 15).

Enlarging the affective as well as linguistic dialogue occurs through the therapeutic couple's trial-by-error "improvisation of relational moves" (Lyons-Ruth & Boston Change Process Study Group, 2001) rather than the therapist's deliberate attempt to structure the treatment. When patient and therapist both sense that they are fitting together in moving toward mutually held goals, the result is often an experience of vitalization that reinforces a growing sense that their shared relationship is a valuable and helpful one. Repeated rounds of relational improvisation tend to create increasingly effective patterns of fitting together that eventually come to compete with the patient's old predispositions and to destabilize them— thus generating the experience of possibility, flux, and disorder that is the (often disquieting) subjective precursor to change.

Whether such shifts in the patient's implicit relational knowing occur

suddenly (in a moment of meeting) or gradually (through ongoing dialogue that is progressively more inclusive and collaborative than the patient expects) their context is always an enactive and intersubjective one. Years ago, Frieda Fromm-Reichmann remarked that the patient needs an experience, not an explanation. One might say the patient needs a relationship more than a reason why.

What is enacted in the therapeutic relationship will be a function of the interaction of the therapist's implicit relational knowing with that of the patient. Focusing on the quality of our participation as therapists is essential in order that we recognize what we may be unwittingly contributing. As we have seen, co-constructed enactments have the potential to provide some of the most vital contexts for transforming our patients' sense of themselves, of others, and of relationships.

But when clinicians unconsciously collude in replaying the patterns encoded in their patient's internal representations, co-constructed enactments can be obstacles to realizing the goals of treatment. Old learning can be locked in place, familiar expectations confirmed, the problematic past repeated; the result can be a therapeutic impasse. Worse still, the patient can be retraumatized. In addition, there is the issue of our stance toward experience: To the extent that enactments fail to attract our thoughtful attention, it's as if we're on automatic pilot—sleepwalking through our role in the interaction rather than awake to it, embedded in the experience rather than reflective or mindful about it.

All this makes it imperative for us to be consistently attentive to the nature of the implicit relationship we enact with our patients. To engage with what they cannot verbalize, we have to tune in as much to the music as the words: How do we feel we're affecting and being affected by them? How does the patient feel he is affecting and being affected by us? What can we infer about his subjective and intersubjective experience—and what do we sense about our own? We must keep in mind that every verbal exchange, every interpretation, every intervention is an interpersonal event; each one influences the shared implicit relationship in ways large or small, and often unanticipated—such that our attempts to be helpful (like my overeager effort to "reach" Eliot) can have an impact very much at odds with what we intend or expect.

WORKING WITH EVOCATIONS OF THE UNTHOUGHT KNOWN

A high-powered, rather intellectual executive came to see me, ostensibly at his wife's insistence. She complained that he was tense, distracted, and emotionally unavailable. The patient, whom I'll call Gordon, wasn't sure about this, or about his need for therapy, but he seemed willing to give it a

(brief) try. Three or four sessions into a treatment that appeared to have an increasingly dubious future, I found myself noticing the care with which I was choosing my words. I realized that I was feeling unaccountably anxious, almost as if I were being threatened by a prosecutor and needed my language to be bulletproof.

After some hesitation, I chose to share this experience with my patient. Hearing what I had to say, Gordon was astonished. He said that I was describing *his* experience, not only when he was here with me but also more broadly. He had never before found the words to describe it, but now it seemed to him that he was bringing what he called his "internal landscape" into the interaction between us. In this connection, he disclosed to me that he had a pattern at work of compulsively "goldplating" his performance, out of a vague sense of threat, and added that his mother, a Holocaust survivor, had recently asked him, "Don't you feel anxious? You must be the only Jew there."

As we explored his experience, and ours, over the course of several sessions, Gordon became aware that what drove his own bulletproofing was specifically a fear of judgment and attack, especially in environments he didn't trust to be rational. He thought his mother "had this same anxiety from her experiences" and had somehow transferred it to him. Now it appeared that he had transferred it to me. My vulnerability to feeling threatened allowed Gordon to evoke in me an experience he was at pains to avoid in himself. By "relocating" his unconscious sense of danger, he enabled the two of us to identify/articulate it and then to begin to grasp that, at some level, the feelings he was reluctant to claim as his own were, in fact, originally his mother's.

In suggesting that this patient evoked in me what he was reluctant to know and, hence, unable to tell me, I'm referring to *projective identification*. Conventionally understood, this is the process through which we project onto (or into) another what we cannot bear in ourselves. Then we relate to the other in such a way that he comes to identify with what we have projected. Projective identification, while usually considered a mechanism of defense, is also a mode of nonverbal communication.[7]

As Melanie Klein originally conceived it, projective identification was essentially the *fantasy* in the minds of infants and psychologically primitive adults that they could somehow relocate parts of themselves in others. The psychoanalysts Winnicott and Bion are generally credited with "interpersonalizing" Klein's insight. They realized that what Klein had regarded as an exclusively internal phenomenon was in fact an interpersonal one: All of us—from birth onward—actually evoke in others experiences that we are unable or unwilling to claim as our own.

Bion (1962) theorized that "normal projective identification" was the single most important medium of communication in infancy. Affects that

were overwhelming were projected by the infant into the receptive mother, who contained and processed them before returning them to the child in a modulated and "digestible" form. The observations of infant–parent research tend to confirm Bion's theory—while adding a crucial emphasis on bidirectional influence and co-construction.

Stephen Seligman (1999), a psychoanalyst and researcher at the University of California, has suggested that a realistic understanding of infant–parent relationships must take into account the *parent's* projections as well as those of the infant. In these and other close relationships—such as marriage and psychotherapy—adults clearly make use of projective identification. Bion (1967) actually argued that projective identification was the most significant form of interaction between patients and therapists. What I emphasize in subsequent chapters is the complexity of projective identification: first, the fact that it is bidirectional; and second, that as therapists, we must be wary of assuming too readily that what we feel the patient has evoked in us belongs to the patient alone. Usually human beings need a hook to hang their hat on.

Precisely how we evoke own experiences in others is a matter that has been clarified somewhat by contemporary research in a variety of fields. It now appears that the transfer of internal states from infant to parent (and vice versa) as well as from patient to therapist (and vice versa) is mainly accomplished through the medium of body-to-body communication. You might say that we become what we behold: When we perceive emotions in others, we feel these emotions in ourselves.

As previously mentioned, newborns as young as 42 minutes will imitate the facial gesture of a model who opens her mouth or sticks out her tongue (Meltzoff & Moore, 1998). At two-and-a-half months, infants will react to their mothers' displays of emotion with corresponding affects of their own (Haviland & Lelwica, 1987).[8] In related research, Dimberg et al. (2000) showed adult subjects a neutral video in which 30-millisecond sequences of a smiling face and an angry face had been embedded. When exposed to these subliminal segments, the experimental subjects reflexively shifted the micromusculature of their own faces to conform to the expressions they (unconsciously) beheld on the faces in the video.

Apparently we are constructed by evolution to reflexively imitate the facial behavior of those with whom we interact. But what does imitation have to do with the transfer of internal states? Duplicating the facial behavior of another is not the same as participating in his emotional experience. Or is it?

Paul Ekman,[9] the world's preeminent investigator of the phenomenology and psychophysiology of facial expression, has discovered that facial muscle reactions not only *express* emotions but also *activate* them. When we deliberately assume the facial expression associated with a particular

emotion, our physiology and pattern of brain activation change in conformity with it.[10] Ekman's research coupled with the imitation studies suggests that in fact we often have access to such states in others whether we choose to or not. For when—unconsciously and involuntarily—we duplicate the facial expression of another person, we also set up within ourselves an emotional response that resonates with, matches up, or corresponds to the emotional experience of that person (Ekman, 2003; Ekman, Levenson, & Friesen, 1983).

This may be how as therapists we have the potential to know "from the inside out" what our patients are experiencing. What they cannot put into words, they convey through face-to-face communications that evoke their emotion in us. Not surprisingly, Ekman believes that the "music" of the voice (tone, rhythm, contour) both communicates and activates emotion just as the expression of the face does. Call it projective identification or nonverbal communication, the fact is that our patients will activate inside us resonances of their own experience.

The crucial point here is one at the very center of the intersubjective, relational approach to psychotherapy: *To access what our patients cannot put into words, we must tune in to our own subjective experience*. Later, I explore in detail how contemporary relational theory can help us to utilize our own subjectivity to identify, understand, and make good use of the patient's evocative influence. For now, I will only say that to receive the patient's nonverbal communications we must learn to recognize their reverberations inside ourselves.

Once we do so, it may be vital at certain times to deliberately disclose to our patient what we believe has been evoked in us. At other times we may use our awareness of what has been evoked to develop and convey a deeper understanding of the patient's unspoken experience. At still other times, patients may need to see us successfully struggle to bear experiences they have found unbearable. None of this is possible without understanding that our patients will often evoke in us what they cannot communicate through language, except perhaps the language of the body.

WORKING WITH EMBODIMENTS OF THE UNTHOUGHT KNOWN

A woman patient was acutely uncomfortable whenever the possibility arose of a silence between us. In exploring the details of this experience, she said that if there were no conversation then we would simply be looking at each other. And if that were to occur? I inquired. Then we'd each just be looking at the other's body, she answered. It'd be like we were just two bodies here. This apparently provoked for her the very troubling question of the relationship between our bodies—also known as the issue of sexuality.

We cannot exclude the body if psychotherapy is to make room for as much of the patient's experience as possible. The "talking cure" is likely to be significantly less inclusive, less integrative if it is only a conversation between talking heads. Bodily sensation is always the substrate of emotion: To a considerable extent what we feel physically is what we *feel* emotionally.

Preverbal experience, identified by attachment research as so influential, is largely, of course, bodily experience. And as I've indicated previously, it is body-to-body communication that provides the evocative subtext of the spoken dialogue in psychotherapy. Although much of the impact of this communication registers outside conscious awareness, it is also true that it can be very hard to find what we fail to look for. Clinicians cannot afford to ignore the body—neither their patient's nor their own—because the body often receives and transmits what has not or cannot be put into words.

The impacts of acute trauma as well as disorganized attachment are frequently somatic. A patient of mine who was chronically traumatized in childhood finds herself alternately overtaken by physical pain or anesthetized to it—as if the internal signals were either deafeningly intense or barely audible. She feels at times a prisoner of her own body and at times as if she has no body of her own. She has difficulty knowing whether her physical suffering might not really be a stand-in for her emotional suffering.

Invariably patients like this—who oscillate between overwhelming hyperarousal and numbing dissociation—have enormous difficulty with affect regulation. They have trouble translating somatic sensations into feelings they can articulate and use to guide appropriate action. The ease with which they can be autonomically triggered makes it difficult for them to think and feel; instead, they deny and dissociate. Unsurprisingly, neurobiological studies show that patients with a history of trauma have increased reactivity in the amygdala and correspondingly *diminished* activity in the prefrontal cortex (Rauch et al., 2000; Shin et al., 2004). For such patients, "the body keeps the score" (van der Kolk, 1996, p. 214).

It's as if the body remembers too well the agonies it registered in the past—and now reacts as if everyday difficulties might be life-threatening disasters. Much of the work of psychotherapy with such patients involves the effort to recognize, tolerate, and label somatic states so that bodily sensations can be linked with emotions and emotions with the contexts that provoke them. With these patients the path to affect regulation and the integration of dissociated experience usually begins with the body.

In contrast to patients who switch between sympathetic nervous system hyperactivation and parasympathetic deactivation are those in a dismissing state of mind with respect to attachment. Such patients can truly seem like talking heads and rather unexpressive ones at that, appearing stiff in posture and impassive of demeanor, their voices having little inflection.[11] Therapists with inhibited, deactivating patients like these may need to be

especially deliberate about attuning to their own bodily sensations—of tension, constriction, sleepiness, and so on. Often the reverberations of the patients' own disavowed emotions, or the defenses against them, will register first in the body of the therapist.

A clinician colleague told me that once he had felt a sharp ache in his chest while working with a "real Marlboro man of a patient." This patient had shown little affect over the course of several years of treatment. The therapist sat silently with the aching sensation in his chest and realized that it was a bodily echo of feelings he had had as a lonely adolescent. He decided to share his experience with the patient. When he did so and then asked if the patient had ever felt a similar sensation, tears welled up in the man's eyes and he began to talk for the first time about his own boyhood feelings of aching loneliness—feelings he had never been able to share or overcome.

The body, to paraphrase the psychoanalyst Otto Kernberg, is a geography of personal meanings. To get at these meanings we have to make room for the somatic self, bring our attention both to what the patient's body reveals and to the patient's relationship to her body. We also have to attend to the sensations of our own body—for often they represent resonant physiological responses to what is occurring within the patient. Finally, as indicated in the vignette that opened this reflection on the body in psychotherapy, we have to attend to the relationship between the two bodies in the room. These are all routes to recognizing, engaging, and, if all goes well, modifying the impact of problematic formative experiences for which as yet our patients have no words.

Focusing on the nonverbal domain can allow us to connect with facets of the patient's self that have never been integrated and cannot be articulated. By becoming aware of what the patient enacts with us, evokes in us, or embodies, we have the opportunity to begin to know something about the patient's "unthought known" while often learning about ourselves in the process. Attending to the relational, intersubjective, and affective undercurrents of the therapeutic interaction can help make room for experience and awareness the patient has previously had to disown. And ideally our responses to the patient can enable that experience and awareness to deepen.

NOTES

1. Note that the research evidence should not be misconstrued to suggest that the trajectory set by our first relationships is unalterable. Working models have the potential to be updated; early experience establishes stable patterns, not rigid structures.
2. Thus deprived of the capacity for expressive language, people who are traumatized may experience "speechless terror" (van der Kolk et al., 1996).
3. Individuals traumatized in childhood have been found, in some studies, to have smaller

left hippocampi and diminished left-brain development, in general, when compared with healthy control subjects. Correspondingly, when adults with a history of abuse were asked to recall a disturbing early memory, their hemispheric activity showed a radical skew to the right; when recalling a neutral memory, the skew was way to the left. In a control group, by contrast, hemispheric activity was balanced, regardless of whether the memory was disturbing or neutral. Moreover, the volume of the corpus callosum—the brain's main channel of information exchange between its two hemispheres—was found to be significantly smaller among traumatized individuals than among controls without such a history. Trauma thus appears to impede neural as well as psychological integration—isolating the emotional right brain from the verbal resources of the left.

4. It perhaps determines the usual choice of mother as the primary attachment figure because, as Main (1999) notes, the maternal voice to which the newborn orients was such a familiar feature of the intrauterine "soundtrack."

5. Together with the Freudian *unconscious* produced by repression, this implicit *nonconscious* (Stern, 2004; Siegel, 1999) is probably what Bollas had in mind when he coined the term the "unthought known."

6. The self psychologist Michael Basch (1992) has written that "the patient subtly causes the therapist to resonate autonomically with the patient's unconscious" (p. 179).

7. In this connection, Schore (2003) writes: "Freud began to model the state of mind of 'evenly suspended attention' in which one could receive the unconscious communications of others. I suggest that if Freud was describing how the unconscious can act as 'a receptive organ,' Klein's conception of projective identification attempts to model how an unconscious system acts as a 'transmitter,' and how these transmissions will then influence the receptive functions of another unconscious mind" (p. 59).

8. Mothers in face-to-face interactions with their infants were asked to adopt a variety of facial expressions: In response to a show of joy from their mothers, the infants' own joy appeared to be heightened and their "mouthing" movements decreased; in response to the mothers' sad face, the infants appeared subdued and mouthing increased; in response to their mothers' angry expression, the infants showed anger and their bodies stilled (Haviland & Lelwica, 1987).

9. Ekman initially won renown for demonstrating cross-culturally that every basic emotion (sadness, anger, fear, surprise, etc.) is associated with a signature pattern of facial muscle reactions: enjoyment, for example, is reflected in the smile but also crucially in the involuntary engagement of the muscles around the eyes.

10. Illuminating the process, Ekman quotes from *The Purloined Letter* in which Edgar Allan Poe, writing in the persona of a detective, explains how he deliberately gains access to the internal states of others: "When I wish to find out how wise or how stupid or how good or how wicked is anyone, or what are his thoughts at the moment, I fashion the expression of my face, as accurately as possible, in accordance with the expression of his, and then wait to see what thoughts or sentiments arise in my mind or heart, as if to match or correspond with the expression" (Poe, cited in Ekman, 2003, p. 37).

11. Ekman's research suggests that such inhibition of the body actually inhibits the subjective experience of emotion in infants as well as adults.

CHAPTER 9

The Stance of the Self toward Experience

Embeddedness, Mentalizing, and Mindfulness

The investigations of Main, Fonagy, and others confirm that the capacity to reflect coherently upon experience—rather than being embedded in it or defensively dissociated from it—is a marker of both our own attachment security and our ability to raise children (and perhaps patients) who will also be secure. As in the Adult Attachment Interview of a secure adult, this capacity for a "reflective" or "mentalizing " stance (I use the terms interchangeably) is manifested in a coherent account of experience that, in turn, reveals a coherent self. By that I mean a self that (1) makes sense rather than being riddled with inconsistencies; (2) hangs together as an integrated whole rather than being fractured by dissociations and disavowals; and (3) is capable of collaboration with other selves. Following the lead of Daniel Siegel (2006), I would suggest that a coherent self is also one that is stable, adaptive, flexible, and energized.

As psychotherapists, we aim to help our patients to live, more and more, from within such a coherent self. Our task is to co-create a relationship with our patients that allows them to make sense of their experience, to feel more "together," and to relate to others more deeply and with greater satisfaction. Central to this task in the model of psychotherapy I am proposing is the therapist's mentalizing stance that fosters the patient's own

capacity to mentalize. For mentalizing—implicitly and explicitly—is key to integrating the dissociated experiences of the patient that have been accessed through a focus on the nonverbal realm.

Nothing predicts an adult's capacity to raise securely attached children better than the ability to freely access and collaboratively reflect upon attachment-related memories and to construct and present a coherent narrative of early attachment experience. Recall the AAI research revealing that it is this ability that distinguishes secure adults from those with suboptimal attachment experiences. Dismissing adults cannot freely access attachment memories; their narratives are rigid and incomplete. Preoccupied adults cannot collaboratively reflect; their narratives are chaotic and confusing.

There are, however, *some* individuals with those kinds of experiences who can, so to speak, jump the tracks of their developmental trajectory to produce coherent narratives and raise secure children. This empirical finding concerning "earned security" is a momentous one with very encouraging implications for psychotherapy. Quite simply, it confirms that individuals can potentially transcend the limits of their history—breaking the chain of disadvantage that transmits insecurity and trauma from one generation to the next. What turns out to count as much as, and sometimes more than, our formative experience is our stance toward that experience.

Taking this conclusion as my starting point, I find it very useful clinically (as well as personally) to think in terms of three primary stances toward experience: We can simply be *embedded* in experience, we can have a *mentalizing* and *reflective* stance toward experience, or we can be *mindful*.

Much of the time, without being aware of it, many of our patients are too embedded in problematic experience—too identified with what they believe and feel—to be able to envision alternative views of that experience. To help them access its *multiple* levels rather than play out the one-dimensional version in which their self-protective/self-defeating credulity keeps them trapped, we must tune in to the nonverbal domain. And to do that effectively, we must be able to mentalize—that is, we must be able to find our way to an intuitive grasp of the mental states that underlie our patients' present experience. This is *implicit* mentalizing and it allows us to reach, resonate with, and respond in an attuned fashion to, experience in the here and now for which our patients may as yet have no words. Then, having accessed this unspoken experience that has been dissociated or disowned, we must be able to reflect on it with the patient in order to further its integration. This requires *explicit* mentalizing, which enlists language to help patients make sense of their experience by situating it in the context of the lived past and the anticipated future as well as the present moment. Mentalizing implicitly and explicitly, we gradually enable our patients to do the same.

Psychotherapy in all its forms has been seen to involve a relationship that kindles or disinhibits the capacity of the patient to mentalize (Fonagy et al., 2002; Holmes, 2001). As we will see, psychotherapy has further been understood as a process that cultivates the patient's capacity to be mindful (Martin, 1997; Germer et al., 2005). Mindfulness is defined as "bare attention"—that is, the "clear and single-minded awareness of what actually happens to us and in us, at the successive moments of perception" (Nyanaponika, 1972, p. 5). Baer (2003), reviewing the literature on mindfulness training as a clinical intervention, describes it as "the non-judgmental observation of the ongoing stream of internal and external stimuli as they arise" (p. 125). Like the mentalizing stance, a mindful one may well have the potential to enhance integration, emotion regulation, and security of attachment. But before addressing the therapeutic implications here, I want to say a few words about each of the three stances toward experience.

EMBEDDEDNESS

When embedded in experience, it's as if we *are* the experience as long as the experience lasts. Whatever we sense, feel, and believe at any given moment, we simply take at face value. In many circumstances, of course, such a stance may be just what is called for—say, when we're immersed in the pleasures of music, or skiing, or making love. In others, anything *but* such a stance puts us at a critical disadvantage: Second-guessing our sense of danger can be hazardous when, for example, we find ourselves in the path of an onrushing truck. If, however, a stance of embeddedness is regularly our *only* option, our experience of ourselves and others is likely to be very problematic.

Within such an unreflective frame of mind, somatic sensations, feelings, and mental representations that might provide *information* about reality are felt instead to *be* reality. Here—and this is the crucial point—there is only a single perspective on experience, a single view, as if there were no interpretations but only perceptions, no beliefs that are not also facts.

Unavoidably, this complicates the task of regulating emotions and making good use of them. For if every feeling is a pipeline to the truth, we have neither the rationale nor the capacity to put the brakes on what we feel—and, as a rule, unmodulated feelings serve poorly as appraisals of reality and guides to action. When feeling frightened, for example, the circumstances that seem to have evoked our fear are regarded—*unquestioningly*—as realistically dangerous. Of course, such an appraisal only amplifies our fright. Thus embedded in experience we run the risk of crying "fire" in a crowded theater. In instances like this one the internal world trumps external reality, regardless of the "facts of the case."

Conversely, when we're deeply embedded in our experience, it can be hard to draw a boundary that differentiates events on the outside from how they register on the inside: Here, whatever happens to us is felt in some way to be who we are, and that feeling is too compelling to question. Thus, the stance of embeddedness is akin to the mode of *psychic equivalence* (Fonagy et al., 2002), in which our subjective experiences of the internal world and external reality are simply equated. Locked into this way of being, we are trapped in what Melanie Klein called the *paranoid–schizoid position*, where splitting predominates and the self is felt to be the object of experience rather than an initiating, interpreting subject.

Confined to such a stance we have neither the incentive nor the mental space to deliberately think about our experience, both because there is no sense here of the subjective, rather than objective, nature of that experience *and* because unmodulated feeling simply drowns out thought. Moreover, a stance of embeddedness undercuts our capacity to respond *implicitly* to experience—our own or others'—in light of underlying mental states. When this stance is our default option, we're on automatic pilot and, as such, all too constrained by outdated working models and habitually structured patterns of thinking, feeling, and doing.

MENTALIZATION

A mentalizing stance creates the potential for affective, cognitive, and behavioral flexibility, in large part because it allows us to envision multiple perspectives on any given experience, enhancing the likelihood that preexisting models can be updated and habitual patterns "deautomatized." This openness, together with the self-interrogating quality of the mentalizing stance, is instrumental in generating the AAI narratives of secure adults that are coherent rather than rigid or chaotic.

Mentalization makes possible both our conscious efforts to make meaningful sense of our experience and our nonconscious responsiveness to experience on the basis of the feelings, desires, and beliefs that underpin it. In so doing, the mentalizing stance enhances our ability to identify and modulate our affects, so that they do indeed serve their primary function— namely, to help us evaluate our experience of the world and, on the basis of such evaluation, to guide our actions in an adaptive fashion.

Suppose, for example, that we've been gripped by the impulse to withdraw from a close friend who has come to seem newly needy and insecure. With a mentalizing stance we might be moved to wonder about our desire to pull away rather than take our feelings entirely at face value and be driven to act on our impulse—perhaps becoming aware that our friend's apparent vulnerability is an uncomfortable reminder of our own. Aware-

ness of this kind depends on the ability not only to deliberately reflect but also, more fundamentally, to know implicitly that experience has interpretive depth. In other words, experience (such as feeling put off by a friend's insecurity and wanting to withdraw) has meaning that can only be fully grasped in the context of underlying mental states (such as our own anxiety about being vulnerable and a resulting tendency to exaggerate the vulnerability of others).

Attachment theorists have focused attention on various aspects of the mentalizing or reflective stance. Main (1991) emphasizes the capacity for metacognition—thinking about thought—that is grounded in the recognition of an *appearance/reality distinction* (things may be other than they seem), *representational diversity* (different people may have differing perspectives on the same reality), and *representational change* (one's views of reality may well shift at different times and in different contexts). Fonagy, like Main, stresses the capacity to maintain multiple views of a single situation; he also emphasizes what he refers to as *mind reading* (2001) or *mind-mindedness* (1991), asserting that the essence of mentalization is the ability to read or interpret people's behavior and experience in light of underlying mental states. Jeremy Holmes (1996), integrating the contributions of Main and Fonagy, highlights what he calls *narrative* (or *autobiographical*) *competence,* which is the capacity to be conscious of one's psychological life over time, to differentiate between one's own feelings and those of others, and to grasp the representational nature of thinking itself.

MINDFULNESS

To be mindful is to be right here, right now—capable of being fully present in the moment, receptive to whatever experience should arise, yet caught up in no particular aspect of experience. To be mindful is also to be aware of experience without judging or evaluating it. This state of open, alert presence and nonjudgmental awareness is ordinarily cultivated through meditation. The ultimate aim of such practice, however, is not to achieve a mindful state while meditating but, rather, to exercise—and thereby strengthen—the capacity to be mindful as we go about the daily business of living our lives.

A personal illustration: After an astoundingly stressful morning, I walked into a case conference that I've led for many years. Ordinarily I looked forward to meeting with the therapists in this group, but today—feeling cut off, anxious, and irritable—I simply did not want to be there. Going through the motions seemed to be the best I could manage. Too embroiled in my own angry tension to usefully reflect, it occurred to me to try to summon a mindful stance. I took a few deep breaths and resorted to the mental trick of imagining that my *present* experience—in this case, relating

to a number of therapists, many of whom I'd known fondly for years—was also the *last* experience I would ever have. It may sound a bit dark, but this sleight of mind often returns me—sometimes as if in a flash and with a resounding "whomp"—to the often precious here and now. With the benefit of several conscious breaths and my "thought experiment" I landed with both feet in the present moment, feeling isolated no longer and quite content to be exactly where I was. Shifting from a stance of embeddedness to one of mindfulness seemed to "change everything."

The mindful stance toward experience, like the mentalizing stance, confers significant benefits. In the overview, it appears that the practice of mindfulness can help us to modulate difficult feelings, diminish self-imposed suffering, adapt to life's challenges more skillfully, and experience more deeply the joys that life affords us (see Baer, 2003; Lazar, 2005; Martin, 1997; Segal, Williams, & Teasdale, 2002).

Much of the formal research has focused on the impact of meditation on the body, demonstrating that such practice lowers the usual indices of stress: It reduces not only glucocorticoid (stress hormone) levels but also heart rate, oxygen consumption, and so on (Sapolsky, 2004). In addition, while stress undercuts the competence of the immune system, mindfulness meditation has been shown to strengthen it (Davidson et al., 2003). In the same study, novice meditators[1] showed over time a heightening of activation in the left prefrontal region of the cortex that is associated with positive emotion and amygdala inhibition. They also gave first-person reports of diminished anxiety as well as an increase in positive feelings; the greater the leftward tilt in prefrontal activity the more positive, and the less negative, feelings they reported.

Studies of highly trained meditators with many years of practice show even more dramatic results. One subject, a Tibetan Buddhist monk, defied researchers' expectations when he showed no visible evidence of a putatively impossible-to-inhibit startle reflex in response to the sound of a gunshot; the leftward tilt in his prefrontal activity was off the charts (three deviations from the norm). He was also spectacularly adept at reading the microexpressions of the face that, according to Ekman, reveal the emotional reality of other people (Ekman, 2003; Goleman, 2003).[2]

A burgeoning research literature (see Walsh & Shapiro, 2006) suggests that mindfulness and meditation may have some very salutary effects in relation to a wide range of physical conditions (e.g., hypertension, asthma, premenstrual syndrome, and type II diabetes) and psychological problems (e.g., depression, obsessive–compulsive disorder, anxiety, and phobias). There are different ways to explain how mindfulness practice produces these effects. At a physiological level, such practice appears to diminish the autonomic reactivity and sympathetic nervous system hyperarousal that are provoked by amygdala-based emotions such as fear and anger. At a psychological

level, it seems to facilitate calmness, self-knowledge, and self-acceptance, as well as the deautomatization of habitual patterns of thinking and feeling. And as I've proposed, it may contribute over time to the creation (or consolidation) of an internalized secure base. Finally, there is growing evidence to suggest that mindfulness enhances empathy (Morgan & Morgan, 2005)—a finding consistent with the conclusion that meditation strengthens mentalizing (Allen & Fonagy, 2002). Clearly, mindfulness has an important role to play in psychotherapy.

FROM EMBEDDEDNESS TO MENTALIZING

All of our patients are embedded in experience some of the time and some of our patients are embedded in experience all of the time. The latter are prisoners of the moment, trapped by internal and external circumstances that feel intractably "real." Like infants and young children, though for very different reasons, these patients (who often have borderline level ego strength, PTSD, and/or major depression) are unable to maintain *multiple* views of any given experience. Their one-dimensional perspective leaves no mental space for interpretation; consequently, they have enormous trouble making sense of their own experience or that of others on the basis of mental states. Locked into such a stance, moreover, they have little capacity to identify, modulate, and effectively express the feelings evoked by experience, especially painful experience.

Most of our patients (and most therapists) find themselves similarly embedded in experience at times, but more rarely and usually only in the face of significant distress. Thus for most of us what I'm calling embeddedness is context dependent, such that there are some events, some relationships, and some events *in* relationships that leave us feeling completely swallowed up. Swamped by overwhelming emotion, we can feel utterly unable in such contexts to get our head above water, so as to stand outside the experience and think about it with some part of ourselves.

Whether in childhood or psychotherapy, the movement from a rigidly embedded stance to the flexibility of a mentalizing and reflective one usually occurs in the setting of close relationships. Roughly the same ingredients of these relationships that promote security of attachment also foster the capacity for mentalizing. As discussed in Chapter 4, the bridge from embeddedness to mentalizing is built on a foundation of affect regulation, recognition of intentionality, and symbolic play.

In healthy enough development the mentalizing stance of the young child is coaxed into being through the sensitive responsiveness of her caregiver. Such responsiveness is itself entirely dependent on the caregiver's ability to mentalize—that is, to interpret the child's largely implicit, nonverbal

cues as communications about mental states. Much the same can be said of psychotherapy in which our own empathic attunement to the patient's communication arises largely out of our capacity to mentalize. Indeed it is mainly in the context of an intersubjective relationship of increasingly secure attachment—supported by the therapist's essential focus on the non-verbal dimension that is enacted, evoked, or embodied—that the mentalizing therapist activates the patient's own mentalizing potential.

Healthier patients and their therapists may well be able to reflect quite consistently on their mental states together until one partner or the other stumbles into experience that is emotionally overwhelming. When mentalizing is thus derailed (say, in the course of a disturbing enactment) or when the potential for mentalizing has not yet been kindled, then the patient—and sometimes the therapist—can be caught up in the embedded, one-dimensional mode of psychic equivalence in which the mind and the world are conflated. It is worth taking a look at how children make this equation between internal states and external reality—because we so regularly see variations on the theme with adult patients in an embedded stance.

In a well-known experiment (Gopnik & Astington, 1988) children between the ages of three and six were shown a tube of M & Ms and asked what they thought was inside it. All replied, "M & Ms" and presumably all were disappointed when shown that the tube actually held nothing but a pencil. Asked a moment later to predict how a friend seeing the M & Ms container would answer the same question, most responded, as if it were entirely obvious: "A pencil." More striking still, when asked to recall what they themselves had thought was in the M & Ms tube when they were first shown it, most had the same answer: "A pencil."

This "false-belief" test clearly demonstrates the difficulty children have (particularly before the age of four or five) keeping in mind more than one view of experience. In the language of metacognition they have, at best, a tenuous understanding of representational diversity and change: That is, they can imagine neither that their friend might have a different perspective than they do nor that their own perspective might have changed. In this study as in life, young children—and adults embedded in experience—can have extraordinary difficulty keeping the internal world from being equated with, and in some sense nullified by, the external reality.

But, of course, psychic equivalence works both ways. A colleague told me that, as she was about to give her nearly two-year-old son a bath, he cried out in protest, furious to be put in the tub against his will. Apparently gripped by rage, he bit her, and then cried out once again, "Momma *bited* me!" Here the internal world—of anger, then fear—trumped the external reality such that they became one.

One of the perils psychic equivalence drags in its wake is the all-too-easy projection of what is felt inside (fury, terror) onto the outside, creating

in the process the experience of a very dangerous world. Adult patients embedded in their experience, such as those we might describe as borderline, are vulnerable to exactly this sort of danger. They equate feelings with reality and react as though threatened when their own feelings are projected onto others: feeling angry, for example, but also ashamed in response to the therapist's misattunement, they may well decide that the therapist is ill-intentioned, and perhaps ill-equipped to be helpful.

Largely it is danger of this kind that propels both children and adults into the refuge of what Fonagy calls the *pretend* mode. When we turn away from physical reality to dwell in the pretend realm—when we get lost in play or fantasy—we *decouple* the inner and outer worlds rather than equating them, thus liberating ourselves through imagination from the oppression of mental states that feel all too real. If, for children and adults alike, experience in the embedded stance of psychic equivalence simply is what it is—sometimes frighteningly so—experience in the mode of pretense is what we *want* it to be.

To make this more vivid: The other morning, my four-year-old woke me up, asking that I tie a knot in the towel he wore like a cape around his shoulders. After complying, I committed the *faux pas* of inquiring whether he was still my son or had now become Superman. "Dad*dy!*" he complained, the accent on the second syllable a clear note of reproach. Then tearing out of the room he cried, "Neither, I'm Batman!" A little later, descending the stairs, I picked up his "cape" off the landing. Ever the psychologist apparently, I couldn't resist asking him over breakfast, "Are you my son now or are you Batman?" With a broad smile he answered, "I'm Batman. *Sometimes I wear a costume to be Batman.*"

Symbolization in the pretend mode represents a momentous developmental advance beyond embeddedness or psychic equivalence. When symbolizing, we make one thing stand for (or refer to) another, while recognizing that the symbol and what it symbolizes are two separate entities. Putting on the towel (symbol) that stands for Batman's cape (the symbolized) allowed my son to "be" Batman without actually believing that he *is* Batman—in other words, he is able in symbolic play to have two perspectives on the same experience and to grasp the appearance/reality distinction. In the mode of pretend, we have the opportunity to exercise a rudimentary version of three components of mentalizing—we can symbolize, maintain multiple perspectives, and know the difference between appearance and reality. In a sense, we can mentalize just so long as we're pretending.

Fonagy, too, tells a Batman story about his four-year-old son (Allen & Fonagy, 2002), recounting that on one of his trips to a conference abroad he went to great lengths to fulfill the boy's request for a Batman costume. When Fonagy brought it home, his son put it on, and took one terrified look at him-

self in the mirror, before bursting into tears and insisting that the costume immediately be put away. Moments later, securing an old skirt of his mother's to wear round his shoulders, he happily pretended to be Batman.

In the mode of pretense, experience can be what you want it to be—but only as long as the wolves of reality are kept sufficiently distant from the door. When Fonagy's son saw an image of himself in the overly realistic costume, he looked *too* much like Batman and felt that he *was* Batman. The pretend mode—with its security-enhancing potentials for symbolization, the appearance/reality distinction, and the taking of multiple perspectives—collapsed into psychic equivalence.

Of course, the same kind of collapse can occur in therapy. Recently, for example, I became aware over the course of several sessions that a woman patient with whom I had long enjoyed a good working relationship now seemed unusually anxious with me. Exploring her anxiety revealed that she had been troubled by questions about the nature of my feelings for her—and my "boundaries"—ever since a session in which I had not only been complimentary about her appearance but also had touched her shoulder as she left my office. This episode (about which more will follow) illustrates the fragility of the (protectively) "pretend" or "as if" quality of the therapeutic relationship.

In the face of a therapist's misattunement and a patient's vulnerability, the "play space" of therapy can quickly become all too frighteningly real, and along with the collapse into embeddedness can come the disruption of affect regulation. For when internal experience seems suddenly no different than external reality (when, for example, our fear is felt to be unquestioningly reality based), we may well feel overwhelmed, as if confronting alone a dangerous, no-exit situation.

The tales of two four-year-olds and one adult in therapy are intended to illustrate how the mode of pretend takes us part way—but only part way—from embeddedness to mentalizing. While psychic equivalence is too real, pretense is simply not real enough and, as such, is comparatively fragile. Yet it's a vital waystation, because the pretend mode affords us real access to mentalizing abilities that are simply out of reach so long as we're embedded in experience.

Children perform at a much higher level on the kind of false-belief test described earlier if the task is framed as pretense. In contrast to the "real version" of the task that challenged the capacities of many four-year-olds, the pretend variant proved a breeze for almost every three-year-old (Gopnik & Slaughter, 1991). As the influential developmentalist Lev Vygotsky put it, "In play the child is always above his average age, above his daily behavior; in play it is as though he were a head taller than himself" (cited in Fonagy et al., 2002, p. 261). While pretending, the child can exercise and strengthen important mentalizing skills.

The same is true of the patient in psychotherapy. The therapist who maintains the "frame" of the treatment—that is, the boundaries—creates a kind of transitional space in which there can develop a therapeutic relationship that is pretend as well as real. This duality is probably what Freud (1914/1924b) had in mind when he spoke of transference as an "intermediary realm between illness and real life" into which the patient's dissociated impulses could be admitted "as to a playground" (p. 374). Because the stakes here are not quite as high as they might be in another important and intimate relationship, the patient can afford to risk more, very much like the child at play. The pretend aspects of psychotherapy—along with the therapeutic relationship as a secure base—provide a degree of freedom and safety that may allow the patient more freely to imagine, think, and feel.

Yet imagining cannot take us all the way to mentalizing because the associated sense of freedom and possibility so easily evaporates—along with the ability to regulate affects—once pretense is confronted with reality. Think of Fonagy's son and the fear he felt when confronted with the all too real image of himself as Batman. Or think of patients in a narcissistic rage who "lose it" when their vitally sustaining but vulnerable fantasies about themselves are challenged by external realities—such as others' responses to them that are out of keeping with their own needs.

Whether in childhood or psychotherapy, we make it all the way from embeddedness to mentalizing only when given opportunities to integrate the "nonmentalizing reality-oriented" mode of psychic equivalence with the "mentalizing nonreality-connected" mode of pretend (Fonagy et al., 2002, p. 266). Such integration frees the mind from the tyranny of brute facts (including, especially, mental states *felt* to be facts) but without leaving factual reality behind.

Neither equating the mind with the world nor dissociating the mind from the world, this synthesis of "groundedness" and imagination allows us to respond to experience in light of the *relationship* between internal states and external realities. Think of it this way: When we are embedded in experience, that experience is "known" to be real, and therefore we feel compelled to act; when we are pretending, experience is known to be unreal, so no real action is necessary. When we are mentalizing, however, we can ask ourselves just how real or unreal our present sense of our experience actually is. We can wonder, in other words, just how our internal state currently relates to the external reality—and then, with greater freedom and more reliable information, we can choose how (or if) to act.

The ability to wonder in this way results from a *benign circle* involving experiences of secure attachment that foster, in turn, affect regulation, optimal arousal, and mentalizing (Allen & Fonagy, 2002). In this synergistic process, the ongoing relationship with a sensitively responsive caregiver (or empathically attuned therapist) provides the experience, and eventually the

expectation, that affects can be regulated and arousal maintained within the "window of tolerance" (Siegel, 1999). The resulting sense of a secure base makes it possible for the child (or patient) to explore: to look into the face, the mind, and the heart of the caregiver (or therapist) and to find there a reflection of himself as an "intentional being" whose behavior makes sense in light of the feelings, wishes, and beliefs that are its context.

When behavior, especially nonverbal behavior, is responded to in this way—in light, that is, of underlying mental states—it generates in the child (or patient) a gradually heightening awareness of multiple levels of experience and multiple perspectives on experience. It engenders, in other words, a mentalizing stance toward experience. In turn, the capacity to mentalize fosters a growing ability both to regulate affects and to experience the attachment relationship as a secure base. This is the benign circle that makes possible psychological growth, integration, and the emergence of an *internalized* secure base, whether in childhood or psychotherapy.

STRENGTHENING THE REFLECTIVE SELF
AND FOSTERING INTEGRATION IN PSYCHOTHERAPY

Main's work on metacognition and Fonagy's on mentalizing strongly suggest that the child needs attachment relationships not only for the protection and felt security they afford but also to provide the intersubjective context in which his reflective capacities can develop. The first stage in this process involves affect-regulating interactions with the attachment figure that teach the child about feelings. Because emotion is at the core of the developing self, interactions like these that *effectively* regulate affects make possible the integration (rather than dissociation) of the child's many emotional experiences and, thus, the child's growing sense of a coherent self.

Like the developing child, a patient in the quintessentially intersubjective context of psychotherapy has the opportunity to learn (or be reminded) that feelings can be recognized, shared with others, reflected upon, and potentially altered. In the model of psychotherapy as transformation through relationship, the secure base and the therapist's focus on nonverbal experience permit the patient's dissociated feelings to surface and be recognized. And once such disowned feelings emerge and are felt, they have the potential to change—that is, to be accepted (bitter anger about the past may soften into regret) and/or transformed (needs once disavowed may be "owned" and gratified). The relationship that makes room for emotions previously denied, and the therapist who helps the patient to bear and understand them, also make their integration more feasible.

But the patient in psychotherapy, like the young child, may have an

impossible time knowing his internal states—or even knowing that he *has* internal states that can be known—until these are recognized by another. Let's take a look now at how the other—parent or therapist—can make the knowing, naming, and reflecting on such unrecognized internal states possible.

I'll focus first on this process as it unfolds in childhood, while making bridges to psychotherapy along the way. Then I'll present some clinical material that illustrates how what we know about the developing child—her need for a mentalizing other to help regulate her feelings, her use of symbolic play and language in moving from embeddedness to mentalizing—can illuminate the integrative process of psychotherapy.

As you will recall, Fonagy and his colleagues observe that infants and young children initially learn about their feelings through experiences of mirroring that are both contingent and "marked." A child in distress, for example, may be soothed when his mother is able to resonate with, reflect upon, and accurately mirror his internal state back to him—but with enough of a difference so that *her* display of feeling is "marked" as a response to *his* internal state rather than an expression of her own. Moreover, for such mirroring to foster the child's ability to regulate as well as recognize his affects, it must be accompanied by an attitude or action suggesting that the distress can be coped with—certainly by the caregiver, but also potentially by her child.

Another episode from my personal archive will illustrate how this process can work. When my daughter was just shy of 18 months, I happened to be the parent who woke in the middle of the night to her frantic cries of "Mommy! Mommy!" When from her crib she saw *me* opening the door to her room, she yelled furiously, "Bad Daddy! I hate you! Get Mommy!" This was hardly the reception I hoped for at three in the morning and I felt myself growing tense. Trying to be heard over her tearful screams I told her—no doubt with quite an edge—that Mommy was sleeping and that I was not going to wake her. At the side of my daughter's crib, however, I found myself softening as I suddenly understood (or rather *felt*) the irrefutable logic of her behavior: Clearly she believed that if she were angry and loud enough, then she would get me to get her mother. All this went through me in an instant, but I can see in retrospect that it enabled me not only to calm myself, but also (unthinkingly) to mirror her rage, with an exaggerated "mean face" and a little accompanying growl to mark my show of feeling as "pretend," and then to segue from the growl into a long and sympathetic "awwnhhh" as if to reflect the needy disappointment beneath her anger. Then I put the mime into words telling her that, of course, she was angry because she so wanted mommy and daddy wouldn't go get her. Whereupon I heard her, through her tears, trying to say something I couldn't initially make out. When I did, it was: "Daddy, help me feel better." Fol-

lowing which we shared an emotional hug and a song, before I put her down in her crib for the night.

While I couldn't interview my daughter to get her take on this interaction, I'd like to believe that it was one that helped her to know her feelings and to begin to regulate them. How? By seeing herself as I saw her—in other words, by seeing herself in the mirror of my mentalizing responses to her as an intentional being whose behavior expressed feelings and wishes that were knowable, namable, sharable, and *changeable*.

Several mutually reinforcing aspects of the interaction are important to highlight because they bear directly on our work with patients. First, it was only once I managed to find a reflective stance and so succeeded in regulating my *own* feelings that I was able to grasp and mirror back to her what *she* was feeling. Second, it was only when I understood her affects in light of her intentions that I was able to make sense of them. And third, it was precisely this "mentalizing" of her emotional experience that allowed me to get a grip on my own, so as to be able to be of help to her.

To activate a similar process in psychotherapy, we must be able not only to respond emotionally to the patient but also to reflect on emotion—our own and the patient's—so that rather than simply being gripped by feelings we can try to make sense of them. (Needless to say, this sort of responsiveness can, at times, be very difficult to summon, and it usually requires that therapists themselves have considerable experience as patients.)

More of the symmetry between the activities of the mentalizing clinician and the mentalizing parent will become apparent as I review what is currently understood about how children come to know, regulate, and integrate their emotions. Critically, this kind of development can only occur in the context of a relationship with an attuned other. Until children experience such a relationship, they may not "know" what they feel but only that they feel it (Coates, 1998). In order to turn their "raw feelings into symbols" (Holmes, 2001), children need intersubjective, affect-regulating interactions in which they can come to know themselves in the process of being known by another. Precisely the same can be said of patients in psychotherapy. For children and patients alike, it is their interaction with an attuned and sensitively responsive other that makes possible the development of a reflective self.

The experience of contingent and "marked" mirroring—and emotional attunement more generally—allows children to develop *representations* of their affects through associating them with the initially (mainly) nonverbal and eventually verbal responses of the attachment figure. First at the nonverbal level, the attuned parent "names" the child's feelings through bodily behaviors—facial expressions, tone of voice, gestures, and the like—that communicate an empathic recognition of the child's inner experience. Thus the first representations of the child's internal states are found in the

mirror of the mother's responses. Winnicott (1971a) probably had this in mind when he wrote: "What does the baby see when he or she looks at the mother's face? The baby sees himself or herself. For the mother is looking at the baby and what she looks like depends on what she sees there" (p. 112).

Of course, parents also draw on spoken language to help their children to represent feelings. Using words such as "sad" or "angry" to label their child's affects, parents generate an emotional lexicon that becomes more serviceable as the child hears others using these words to describe affects (a crying friend is said to be sad) and as she begins to do the same (finding her understanding of the words confirmed or corrected). A similar version of these nonverbal and verbal processes unfolds in the patient's relationship with the therapist, allowing emotions to be felt and then to be represented in increasingly nuanced and self-knowledgeable ways.

Critically, feelings (and other mental states) that can be represented—especially by words—are more easily identified, shared, reflected on, and modulated. Hence the enormous significance in childhood *and* psychotherapy of affect-regulating relationships in which this ability to be articulate about feelings can develop. As Fonagy puts it, "Language is the representational medium *par excellence* for mentalizing explicitly" (Allen & Fonagy, 2002, p. 29). Emotion is the target of much, if not most, of this explicit mentalizing. The talk in the "talking cure" thus has the potential to strengthen the patient's ability to regulate and integrate her emotions. (For this potential to be realized these emotions must come alive in the here and now of the therapeutic relationship. Otherwise the talk is probably only talk.)

Beyond their role in these affect-regulating, affect-representing interactions, parents strengthen the child's mentalizing when they observe, participate in, or comment on the child's symbolic play. Here the parent's verbal and nonverbal responses to the child's "pretend" experience provide an additional perspective—an adult perspective—that helps link the inner world of imagination to the outer world with all its constraints and possibilities. Similarly in child psychotherapy, the clinician implicitly or explicitly offers views of the child's play that both resonate with and extend the child's own views.

In the treatment of adults, we do something very similar when we offer our patients empathy and interpretation—in response, of course, not to their play but, rather, to their experience of the relationship we share. The transference–countertransference situation always has elements of "pretend" as well as actuality that help make room for a wide range of emotional experiences and states of mind, including some that have been defensively excluded from the patient's ordinary sense of herself. The paradox of pretend is that by virtue of our relationship with the patient being

less real it can potentially be more real—emotionally deeper, more authentic, and more inclusive.

When we help to access, illuminate, and bridge the patient's various emotions, states of mind, and levels of experience (explicit and implicit, symbolic and nonsymbolic) we are strengthening the patient's capacities both for affect regulation and for mentalizing. In the process, we facilitate the integration of experiences the patient has previously felt the need to dissociate or disown. And in so doing, we contribute to what has been called "the pinnacle of explicit mentalizing, namely, the ability to make sense of oneself and others in terms of a coherent autobiographical and biographical narrative" (Allen & Fonagy, 2002, p. 29).

STRENGTHENING THE REFLECTIVE SELF: AN ILLUSTRATION OF THE CLINICAL PROCESS

"Rebecca" is the patient I mentioned previously (p. 142) who became anxious when I complimented her on her appearance and, later, touched her shoulder lightly as she left my office. In reviewing how the two of us dealt with the emotional fallout from that very disturbing encounter, I hope to convey how the benign circle of attachment, affect regulation, and mentalizing actually operates in psychotherapy.

More specifically, I will be clarifying how I think about and conduct myself in relation to four continuously interweaving and overlapping facets of clinical work. First is the patient's shifting stance toward experience, which determines, to some extent, the nature of my clinical choices in each session. Next is my sustained focus on, and use of, the nonverbal domain—the evoked, enacted, and embodied—to surface the patient's implicit and dissociated experience in the immediacy of the here and now. Then there is making the implicit explicit: Recognizing and naming her experience in the moment makes room for it and, as such, fosters its preliminary integration. Finally, to further integration, there are my efforts in dialogue with the patient to make sense of her experience—that is, to connect its disparate elements so as to give this experience a meaningful context in terms of her remembered past, lived present, and anticipated future. The sum of these efforts involves what the psychoanalyst Roy Schafer (1992) calls "retelling a life." When all goes well enough, this process generates a coherent life story or narrative that can anchor and deepen both the patient's sense of wholeness and her capacity to love.

Bear with me briefly while I set the stage. Rebecca is a physician in her early 30s who sought psychotherapy feeling enormous insecurity in the wake of her divorce. Though she was extremely bright, vivacious, and appealing, she couldn't imagine that anyone would be interested in her. Super-

ficially confident, she was racked intermittently by a nameless misery that left her overwhelmed and sometimes sobbing. She was confused by her emotions and vulnerable to being blindsided by them. Consequently she felt she stood on a shaky foundation.

Little by little, we came to recognize together how hard it was for her to experience the world from *inside* herself and to feel like the author of her own life; instead, she customarily saw herself as if through the eyes of others and lived mainly in relation to others' expectations and needs. We gradually began to understand that her difficulty in knowing her own mind had developed out of the necessity in childhood to devote her primary attention to the mind of her mother.

Unpredictably available, and too often in a rage, this formidable and charming woman was someone whose love Rebecca had deeply craved and whose disapproval was terrifying. To adapt, she had toed the line, functioned as a peacemaker, and excelled in ways that mattered to her mother. Yet for all her achievements and her compliance, she had nonetheless often felt that to her mother she was, at best, secondary and, at worst, burdensome.

On top of her feelings of longing and intimidation in relation to her mother, Rebecca felt unseen by her father, whose attention she believed had been captured and monopolized by her older sister. Lacking the genuine security of authentic connection, she had felt lonely in her family and unsupported, uncertain of her desires and inhibited in the assertion of her needs.

Keep in mind that this narrative emerged over the course of a couple of years of therapy and reflects an awareness that Rebecca could not have articulated when our relationship began. This relationship and the understanding it fostered slowly made it possible for her to know her needs and to assert them, as if feeling that—perhaps—she could now claim for herself the right to a life of her own.

Several years into treatment, Rebecca married again, this time very happily to a man who, by her own account, was unconditionally loving and supportive. She had begun to feel troubled about the sexual dimension of their relationship, however: Specifically, she was put off that he seemed always to be coming on to her, while she could only sporadically connect with her own desire. In addition, she was disturbed and puzzled whenever she became aware of her emotional withdrawal after having experienced a period of closeness with her husband.

The Shifting Stance toward Experience

For many weeks, Rebecca said nothing at all about how shaken she had been by my misattuned touch. She apparently believed unquestioningly that she couldn't safely say a word about how my behavior had unnerved her.

This, in spite of several years of apparently open exchanges between us that might have raised at least the possibility of an additional perspective—in particular, that our relationship might be safe enough that she could tell me she felt unsafe. Clearly Rebecca could find herself at times embedded in her experience, in this case her very troubling experience of the relationship between us.

At other times, Rebecca could see that her therapy had a partially "pretend" quality: Our relationship was, as she put it, "a real one that was also artificial." While her sense of this relationship as a secure base was real enough, it was also the relationship's "artificiality" that made it possible for her to experience some of the same freedom that permits a child at play to mentalize. In the protected sphere of pretend, Rebecca could allow herself a wider range of feelings, thoughts, and impulses in our sessions than she could outside them—and she could reflect on these mental states rather than simply experiencing them.

Yet the safe psychological space created in the pretend mode could collapse when contradicted by an experience too out of keeping with the pretense. As long as she had seen me garbed only in the costume of the good father, so to speak, the threat I represented—the threat of sexuality or closeness—could be relegated to the periphery. But when I complimented and touched her, the reassuring pretense gave way to a sense of danger that seemed all too real.

Rebecca attempted over a number of sessions to restore and maintain the pretense that she felt entirely safe with me. But as so often happens in interactions like these, her nonverbal communication revealed what she felt too unsafe either to disclose to me or to fully acknowledge to herself. This revelation was the first step in enabling her to consider with me the meaning of what had occurred between us. Over a sequence of several subsequent sessions, Rebecca's stance toward her experience shifted between embeddedness and pretend—and gradually moved in the direction of mentalization.

The Nonverbal Route to Implicit/Dissociated Experience

The first session of the sequence began with a longish silence broken by Rebecca's remarking a bit nervously that she has nothing much on her mind, nothing special to talk about.

> When I ask how that is for her, she answers that it makes her uncomfortable. "How so?" I inquire. To which she replies, "Then we'd just be looking at each other." "And if we were looking at each other?" "I don't know. It just makes me uncomfortable. You know?"
> She quickly segues into an account of two parallel experiences—

the first with a woman friend whom she keeps at arm's length, without quite knowing why, the second with her husband. They had just gotten back from a romantic weekend away: great sex the first night, and then when he was seductive in the morning she pushed him away. She doesn't know why. There could have been a fight then, but they steered clear of it and the rest of the weekend went all right—though she says she can't stop trashing the two of them because they did nothing but lie around, watch videos, go out to eat, and make love. Hearing this, I apparently have a look about me that says to her something like: "Mmm, that sounds nice!" She fixes her eyes on me then, saying, "You and my friend obviously think the same way about this kind of thing. I don't know what's wrong with me that I can't appreciate it. You know?"

And now there's another silence.

Tuning in to the music here rather than the words—that is, to the non-verbal dimension of our interaction—I'm aware of feeling inside myself a tremor of anxiety that may mirror hers. I also sense a bit of annoyance as I notice (not for the first time) her repetition of the phrase "You know?" delivered quite pointedly and with a slightly frowning, quizzical expression on her face. I'm aware, too, of a different kind of "you know" that has come to punctuate her speech like a nervous tic in recent weeks, perhaps betraying her discomfort. But the more pointed "You know?" seems to carry the implication that as her therapist I don't know, don't understand, and perhaps can't be trusted to do either as previously I could. Now there gels in my mind the overdue recognition that our relationship in the past few weeks (or might it be longer?) has had a vaguely uncomfortable and superficial feel, quite at odds with the ease and depth I usually associate with our interactions. Guessing that my experience is related to hers, and hoping to reach beyond the words to the implicit, as yet unverbalized, level of the present interaction, I wonder aloud what she's feeling now, in the silence.

She tells me she's that she's uncomfortable just as she was earlier, and that there's something about our silently looking at each other that makes her a little anxious. I tentatively share my sense that she may actually have been feeling quite uneasy here for some time, not just in this session, but perhaps for several weeks, and maybe more.

She half sighs, half groans in response and looks away. I ask her, "What's the sigh, or is it a groan?" She says she thinks she knows what's happened, but she's not sure she can talk about it. After saying in a softer tone, "I can see how hard this is for you," I ask if she knows what might be making it so difficult for her to talk to me about something that's so clearly troubling her.

What emerges is her worry that I'll be devastated by what she has to say, though she thinks I've probably heard these kinds of things be-

fore. Eventually she lets me know of the "confusion and upset" that were triggered perhaps a month earlier when I complimented her and touched her on the shoulder. Up to that point, in all the time she'd worked with me, she says, I had never before touched her. When I did, it seemed suddenly to call everything about our relationship into question. Saying this, her eyes fill with tears.

The focus on nonverbal (or paraverbal) signals in the session—my anxiety and annoyance, my sense of the flatness of the preceding sessions, Rebecca's repeated "You know?" with the accompanying body language, and her sigh—were all routes to vital and troubling, but implicit and perhaps dissociated, experience. All my subsequent interventions in this hour were aimed at making as much room for that experience as possible. In so doing, I communicated implicitly and explicitly that her experience here was a priority for me. This openness to, and genuine interest in, her emotions and thoughts, her anger and suspicion, seemed to enable her to feel safe enough with me to delve into her experience more deeply.

Making the Implicit Explicit

Surfacing implicit experience in psychotherapy is crucial if we are to accommodate what our patients may have long felt the need to exclude from their relationships, their sense of themselves, or both. Sometimes the accessing of such disowned or dissociated experience is not only necessary but also sufficient—in and of itself—to effect therapeutic change. More often, I suspect, it is necessary in addition to explicate the implicit by putting the experience into words.

> Vaguely recalling the moment that had so unsettled Rebecca, I could have disclosed my sense that I had probably been feeling close to, and concerned for, her then—and that my gesture as well as my earlier compliment had probably arisen from my (unconscious) desire to actively convey that I was with her. However, I felt that such a disclosure would have been a premature encroachment upon her experience. So instead, wishing to make space for that experience, but also to reassure her (and thus perhaps protect both of us from her fears about me), I let her know that I'm actually feeling relieved to be talking now about something that's clearly been so disturbing to her and so difficult for her to share with me. I also tell her that one of the signals to me of her distress was the repetitive "you know" that hadn't previously been part of her speech pattern, at least not that I'd noticed—but that I haven't heard her say "you know" since she told me how I had upset her.
>
> Hearing these words, she begins to sob. As she settles, I ask if she can tell me what her tears are about. She says it's sadness: sadness that she has to be so held back, that she so needs for things not to be too in-

timate here and that, as we talk, it feels more intimate, and that troubles her: "I have to keep therapy compartmentalized. I need to keep you at arm's length. I know therapy is artificial, it's not quite real. It is and it isn't. But then with your compliments and your touching me it just got too confusingly real."

"And that made you enormously uneasy."

"Yes it did. I didn't know if we were going to be able to continue. Like suddenly I didn't know what your intentions were, or what kind of relationship we actually had."

"And making it even worse, I think, was your feeling unsafe to talk about what I had done and how it had affected you."

What is being named here, of course, is her implicit experience in relation to me of feeling threatened and mistrustful. Her difficulty being explicit—even now—about the specific danger I represented is a measure of how endangered she felt. Not until the next session could we put words to this danger and how she had dealt with it.

Rebecca begins the hour with a kind of joke—"Are we OK with each other now?"—spoken with a cocked head and back-and-forth gesture of the hands at chest level, palms facing inward. I laugh with her, but then suggest that her humor probably reflects her sense that the conversation we began last time is unfinished. She says it was very disturbing then, and still is today, to be talking in such a way that I might think she's impugning my integrity.

I say, "So for you to tell me I was being seductive would have been to impugn my integrity?"

"Something like that. How could I say you were coming on to me without calling your integrity into question? And I didn't know if you were. It felt that way, but I couldn't tell. I mean, at some level I knew you weren't, you've helped me in a million ways and never given me reason to doubt your concern for me. But then you'd never touched me before, so . . . I just tried to pretend that it hadn't happened or that it didn't matter to me."

"But of course it did matter—so much so that you weren't sure you were going to be able to continue with me. And you couldn't say a word about it."

Deeper levels of Rebecca's implicit mistrust and fear are gradually being made explicit—first, the suspicion that my compliment and my touch had an exploitive intent; and second, the doubt that I could hear her suspicion without becoming impossibly defensive.

I tell her there's something I don't fully understand: "If you'd been able to say you were worried that I was coming on to you—and I actually

was coming on to you—wouldn't that simply be taking care of your-self rather than impugning my integrity? It would be as if I'd been caught red-handed." "Of course it would," she answers. "But all that's assuming you would be honest." A little caught off guard at the extent of her mistrust, I say, "And that seems to be a very hard assumption for you to make . . . I guess we're both seeing how difficult it is for you to trust me."

A little later I make some of my own experience explicit when she asks me why I'm so determined to keep discussing all this: Is it because I think there's something valuable to be mined here, something for her to learn? Or is it because I'm concerned that I've done something wrong and want to get clearer about that?

I begin by saying I believe there's a great deal of importance to what we're exploring together. Then I add that I'm always more than open to learning about my part in what goes on between us. Virtually in midsentence, however, I have the sense that my words feel somehow canned and inauthentic and fit poorly with what the moment between us seems to call for.

So I take what feels like a "truer" tack: "I have no doubt that I would be self-critical if I felt that what's gone on here had damaged our relationship in some irremediable way or if I felt that I'd acted out some unconscious and destructive impulse. But the fact is, I don't. At this point I can't remember all the details of what occurred, but I do recall feeling close to you as the session ended and given that you seemed to be going through something that was very difficult for you, I suspect I was trying—pretty clumsily as it turned out—but trying, in any case, to communicate that I was with you."

Rebecca replies that it's a huge relief to be hearing me saying all this. "How so?" I ask. "It just gives me more room to think about my side of what's been going on here." She's quiet for a few moments be-fore she asks in a tone of anguish and pleading, "Why should all this be so incredibly threatening to me?" And then she begins to struggle to answer her own question.

Rebecca's response here is in keeping with my sense that the therapist's deliberate self-disclosure can sometimes help the patient to feel less embedded in her own emotional reality. Perhaps in articulating a different viewpoint, the therapist opens the patient to considering more than one perspective on her experience—a hallmark of mentalizing.

Beyond the nonverbal behavior that signals our indispensable reso-nance and attunement, patients like Rebecca—in order to feel that we are with them and that they are understood—almost always need contingent responses that are conveyed in spoken language. When patients can read our mind in our words as well as in our face, they are helped to experience their relationship with us as one that can accommodate what they may pre-viously have felt the need to dissociate.

When we use language to name the unnamed, w/
bear and communicate their own unbearable feelings
teractive regulation of our patients' distress streng*
tolerance and their experience of the therapeutic *
base. As we are about to see, such interactive r*
mentalizing.

Making Sense of Experience: Interpretation, Mentalizing, and Narrative

Though the reality of clinical work is rarely optimal, let me sketch for illus-
trative purposes an optimally therapeutic version of the process I've been
describing. Having created both a secure base and a transitional space in
which the patient can have experiences with us that feel neither as if they
are "only transference" nor as if they are simply "real"—Freud (1914/
1924b) called it an "intermediate realm" (p. 374)—we read nonverbal signals, inside ourselves and from the patient, in order to access in the here
and now the patient's implicit experience. (Paraphrasing Damasio, we are
helping the patient to connect with the *feeling* of what is happening—with
the emotional and bodily dimensions of that experience.) Having touched
the perceptible edge of the patient's internal working model or implicit narrative, we try to make the implicit explicit. Only then do we finally attempt
with the patient to reflect on that experience in order to make sense of it.

The theoretical sequence I've sketched makes possible a process
through which experience that was previously *only* felt—or not felt at all—
can be lived out in the setting of a relationship in which that experience can
be understood and given a new context. Implicit and explicit experience
that is safely shared is changed. This is *representational redescription*
(Karmiloff-Smith, 1992), whereby the functional, influential past (though
not, of course, the historical past) is altered, making available new possibilities in the present (Stern, 2004). Ultimately our aim is to enable our
patients to generate a coherent narrative about their life that reflects their
experience of a coherent self. This was my aim with Rebecca and interpretation was an important part of realizing that aim.

> When Rebecca plaintively asked why my touch had so threatened her,
> she was clearly no longer embedded in her experience or involved in a
> pretend exploration decoupled from reality: "I know I like men to be
> attracted to me, but it's as if I just want to be seen and not touched. I
> don't want anyone to get too close. So whenever someone comes on to
> me I usually just turn the whole thing off. I guess I'm talking about the
> past, but even now with my husband I just immediately withdraw. So
> was something like that going on with you? That must have been part
> of it, that automatic pulling back when someone comes on to me. But
> it feels like there's something missing here, something I'm not getting
> to."

To which I respond with the following interpretation: "I think I know what that something might be. I suspect that when I complimented you and touched your shoulder and you felt disturbed, you didn't quite know why. You explained it to yourself by deciding that I was being seductive, not that I was feeling close to you or supportive. And the thought that I was coming on to you pretty much undid any sense of closeness here between us, closeness that I think you both value and fear."

She says, "I think that's right, it feels right" and brings up instances of withdrawing when she gets signals that someone is interested in being close to her, be it a close woman friend or her husband. Responses like these have puzzled her, though she says that growing up she got to be very good at being alone. Here she becomes tearful and—when I ask what's going on inside her—says that she just got a very moving image in her mind of being a boxer and having me, and her husband, and her woman friend "in her corner, on her side."

In the next and final session I'll draw from, Rebecca says that our last conversation opened her heart, but that it didn't stay open. She was making love with her husband on the weekend, feeling an extraordinary intimacy, as if they were on the verge of recommitting to one another. And then she "just shut down, closed up, and dried up." She felt herself doing so almost as if deliberately. Several days later, she was feeling upset, and she told him she just wanted to sit on the couch by herself and read—as a way of preempting what she imagined might be a sexual overture from him.

Some part of her, she says, wants to trust and be close to him and be comforted, but there's another part that won't let her: "It's like there's this little girl inside me who's angry and hurt and spiteful and just wants to go off and be by herself. I've actually found myself thinking about just ending it with my husband and getting a place alone and making it exactly like I want it to be, without having to check whether this painting or that weaving can go over the fireplace or not. That little girl is just so angry. It's like there's this part of me that wants to open up and she just won't let me."

I say, "I can see why she's angry, feeling that she can't do what she wants unless she's alone. Which is also what I think you feel much of the time. She's obviously incredibly important to you." In a tearful voice—sad, but also a little wistful—Rebecca says, "She's been a good friend for a long time."

And now here's Rebecca's interpretation. She says, "It's like she's always been there, almost like the guardian of my real feelings, all the hurt and anger and all the wishes I had to pretend I didn't have, because there was no one there in my family to have them with. But she kept them."

"And is there still no one to have them with?"

"I know I don't have to be alone now, but it's as if I can't quite believe it. Or don't want to. I mean, it's like I cling to my mistrust—the idea that you're coming on to me or that my husband's only interest in

me is sexual. At some level, I know all of that's not true. I have the love and support that I've always wanted, but for some reason that's almost harder than not having it. So I get envious of other people even when I actually have everything that I envy them for. God, it's just so crazy, and so sad."

Helping patients change their stance toward their own subjective experience depends, in part, on our explicit mentalizing (i.e., interpreting) that make connections between different elements of that experience. Such connections are essential to the integration of dissociated states of mind—in Rebecca's case, a state of overcredulous trust on the one hand and stubborn mistrust on the other. Without this integration, neither a patient's sense of self nor her autobiographical narrative can be made coherent.

Rebecca's narrative involved the implicit knowing that autonomy and intimacy were mutually exclusive. In one part of this narrative, Rebecca could have no voice—no independent will—if she let herself be close to someone who mattered to her: hence, her silence regarding my touch and her difficulty rejecting her husband's overtures. But in a separate part of this narrative, she could trust others to be responsive to her and supportive—only that view had a pretend quality that made it very unstable. Because the narrative is self-contradictory, Rebecca often wound up feeling confused as well as voiceless.

Our work together accessed her contradictory states of mind and made it possible for her to begin to consider the relationship between them. We were also seeing that Rebecca's incoherent narrative poorly represented the possibilities available to her in the present—more specifically, that losing herself precluded both being close *and* getting what she needed. The fact that Rebecca could now *in a single state of mind* experience both her desire and mistrust—and reflect upon them—signaled to me that their integration was now under way.

The kind of relational, emotional, and interpretive process I've sketched not only contributes to the integration of dissociated states of mind but can also help make bridges between feeling and thinking, implicit and explicit memory, and—in the brain—the right and left hemispheres as well as the "higher" functions of the cortex and the "lower" functions of the limbic system and brainstem. These kinds of integration are the yield in psychotherapy of the benign circle of affect regulation, attachment, and mentalizing that fosters, in turn, greater coherence in both our patients' sense of self and their autobiographical narrative.

Rather than any *particular* understanding, it is the experience of a relationship in which the patient feels understood—and inspired to understand herself—that is ultimately most therapeutic. Thus, what we hope to make possible for our patients is the awareness that insight is possible, rather

than any particular insight. Through our implicit and explicit mentalizing we cultivate in our patients the twin capacities for insight and empathy—capacities that, taken together, are more or less the equivalent of mentalizing.

Mentalizing and Mindfulness

Fonagy originally referred to the reflective self as "the internal observer of mental life" (Fonagy et al., 1991b, p. 201). Without such an internal observer, we are simply embedded in subjective experiences that we confuse with objective realities. Unable to reflect on the difference between feelings and facts, we remain blind to the ways in which we habitually construct as well as construe the "reality" of our own experience.

Around both of these matters—the importance of the internal observer and the subjective, rather than objective, quality of mental states—a mentalizing stance can be seen to overlap with a mindful one.[3] The two converge in facilitating the recognition that our subjective experience is largely a psychological construction, and that much of our psychological suffering can consequently be seen as (unconsciously) self-generated. Both have the potential to lift us out of our embeddedness in experience and the quality of automatic responsiveness it imposes.

Yet mentalizing and mindfulness are clearly not the same. The kind of mental activity associated with each is distinct, as are the contributions each can make to psychotherapy. Mentalizing has been compared to using a telescope: It sharpens our view of "distant" experience by bringing the past or the unconscious "closer." Mindfulness has been compared to using a microscope: It gives us a vivid and detailed view of immediate experience that might otherwise remain hidden in plain sight (Rubin, 1996). While mentalizing may provide a key route to the establishment of a coherent self, mindfulness has been seen as key to the transcendence of the self. For mindfulness is the centerpiece of a 2,500-year-old Buddhist tradition in which the aim is to undo the self-imposed suffering caused by clinging to illusory images of self.

MINDFULNESS IN PSYCHOTHERAPY

. . . in most psychodynamic treatments there is a rush toward meaning, leaving the present moment behind.
—DANIEL STERN (2004, p. 140)

The Harvard developmentalist Robert Kegan discusses the "socialized mind," the "self-authoring mind," and the "self-transforming mind" as forms of consciousness associated with successively higher levels of psychological maturation (Kegan, 2000). Kegan's categories trace a progression that parallels that from embeddedness to mentalizing to mindfulness.

Clearly mentalizing helps to free us from the constraints of our family and cultural past as represented in the "socialized mind." Through implicit understanding and explicit reflection, mentalizing enables us to take a step back from our experience and representations, in order to make sense of them, and thus to become increasingly the author and interpreter of our own life.

Rather than making sense of the *contents* of our experience, mindfulness directs our receptive awareness to the moment-by-moment *process* of experiencing. Over time such attention can potentially affect a "Copernican revolution" in which the mind that mediates our experience of the world transforms itself (Engler, 2003).

The authors of a recent book on mindfulness and psychotherapy (Germer et al., 2005) describe mindful awareness as:

- *Nonconceptual.* Mindfulness is awareness without absorption in our thought processes.
- *Present-centered.* Mindfulness is always in the present moment. Thoughts about our experience are one step removed from the present moment.
- *Nonjudgmental.* Awareness cannot occur freely if we would like our experience to be other than it is.
- *Intentional.* Mindfulness always includes an intention to direct attention somewhere. Returning attention to the present moment gives mindfulness continuity over time.
- *Participant observation.* Mindfulness is not detached witnessing. It is experiencing the mind and body more intimately.
- *Nonverbal.* The experience of mindfulness cannot be captured in words, because awareness occurs before words arise in the mind.
- *Exploratory.* Mindful awareness is always investigating subtler levels of perception.
- *Liberating.* Every moment of mindful awareness provides freedom from conditioned suffering. (p. 9)

While moments of mindfulness may arise occasionally during everyday experience, the *practice* of mindfulness involves the ongoing effort—as much in daily life as in meditation—to remember to focus our attention on the present, with all the qualities of awareness mentioned above. The yield of this practice, as I'll shortly explain, is the development of a mindful self that can strengthen, in several different ways, the reassuring sense of an internalized secure base.

Awakening the Mindful Self

Mindfulness and meditation, like psychotherapy itself, must be experienced to be known. Cognitive-behaviorists Segal et al. (2002) write that in order

to research, and make therapeutic use of, mindfulness practices they needed to practice mindfulness themselves. As I mentioned in this book's opening chapter, my own experiential awareness of the importance of a mindful stance initially arose not through meditation but in reflecting on the nature of the reflective self.

As I asked myself what seemed the logical question—"Exactly who is it that is doing the reflecting here?"—I had the sudden, compelling, and slightly vertiginous sense that my self as I ordinarily knew it had imploded. What remained (the answer to my question, I suppose) was no "self" per se but instead only awareness. In place of my usual experience of self—saturated with my history and identity, and taking up a good deal of psychological space—was what felt like a single point of consciousness that took up no space at all. For a couple of weeks or so, I was able virtually at will to reconnect with this newly discovered sense of self—or "no self." As I did, I experienced feelings of well-being and gratitude as well as a much enhanced ability to be present. I also experienced decreased defensiveness, a heightened capacity for empathy and acceptance, and an intense feeling of connection to others on the basis of what felt like our shared capacity for awareness, not to mention suffering.

Eventually I found to my surprise and dismay that I could no longer connect with the state of mind that had previously seemed so effortlessly accessible. In discussion with friends and colleagues, however, I came to believe that meditation actually exercises the "muscle" associated with that particularly mindful state of mind.

Of course, meditation takes many forms. Broadly speaking, two primary approaches can be distinguished: concentration meditation and insight or mindfulness meditation. Germer (2005) compares the focus of attention in the former to a laser light beam and the latter to a searchlight. Concentration is a practice that focuses the mind narrowly on an object of awareness (prototypically the breath) while mindfulness entails a wide-open and choiceless focus on whatever predominates in our awareness from one moment to the next. Concentration is said to foster calm, while the benefits of mindfulness meditation are said to include not only self-understanding but knowledge of the nature of the mind itself (Germer et al., 2005).

Incorporating both of these approaches, the practice to which I was drawn is the same one that has been enlisted in a variety of psychotherapies including mindfulness-based stress reduction (Kabat-Zinn, 1990) and mindfulness-based cognitive therapy for depression (Segal et al., 2002).[4] Usually conducted while sitting still with eyes closed, this practice involves countless repetitions of the same sequence that begins as we *locate* our awareness, by bringing attention to the successive inhalations and exhalations of the breath. Then we observe the thoughts, feelings, bodily sensa-

tions, and sensory impressions that spontaneously arise and "hijack" our attention such that our conscious awareness of the present moment is temporarily lost. Finally, noticing that we have "disappeared" into an absorbing thought, feeling, or sensation, our task is to *label* the experience in which we've been caught up, before we gently *return* attention to the breath and to awareness (Germer, 2005).

At the simplest level, the aim of this kind of meditation is to acquaint us with what it means to voluntarily locate our attention and direct it to our experience of the present moment, while deliberately curbing our tendency to characterize or judge what we're experiencing. Repeatedly remembering to focus on present experience with wholehearted acceptance—and repeatedly losing and regaining this focus—is a practice that has many salutary effects.

Like the internal secure base borne of a relationship of secure attachment, the internal secure base that is nurtured by mindfulness can steady us in the face of difficult experience. But how does this development occur? Consider that a mindful stance is *"welcoming* and *allowing.* . . . It encourages 'opening' to the difficult and adopting an attitude of gentleness to all experience" (Segal et al., 2002, p. 58). The more we can access such a stance, the easier it becomes to locate a calm place inside—"the still point of the turning world" (Eliot, 1943/1991b, p. 180)—because a place of calm acceptance has come to be one that we know. The foundation of such acceptance is compassion for ourselves that emerges as we open to our own painful experience: "Mindfulness offers a way to change our relationship to suffering by surrendering our need to reject it. This is an act of kindness to oneself" (Fulton, 2005, p. 63).

In addition, experiences of mindfulness foster a growing identification with awareness itself, rather than the shifting self-states (positive or negative) that we become aware of. The more strongly we feel identified with awareness, the greater our sense of internal freedom and security. For if the original secure base depended on our certainty about the availability of a protective other, the internalized secure base of mindfulness rests, in part, on the sense that there is no need for protection. The identification with awareness removes (more or less) the felt necessity to protect ourselves by clinging to or avoiding transient self-states that are merely that—rather than actual refuges to be sought or dangers to be averted.

Mindfulness practice also provides an experiential education in the difference between being present with awareness and simply being on the scene. It firms up the sense that attention is a faculty we're in charge of: When we remember to be present, and notice that we're not, we can choose to redirect our attention to the here and now. Gradually such acts of "attentional agency" enhance our capacity to be fully present, which may mean living more and more as if each moment might be our last. Mindful-

ness practice also strengthens our sense of an "internal observer" that can be aware of having thoughts, feelings, and sensations, without being entirely identified with them. In other words, mindfulness contributes to "disembedding" (Safran & Muran, 2000). All these effects have particular relevance for therapists and their patients.

As therapists, we can cultivate our own capacity to adopt a mindful stance, either through meditation or, more informally, through deliberate efforts to "wake up" and direct our attention to here-and-now experience, with an attitude of acceptance. Broadly speaking, if we are able to mobilize such a stance as we sit with our patients, then we are likelier to be able to be fully present—in part, because we are "softening into" rather than resisting our experience. More specifically, a mindful stance can strengthen our capacities for affect tolerance, empathy, and "evenly hovering attention."

We can also use such a stance to inform, illuminate, and enhance specific aspects of the work we do with our patients. In this light, psychotherapy can be seen as a kind of meditation for two in which our task is to help the patient to be able to be mindful of her moment-to-moment experience, without judging it. What we often encounter here are the patient's difficulties (and our own) in being present, aware, and/or accepting. Of course, it is these difficulties that then become the focus of our kindly attention. Losing and regaining this quality of mindful attention, over and over again, can be seen as the meditative practice of psychotherapy.

Finally, we can introduce meditation to those patients for whom it appears likely to be of use. Usually, in my experience, these are patients who need help regulating their affects and/or have difficulty being present in a full or integrated way. While I've taught the rudiments of mindfulness practice to a few patients, most of those for whom I've recommended meditation have sought the supportive structure of a class. (Note that the specifics of how, as therapists, we can use mindfulness in the treatment setting will be discussed in Chapter 17.)

The Therapeutic Action of Mindfulness

The practice of mindfulness clearly fosters the affect regulation that functions therapeutically in a benign circle with mentalizing and attachment. Like a secure attachment relationship, mindfulness can temper the acute reactivity of the amygdala and sympathetic nervous system that marks the emotion processes of insecurely attached individuals—especially those who might be described as preoccupied or unresolved.

As I've mentioned, meditation has been shown empirically to diminish the physiological indices of stressful arousal. I suspect this finding is related to the calming effect of the focus in meditation on the breathing body as well as the meditator's growing confidence in her ability to direct attention

voluntarily. With a strengthened sense of the self as the agent or initiator of attention, we may feel less compelled either to reflexively resist or automatically surrender to the bullying of disturbing thoughts, feelings, or bodily sensations. Instead we may be able to simply *be* with them, rather than push them away (avoidant/dismissing style) or remain entangled in them (anxious/preoccupied style). In addition, the practice of labeling the mental events we experience (whether in meditation or everyday life) can diminish their emotional force, perhaps by enlisting the brain's cortical resources to modulate subcortical emotional responses (see Hariri et al., 2000; Hariri et al., 2003). Repeatedly noting and naming our thoughts, feelings, and sensations—and in meditation, returning attention to the breath and to awareness—can strengthen our ability to "disidentify" from troubling emotional states. Such disidentification enlarges the mental space within which patients and their therapists can attempt to understand these emotional states rather than resist or be dominated by them.

Meditation can also be a valuable adjunct to psychotherapy for some patients who might be described as dismissing. Generally remote from their feelings, these patients often have a difficult time being fully engaged in their own experience. They live as if at a remove, not only from others who might matter to them but also from themselves. Meditation with a focus on the breath can ground such patients in the body—the seat of emotion—and generate a heightened sense of what it might mean to actually be present. I think here of a very analytically minded patient whose experience we have captured with the metaphor of "hovering": He feels as if he perpetually hovers over his life, never landing in his body or his relationships. Meditating for the first five to ten minutes of every session has apparently helped him begin to land in his own therapy.

Like psychotherapy, mindfulness practice inside or outside the clinical setting is a way of getting to know our own mind. Listen to Jack Engler (2003) describe the meditative process:

> Trained moment-to-moment attention to the flow of psychophysical events with a minimum of reactivity will trigger a deautomatization of the psychological operations that register, select, organize, and interpret perceptual and conceptual stimuli by reinvesting them with conscious awareness. As this occurs, psychological functions that were once regulated automatically, without conscious awareness and control, become accessible to awareness. (p. 68)

The process Engler describes can be seen to occur through a silent form of free association that is conducted in a relaxed state. Once again, the task when meditating is to focus on the breath while noting, without preference or judgment, whatever mental events arise in the present moment. Focusing

on our breathing, and knowing that we can redirect our attention to the breath—and with it, our awareness of awareness—helps foster a relatively calm, unguarded state of mind. In such a state, previously repressed or dissociated thoughts, feelings, or sensations can surface into consciousness. But these thoughts, feelings, and sensations may well be experienced differently now because they are surfacing in what Daniel Stern (2004) calls a "present remembering context" that is new (p. 199).

Just as a secure relationship with the therapist can potentially provide a transformative context of this kind, so can the state of calm evoked through meditation. When reencountered in such a state of mind, troubling mental experiences rooted in personal history may be recontextualized in a way that modulates their disturbing intensity and even, perhaps, "rewrites the possible memories of the past" (Stern, 2004, p. 200). From a rather different angle, the therapeutic action here may derive from meditation's effects as a form of progressive desensitization in which our troubling experiences are revisited while we're in a state of mental and bodily ease (Goleman, 1988). In the process, these experiences may be changed in ways that make their integration more feasible.

In addition, meditation as well as everyday mindfulness can help illuminate the very processes through which—on a moment-to-moment basis—our experience and that of our patients is constructed and reconstructed. When mindful, we can "hear" the words that express our thoughts, from whispery murmurs at the very edge of awareness to insistent harangues. We can feel the feelings that grip us temporarily and then fall away. We can experience the bodily sensations and sensory impressions that appear and disappear. We can also note how these various representations of our experience interact: A thought may lead to a feeling or bodily sensation, a sensation to a thought or feeling, a sound to a feeling, and so on. *And we can return to the present moment.*

Following the trajectory of our unfolding experience, we inevitably learn at least two things. The first is that our attention to the here and now is repeatedly found and lost: We can be present or not, aware of awareness or not. The second is that our experience is a fluid construction, reshaped from one instant to the next through a kaleidoscopic interplay of thoughts, feelings, and sensations that crystallize in states of mind that come and go. In this connection, consider that a fundamental tenet of Buddhist psychology is that what we take to be our very *self* is itself ceaselessly in flux—and, consequently, the sense of an intrinsic, permanent or fixed self can only be an illusion.

The Mindful Self and the Reflective Self

Circling back now to the reflective self and the appearance–reality distinction, mindfulness offers a further education regarding the *"merely* repre-

sentational nature" of mental states (Main, 1991, p. 128). For as I've just suggested, the practice of mindfulness provides a window on the impermanent and mutable quality of what we think, feel, and sense. Though a mindful stance differs from a reflective or mentalizing one, the impact of both can be similar—that is, to facilitate the recognition that mental states are only mental states, subjective rather than objective, fluid rather than fixed, something we have rather than something we are. In short, mindfulness and mentalizing alike can function as antidotes to embeddedness.

In addition, mindfulness like mentalizing in its most developed form—"mentalized affectivity" (Fonagy et al., 2002)—fosters integration of the "social–emotional" right brain and the "interpreting" left brain. Just as the reflective self can make possible "thinking about feeling and feeling about thinking" (Target, 2005, personal communication), the mindful self can enable our feelings to be informed by thought and our thoughts to be informed by feeling.

Yet mindfulness also offers something that mentalizing does not. For the *mindful* self is aware of the reflective self—and aware as well that reflecting upon experience is entirely different from being fully present to experience. Through repeatedly becoming aware of awareness, we *"shift the locus of subjectivity from representations of self to awareness itself"* (Engler, 2003, p. 65). In this way, experiences of the mindful self have the potential not only to strengthen the "internal observer" but also to access a deep, and perhaps inviolable, sense of who we are at the center of ourselves. In Buddhist psychology and practice, as I mentioned earlier, a vital aim of mindfulness is to discover that at the core of the self is no self at all, but rather "one continuous flow of aware experience" (Falkenstrom, 2003, p. 1559). In psychotherapy, a close relative of this realization of "no-self" is the gradual divestiture of our emotional investment in reified *images* of self (as utterly self-sufficient, say, or utterly helpless) that constrain our potentials for understanding and growth.

Needless to say, we are not required to choose between a reflective stance (that helps us see the patterns in our experience over time) and a mindful one (that helps us to deeply inhabit our experience of the present moment). In psychotherapy, both stances can be healing, and each may well potentiate the other. Certainly, as Fonagy affirms, mindfulness practice strengthens mentalizing. Ekman's finding that experienced meditators have a highly developed ability to "read the mind in the face" points in the same direction, for mentalizing involves recognizing mental states as these are expressed through behavior. Similarly, it may be that mentalizing, which contributes to affect regulation, empathy, and trust, also makes a mindful stance more accessible.

While the relationship between mentalizing and mindfulness may be somewhat ambiguous, it is unquestionable that both have a valuable and

mutually supportive role to play in our efforts as therapists to understand, engage with, and be of help to our patients. Both can contribute to the internalized experience of a secure base, to integration, and to the opening up of mental space that strengthen our patients' capacities to freely feel, reflect, and love.

NOTES

1. These subjects participated in eight weekly two- to three-hour sessions of meditation instruction plus a one-day retreat.
2. Along with one other very experienced meditator, this monk scored far higher than any of the other 5,000 individuals Ekman tested.
3. Barry Magid who is both a psychoanalyst and a Buddhist teacher, describes the impact of meditation in this way: "Following the breath and labeling thoughts initially leads to building up a stable internal 'observer' who is not buffeted by conflicting emotions or swept up by the flow of association or rumination" (cited in Safran, 2003, p. 279).
4. Dialectical behavior therapy (Linehan, 1993) uses mindfulness techniques inspired by Zen sitting meditation, but it does not employ formal meditative practice.

CHAPTER 10

Deepening the Clinical Dimension of Attachment Theory

Intersubjectivity and the Relational Perspective

The research inspired by Bowlby's original insights has given psychotherapists an empirically grounded framework for understanding human development as a relational process. Attachment theory can thus be seen as a relational theory of development and also, perhaps, of the internal world, defenses, and psychopathology. It is not, however, a *clinical* theory, though clearly it has enormously rich implications for psychotherapy—two of which point directly to the intersubjective, relational perspective as the clinical complement to attachment theory.

First, because development is fundamentally a relational process, psychotherapy must be conceived in relational terms if it is to foster the resumption of healthy development. Second, because of the developmental centrality of nonverbal interaction, psychotherapy must find openings to reach realms of past and potential experience that the patient is unable to access with words.

But exactly what does it mean, clinically speaking, to conceive of psychotherapy in relational terms? And just how do we enable our patients to connect with experience that they cannot put into words? Paralleling the relational emphasis in attachment theory, the so-called "relational turn" in

psychoanalysis provides some extraordinarily useful answers to these questions.

BEYOND ONE-PERSON PSYCHOLOGY

During roughly the same period that Main and Fonagy were investigating the preverbal and relational origins of attachment security, psychoanalysts from a variety of schools were scrutinizing their work with patients in closely related terms. Just as attachment research had documented that the nature of the individual's internal working model depends on the quality of the relationships within which it takes shape, these psychoanalysts observed that the nature of the patient's experience in treatment depended moment to moment on the quality of the therapeutic relationship.

On the basis of clinical evidence (including, in some cases, their own experience as patients) they were recognizing the profound limitations of "one-person psychology." This term refers to the assumption that the patient's thoughts, feelings, and behavior are all fundamentally generated from within—and that therapeutic attention must therefore be concentrated on the internal workings of the patient's psyche.

Clinicians who would eventually be described as relational, intersubjective, or constructivist were arguing, to the contrary, that the patient's "psychic reality" could be meaningfully addressed only in the context of the experiential reality jointly created by *both* partners in the therapeutic couple. Just as Bowlby had pressed for an acknowledgement of the influence on the child's development of the actualities of the parents' behavior, the proponents of "two-person psychology" were now arguing that the patient's thoughts, feelings, and behavior are always (at least in part) a response to the therapist. Along with the therapist's well-intentioned interventions, the actualities of her *inadvertent* participation have an impact on the patient.

In this view, therapists are no more capable than patients of parking their individual subjectivity outside the office door—and their efforts to deny or eliminate the impact of their own unconscious, their vulnerabilities, their theories are not only doomed, but also countertherapeutic. The reality of the therapist's "irreducible subjectivity" (Renik, 1993) disqualifies her as an arbiter of truth whose authority derives from her (supposed) capacity for dispassionate objectivity. Moreover, therapist and patient alike are subject to that inescapable condition of intimate relationships that Stephen Mitchell (1993), Robert Stolorow (Stolorow et al., 1987), and Jessica Benjamin (1990/1999) all refer to as *mutual reciprocal influence*.

The recognition of such influence is at the heart of a paradigm shift in psychoanalysis that is now transforming even mainstream ideas about what

constitutes effective psychotherapy. "Intersubjectivity theory" is arguably the best umbrella term for this new paradigm. As discussed in Chapter 4, intersubjectivity has been defined as the "reciprocal influence of the conscious and unconscious subjectivities of two people in a relationship" (Natterson & Friedman, 1995, p. 1). I would add that while the "inter" in intersubjectivity underscores the reality that the experience of patient and therapist alike is created through their *interaction* (thus, the individual is embedded in the dyad[1]), the "subjectivity" in intersubjectivity highlights the fallacy of therapeutic objectivity and the advantages of assuming instead that the emotionally responsive therapist is always irreducibly subjective. The clinical innovations associated with the new paradigm include the rejection of any standard technique in favor of a sort of therapeutic pluralism, the opening up of the option of deliberate self-disclosure, and the focus on enactments of transference–countertransference not only as a key route to insight and new experience but also as potential barriers to both.

ATTACHMENT AND INTERSUBJECTIVITY: CONVERGING AND COMPLEMENTARY THEORIES

Attachment research both underscores and helps to explain the mutual reciprocal influence patients and therapists inevitably exert upon one another. Intersubjectivity theory does the same, but in addition provides conceptual and technical tools to deal with this influence, which can be a problem but also a potential resource.

Bowlby recognized that in infancy and beyond we unconsciously adapt to those upon whom we depend, whether these attachment figures are good for us or not. This sometimes self-defeating adaptation marks, in many cases, the attachments of adulthood. Needless to say, perhaps, patients and their therapists are dependent upon one another. We know how patients depend on their therapists, but we tend to think less about our own needs in relation to our patients.

Of course, these needs of ours vary. If we are in private practice, we depend upon our patients economically. Beyond this practical dependency, we also have what might be called narcissistic needs in relation to our patients—that is, we have needs to feel good about ourselves, both personally and professionally. Depending on our psychological makeup, we may look to our patients to help us feel competent, useful, benevolent, or powerful, and we may look to them to help us feel more secure.

Reciprocal influence has multiple sources, but need or desire in relation to those upon whom we are dependent is undoubtedly one of them. The dependency of patient and therapist—which is mutual but not necessarily symmetrical—makes for a terrain ripe with possibilities for adapta-

tions some of which have the potential to be helpful and others to be very problematic, particularly when they remain unrecognized or unarticulated. Attachment theory illuminates some of the patterns that this interplay of mutual dependency of patient and therapist can generate.

Intersubjectivity theory not only highlights the inescapability and pervasiveness of mutual reciprocal influence but also offers therapists some approaches that can potentially produce a collaborative response to the collusions (and collisions) that mark every therapeutic relationship. At the heart of these approaches is the recognition that our embeddedness in the relationship generates unavoidable transference–countertransference enactments that reflect the initially unconscious, overlapping needs and vulnerabilities of patient and therapist. Intersubjectivity theory approaches these enactments informed by a radical rethinking of traditional analytic constructs.

The Therapist's Personal Involvement

Redefining transference, countertransference, resistance, and neutrality in relational terms, the theory humanizes the therapist's role and enhances respect for the patient in ways that are conducive to the development of a relationship of attachment. In the new paradigm, we are *always* contributing to what is happening in the therapeutic interaction, as is the patient.

The patient's *transference*, therefore, is never completely divorced from the actual nature of the therapist's participation and, accordingly, the exploration of transference must be grounded in the assumption that the patient's views of the therapist have a plausible basis in the here and now. *Countertransference* expresses the therapist's inescapably subjective, but still informative, response to the patient. Because it partly shapes, even as it may also reveal, the patient's transference, countertransference has the potential both to further therapeutic progress and to hinder it. *Resistance* is similarly seen as co-created in the interaction of patient and therapist; as such, it is reconceived as communication rather than opposition. And as for the goal of therapeutic *neutrality,* that is, the effort to insulate the patient from the influence of the therapist's values or personality: In an intersubjective framework, such neutrality is variously regarded as an impossibility, a misleading ideal, and/or a decidedly temporary achievement of patient and therapist working together to loosen the grip of a particular enactment.

The traditional assumptions promoted the therapist's efforts to restrict to a minimum her *personal* involvement in order to remain a neutral observer of the treatment relationship. At its best, this traditional stance reflected respect for the patient's autonomy. At its worst, it turned the therapist into a remote presence whose emotional unresponsiveness and self-

deceptive claims to an impossible objectivity tended to invite and entrench the patient's negative transference.

The relational approach rests, of course, on an entirely different set of assumptions that lead to a very different stance. In this framework, the therapist is just as much a participant in the relationship with the patient as an observer. Our authentic personal involvement, emotional responsiveness, and unavoidable subjectivity, far from interfering, are essential features of every successful psychotherapy. Our best hope for useful understanding here lies in our willingness to examine not only the patient's subjective experience but also our own, as *together* we create a relationship that may be, in itself, the mainspring of therapeutic change.

Intersubjectivity theory arose as a reaction against one-person psychology and Freud's original prescription that the analyst should function as a blank screen, reflecting mirror, or psychic surgeon.[2] While deriving from legitimate concerns about the power of transference and countertransference, Freud's recommendation that the analyst perform a disappearing act upon his own subjectivity was not only impossible to implement but often also countertherapeutic.[3]

Challenging this monadic approach, the theories of intersubjectivity and attachment converge in placing close and co-created relationships at the very heart of development. The theories also share the understanding that the evolving self takes shape as a function of the thoughts, feelings, and behavior that are recognized and allowed expression in these relationships. Whether in early development or psychotherapy, a more inclusive relationship generates a more integrated internal world, while a relationship that cannot contain a full range of experience promotes in the child and maintains in the adult an internal world marked by dissociation.

Integration, Dissociation, and Multiplicity

What Bowlby and Main call the multiple (i.e., contradictory and incompatible) working models of insecurely attached individuals are essentially the outcome of experience for which their formative relationships made no room—experiences, consequently, that had to be dissociated. Such dissociated experiences are defensively excluded from the dominant sense of self, but in the process they are also preserved, so to speak, albeit in an undeveloped form.

In a well-known article—"The Illusion of Personal Individuality"— Harry Stack Sullivan (1964), the father of interpersonal psychiatry, argued that we have as many different selves as we have different relationships. Here Sullivan foreshadowed the work of contemporary relational and intersubjective clinicians who write in terms of the *multiplicity of selves* and the *socially constructed self*—describing the consequences of develop-

ment in ways that partially overlap with the conclusions of attachment researchers.

In this "constructivist" view, all of us have multiple selves, to each of which correspond different sets of feelings, memories, attitudes, and impulses; at the same time, most of us are also capable of sustaining the "adaptive illusion" of being a unitary self (Bromberg, 1998a). Such a self is fluid, rather than fixed: It assumes a variety of shapes in a variety of interpersonal contexts. (You can probably hear echoes here of the Buddhist view of the self—or no self—that was touched on in the last chapter.) Importantly, this psychology of multiple, constructed selves is consistent with the finding of attachment research that contradictory working models are state dependent: That is, they emerge or are activated depending on circumstances, both internal (say, a depressed mood) and external (say, a real-world setback).

For intersubjective and relational clinicians, the question for health or pathology has to do with the extent to which these multiple selves are, or are not, integrated. Put differently, How open are the lines of communication between our differing senses of self? How easily can a particular patient connect with states of mind that differ from those in which he currently appears to be lodged? With these questions, the theories of attachment and intersubjectivity again converge, for in both there is a focus upon the nature of the self's *access* to its own experience.

In describing the developmental trajectory that results in a failure to integrate multiple senses of self, relational theorists—in agreement with attachment researchers—suggest that experiences which could not be accommodated in our most significant relationships tend to be dissociated and undeveloped rather than repressed. Rather than being defensively "forgotten" they are instead relegated to the very edge of awareness. There they remain as unwanted or disowned parts of the self until, in the context of a new state of mind determined by a different set of circumstances, what was previously peripheral now becomes all too central (Bromberg, 1998a; Davies, 1998; Stern, 2002).

A patient of mine, for example, saw herself as exceptionally generous and considerate, in a way that was absolutely fundamental to her good feelings about herself. As a young woman, she told me, she had had a vision of herself—midway between a fantasy and a belief—in which her unusual "decency" or "goodness" was so in evidence that it might uplift and transform the people with whom she came into contact. Perhaps unsurprisingly, this was a patient whose childhood anger had to be suppressed because it dangerously escalated her father's fury. Now, as a new parent, she is profoundly shaken when she finds that her inconsolable infant son can provoke her own uncontrollable anger. She insists in regard to this behavior: "That's not *me*!" Obviously there's a lot going on here: her distress that her

special qualities as a person are insufficient to soothe her son, her vulnerability to rage when seeing him—like her father—expressing feelings of the kind that she had had to suppress, her trouble feeling like a decent parent when she is also an angry parent. The therapeutic task here has been to integrate—and thus to modulate—this patient's contradictory experiences of herself: the goodness she inflated and clung to as a source of self-respect as well as the anger she denied and dissociated in order to preserve both her safety and her attachment to her father.

"Dissociation," of course, is a term with at least a double meaning. First, dissociation means defensively modifying one's sense of reality. This is what patients are talking about when they describe experiences of spacing out, leaving their bodies, or feeling they don't exist. Second, dissociation refers to a splitting off of experience that is incompatible with how one ordinarily sees oneself—as in the patient above who said of her anger, "That's not *me*!"

Dissociation in this latter sense is a feature of the internal working model(s) that segregate aspects of the self, rather than integrating them. The greater the degree of dissociation, the more contradictory, discontinuous, unstable, and confusing is the sense of self—and the less communication there is among the "multiplicity of selves." At the pathological extreme, we find dissociative identity disorder, also known as multiple personality disorder, in which different selves may be largely unaware of each other's existence. At the opposite end of the continuum are those "islands of dissociation" that mark the experience of even the healthiest among us. Somewhere in between lie the fragmented and "multiple" working models of insecure and disorganized individuals.

If there is a difference in the meaning of dissociation for attachment researchers and relational theorists, it may be this: In the attachment world, dissociation simply does not feature in the psychic structure of secure individuals. Among relational writers, by contrast, dissociation is seen as an inevitable aspect of being human. Because we all have experiences that emotionally overwhelm us we will all necessarily have recourse, at times, to what might be described as "normal dissociation"—that is, a temporary experience of a state of mind in which what we are thinking, feeling, or doing is altogether disconnected from our usual sense of ourselves, however integrated that usual sense of ourselves might be.

As for the clinical implications, attachment research and relational theory share a model of the relationship of development to psychic structure which suggests that psychotherapy should be geared to integrate aspects of the patient's experience that are dissociated and, therefore, often undeveloped. That is, the therapist should aim (like the parent of a secure infant) to create a relationship that is maximally inclusive. Psychotherapy in this light leans heavily on the subjectivity of the therapist as a resource—because the

therapist's subjective experience is believed at times to contain aspects of the patient's experience that have had to be dissociated in the context of previous formative relationships. In this connection, it may be helpful to ask which of our own multiple selves is currently lively in our interaction with the patient—for given the co-created nature of relationships, the answer to the question may help us sense which of the patient's multiple selves we are now addressing (Mitchell, 1997).

RETHINKING TRADITIONAL CONSTRUCTS: DEMOCRATIZING PSYCHOTHERAPY AND HUMANIZING THE THERAPIST'S ROLE

The ideas of Bowlby and his heirs offer a powerful vision of the therapeutic relationship in which the patient can potentially experience the therapist as a new attachment figure. Thus attachment-oriented treatment is modeled, to some extent, on the best parent–child relationships.

Similarly, in what might be described as a shadow version of this model, traditional analytic approaches cast the clinician in a highly authoritative role, the parental overtones of which are exaggerated by the patient's dependency. Further sharpening the differential here is the assumption that the clinician is privileged to see and understand with objectivity while the patient's viewpoint is predictably distorted by unconscious needs, defenses, and fantasies.

Very much in contrast, the new paradigm—by deconstructing the fiction of therapeutic objectivity and rejecting the traditional belief that transference is distortion—might be said to democratize the therapeutic relationship. For reasons I'll explain in a moment, such a "leveling" approach that challenges the therapist's *unearned* authority and gives greater credibility to the patient may well make it more likely that the patient will experience the therapist as both a new attachment figure and a secure base. Simultaneously, this approach diminishes the risk in psychotherapy that the patient will be infantilized.

Note that repudiating the impossible ideal of the therapist as objective observer does not mean that the therapist is without expertise or authority but, rather, that this expertise and authority have a different basis. Specifically, the therapist is—or can learn to be—an expert in the process of recognizing, exploring, and transforming the patient's familiar patterns of experience and interaction as these emerge in the context of the therapeutic relationship.

From an intersubjective perspective, this process hinges not only on therapist's sensitivity to the patient but also on the therapist's ability to recognize, reflect upon, and, when desirable, to change her characteristic ways

of participating in the relationship. Such "self-reflective responsiveness" (Mitchell, 1997) can be facilitated by relocating traditional one-person constructs like transference in a two-person context, where they can be used to illuminate the patient's ways of being in a relationship, the therapist's ways of being in a relationship, and the interaction between the two.

Transference Redefined

When Freud discovered that past relationships shape present ones—including, very importantly, the patient's relationship with the therapist—he gave us an extraordinarily powerful clinical resource. For it is clear that through transference our patients have the potential to experience, understand, and transform their most problematic patterns of relating to themselves and others. When old difficulties too painful to resolve reemerge with the therapist, the patient has a second chance to work through troublingly familiar scenarios, and now perhaps resolve them.

In the original conception of transference, the patient displaced onto the therapist feelings, thoughts, and behavior that had previously been experienced in relation to significant figures from childhood. These contemporary expressions of the patient's past were thought to unfold according to a logic exclusively determined by history and entirely divorced from the impact of the therapist's actual presence. In this model, the therapist served as a blank screen on which the patient's transference was projected. Thus, transference was seen as distortion on the part of a patient incapable of accurately perceiving the therapist as a real person.

From a relational perspective (see Aron, 1992, 1996; Hoffman, 1983, 1996, 2001; Mitchell, 1993, 1997, 2000; Renik, 1993, 1999a, 1999b, 1995), the inescapability of mutual influence renders preposterous on its face the notion that the therapist could somehow function as the equivalent of a featureless mannequin the patient dresses in transference (Winer, 1994). As for the allied belief that the patient's viewpoint on the clinician's motives and attitudes is predictably unreliable, Gill and Hoffman (1982) conducted research which demonstrated unequivocally that patients' perceptions of their analyst's countertransference were often more accurate than their analyst's *self*-assessments.

The goal of analytic anonymity is very problematic in light of the fact—self-evident to the patient—that the therapist's personal characteristics have an impact on the relationship. Similarly problematic is the denigration of the patient's judgment implicit in the equation of the patient's perceptions of the therapist with distortion. These traditional assumptions concerning transference can easily undermine the potential for the therapist to be experienced as a secure base. Sometimes they evoke compliance, generating what can amount to pseudotherapy. Sometimes they evoke rebel-

liousness (or another negative transference) that may be intensified when the therapist responds interpretively, adding "insight" to injury.

Within an intersubjective framework, transference is no longer regarded as distortion because the patient's perceptions of the therapist nearly always have a plausible basis. Instead, transference is seen as a kind of rigidity reflected in the fact that among many credible interpretations of the therapist's behavior, the patient seems compelled to believe just one. Transference is thus a matter of selective attention and sensitivity. Rather than being divorced from the actualities of the therapist's persona, it is seen to express the patient's drift toward a habitual way of experiencing a relationship. Importantly, transference in this framework is not only construed but also constructed: Clinical experience confirms that patients frequently behave in ways that elicit confirmation of their particular interpretations of interpersonal reality (Aron, 1996; Gill, 1983; Mitchell, 1993; Renik, 1999a, 1999b).

It is nearly always a mistake to consign the patient's ideas about our attitudes or motives to the realm of unfounded fantasy, just because those ideas depart from our self-perceptions. Others may know us in ways we cannot know ourselves. Because we too have an unconscious, it is vital both to be skeptical about the extent of our self-awareness at any given moment and to regard the patient as a potentially helpful collaborator in identifying aspects of ourselves of which we are unaware (Hoffman, 1983; Aron, 1991, 1992).

With regard to technique, we can best begin by emphasizing what is plausible (or simply accurate) in the patient's transference view. Such a respectful response is essential if the patient is to trust that the therapist is open to the patient's thoughts and feelings, regardless of how discomfiting they may be. This kind of openness fosters the inclusiveness that makes possible the integration of dissociated experience. It may also facilitate an exploration that leads to insight and a collaboration that constitutes, for some patients, a corrective emotional experience.

In attempting to make as much room as we can for the patient's transference reactions, it can be very helpful to wonder aloud about exactly what it is in our behavior or attitude that may have led to the patient's "interpretation." Sometimes the most effective approach to identifying and understanding the patient's experience of the therapist is to encourage the patient's conjectures about the therapist's experience of the patient. In other words, to grasp the patient's transference we may need to hear his or her ideas about our countertransference. Finally, because patients can be quite reluctant to express directly what they actually think and feel about us, it is often illuminating to listen to their communication about extratransferential experience as a coded or metaphoric commentary on their experience of transference.

For example, a patient told me how angry she had been the day before when her internist failed to take her medical complaints seriously. In listening to her describe the experience with her physician, I began to suspect that she was also angry with me. Raising this possibility with her, I learned that she was indeed quite put out with me, on account of her sense that I believed her problems were trivial. As we were exploring this impression of hers, she suddenly asked me what my response to her complaints *had* been. Feeling a little off balance, I nonetheless shared with her what I was just now becoming aware of—the disquieting fact that I'd had trouble really *feeling* her suffering and responding to it with the seriousness it deserved. I told her that this response might well have to do in part with something in me that I needed to understand better, but also that it might be related to the sense I'd had that in conveying her unhappiness to me she often seemed to feel the need to minimize or deny it. What followed was a painful but ultimately productive exploration of her role and mine in generating an interaction that was troubling to both of us.

As this vignette suggests, the new paradigm not only encourages a welcoming, respectful, and empathic stance toward the patient's communication of transference experience, but also makes room for us to disclose our countertransference experience to the patient when doing so seems likely to be of use.

Countertransference Reconsidered

Countertransference reactions are among the key data emerging from what Freud (1912/1924) called the "receptive organ" of the analyst's unconscious as it as it turns "towards the transmitting unconscious of the patient" (p. 328). As such, they provide vital access to the patient's dissociated experience. While classically conceived as an occasional or episodic impediment arising from the psychological shortcomings of the therapist, countertransference in the new paradigm is an ongoing feature of the relationship with the patient and another "royal road to the unconscious."

For all its real potential to inform—specifically, to illuminate even as it influences the patient's transference—countertransference can also interfere, in keeping with its original sense as a hindrance. Because the relationship between patient and therapist is co-created, both partners are in a position to introduce obstacles to the free flow of experience and exploration. The therapist's dissociation or difficulty being present, for instance, can bar the door to the patient's dissociated experience. Thus, a *totalistic* conception of countertransference—the therapist's subjective experience both as resource and resistance—assumes an absolutely central role in an intersubjective approach to psychotherapy.

In this framework, attempting to eliminate countertransference is not

only impossible but also undesirable. What Joseph Sandler (1976/1981) calls "countertransference role-responsiveness"—that is, the therapist's tendency to fall in line with the patient's expectations—can prove to be as much an asset as a liability. Because enacting countertransference may be a precondition for recognizing it (Renik, 1993), therapists are well advised to allow themselves the latitude to be moved by the prevailing interpersonal currents. As Dale Boesky has written: "If the analyst does not get emotionally involved sooner or later in a manner that he has not intended, the analysis will not proceed to a successful conclusion" (cited in Renik, 1993, 1999a, p. 417). Becoming entangled in this way—and subsequently clarifying and transforming the entanglement—may be a sine qua non for effective psychotherapy. The authentic, emotionally charged encounters that are catalysts for change depend not only on the patient being deeply engaged but also the therapist (Ginot, 2001; Maroda, 1999).

From this angle, our effectiveness can actually be undermined by constraints adopted to guard against countertransference enactment. Veteran clinicians are often more effective, as Renik suggests, not because they have worked through more countertransference and enact it less, but rather because they are less defensive about countertransference and more confident of their ability to work through their patients' reactions to it. Consider, too, the research showing that adopting a poker face downregulates emotions (Ekman, Roper, & Hager, 1980). Attempting to mute or mask our countertransference responses in order to maintain our incognito may diminish access to the vital subjective signals that let us know our patients at an emotional level.

With regard to intervention, the new paradigm encourages the judicious use of deliberate countertransference disclosure ("deliberate" in contrast to our ongoing unintentional, unarticulated disclosures of who we are). The particulars of giving voice to countertransference—why, when, and how we might choose to disclose our experience to the patient rather than silently utilizing it as information—will emerge as we address the innovations in technique that spring from intersubjectivity theory.

Resistance Reconsidered

The traditional view holds that resistance arises because something in the patient's psyche must be kept from awareness; its origins are exclusively intrapsychic. In the new paradigm, resistance nearly always has interpersonal meaning as well. From this perspective, it can be seen as the outcome of collusion between patient and therapist to ensure that nothing new or threatening will occur. Put differently, the patient's resistance to experience—usually the experience of what is felt to be unbearable emotional pain—is linked to the fear of an unhelpful response from the therapist. So once

again because the therapeutic relationship is co-constructed (the product of reciprocal mutual influence), it is difficult to see how the therapist could *not* be implicated.

In this light, we should routinely consider behavior we have been taught to see as evidence of resistance (such as the patient's lateness, superficiality, distance from feelings) as, quite possibly, a reasonable response to the quality of the therapist's attunement or lack of it. An attempt to clarify the patient's sense of the therapist's role (if any) in evoking the resistance may make it possible to illuminate whatever preexisting expectations or fears underlie the patient's response.

Of course, the term "resistance" itself has inescapably disparaging connotations. Indeed, the traditional view understands resistance as the patient's unconscious *opposition* to the progress of treatment—as if, were he only to know more, the patient would immediately suspend his foolishness and get with the program. But to consider patients as opposing their own best interests, or opposing the therapist, risks giving the therapeutic relationship an adversarial aura; further, it can cast patients as individuals concealing guilty secrets and therapists as morally superior detectives or confessors. Because neither context is likely to encourage patients to say what hasn't been said or know what has previously had to remain unknown, the classical conception of resistance may work as a barrier to exploration and integration

In contrast, writers including Charles Spezzano (1995), a leading relational theorist, as well as Roy Schafer (1983), a mainstream psychoanalyst, have proposed that we view resistance as communication about aspects of the patient's experience that are hard to tolerate and difficult to put into words. Within this perspective, patients will indirectly convey or unconsciously attempt to evoke in the therapist what they cannot bear on their own. In short, attention to resistance as communication can be another route to the awareness and possible integration of the patient's dissociated experience.

Neutrality Reconsidered

As traditionally understood, neutrality is the absence of investment on the therapist's part in one outcome versus another, the subtraction of the influence on the patient of the therapist's personality, values, or theory. In the new paradigm, such neutrality is regarded at best as an ideal—meant to safeguard the patient's autonomy by providing protection from the therapist's undue influence and to make room for the contradictory facets of the patient's conflicts—and at worst as a misleading illusion, unattainable because the therapist's subjectivity can neither be suspended nor concealed, and undesirable because that subjectivity is an invaluable therapeutic resource (Renik, 1996; Stolorow & Atwood, 1997).

Intersubjective theorists have argued that our conscious efforts as therapists to "bracket" our subjectivity actually increase the likelihood that we will *unconsciously* attempt to influence our patients. The patient's autonomy may be more successfully safeguarded when we are willing to acknowledge and study our own subjective responses, as well as investigating their impact upon the patient. In this connection, Renik (1999b) makes the case that therapists are often most helpful to the patient when they "play their cards face up."

The underlying assumption here is that neither the therapist nor the patient can be objective. Each has an idiosyncratic view of reality and the view of neither should be considered authoritative. Aspiring to a classical version of neutrality, we may deny the patient the benefit of a useful perspective. To foster his or her self-exploration effectively we may sometimes need to present our own point of view—not with the aim of having it accepted but rather in order to have it considered.

Neutrality from an intersubjective viewpoint is the shared achievement of patient and therapist effectively working through some interpersonal resistances together. In so doing, they generate a new opening, a sense of spacious possibility, rather than a constricting investment in a particular interpretation of the current relational reality. Such experiences of "neutrality" reflect a temporary liberation from the interlocking constraints of transference and countertransference (Gerson, 1996).

INTERSUBJECTIVITY'S CONTRIBUTIONS TO THE CLINICAL REPERTOIRE

Intersubjective theory has generated significant clinical innovations that enhance our capacity to understand and intervene in the relational domain, which is critical in light of the empirical finding that a relationship of attachment is the primary context within which psychological development occurs. Specifically, these innovations make for therapeutic relationships marked by their inclusiveness, ready repair of disruptions, and effective negotiation of conflicts and difference. They also help therapists to access their patients' nonverbal experience and to strengthen their capacities for mentalizing and mindfulness.

The Dialectic of Enactments

Because transference and countertransference are linked in a relational framework, neither can be understood in isolation. The therapist's attention is most usefully directed to the interpersonal amalgam known as transference–

countertransference; in fact, the focus on enactments of transference–countertransference is at the heart of an intersubjective clinical approach. In the spiral of reciprocal influence out of which enactments emerge, the therapist's participation is no less significant than the patient's. Thus, for therapy to heal, the therapist as well as the patient must be capable of change.

It is important to keep in mind that enactments are not episodic experiences into which we are temporarily plunged. Henry Smith writes that he has a hard time imagining an "enactment-free" interchange in analysis, and cites Dale Boesky who notes, "It is a bit hard to say what is *not* an enactment" (Smith, 1993, p. 96). Still, it is vital to become aware of the enactments that are ongoing in our relationship with each of our patients: To the extent that such enactments can be made conscious they become the key context within which the tasks of therapy are accomplished; to the extent that they unfold automatically, outside awareness, they may function as barriers to insight and new experience.

By way of illustration, consider the following clinical vignette. When Rodney, a middle-aged male patient with a dismissing attachment style, voiced his concern that he was turning everyone in his life—his clients, his wife—into authority figures, I suddenly saw that our sessions together had regularly assumed the same predictable shape: He would lay out for me what he felt were the successes or failures of his week, while I would implicitly encourage him if he seemed in his terms to be making progress; if not, I would attempt to help him do better. Reflecting on this pattern, I realized that I was playing out a scenario with him that apparently expressed not only his needs but mine.

Rodney's concern about his unbecoming subservience to those he treated as authorities gave me an opening, so I raised the issue with him: Wasn't this also the way *we* had been proceeding together? I offered my impression that he seemed to experience me as a kind of guide or even guru who monitored his efforts and offered needed direction. I added that when he successfully made use of this direction, I suspected that he felt rewarded—but when he could not, perhaps he had felt unsupported.

Notice that until this moment, I had been playing my part in the scenario unthinkingly, perhaps enjoying the role too much to become entirely conscious of it. Therefore, insofar as Rodney experienced our relationship as parallel to the others he referred to, his implicit view that I was presenting myself to him as an authority figure was not a distortion but a reasonable response to my stance. Even in talking to him about all this, I could not escape the authoritative role he characteristically ascribed to me and I characteristically assumed.

In reaction to my intervention, Rodney said, very much in keeping

with the enactment: "So you're telling me this is something to be avoided?" To which I responded, "Perhaps this is more of the same?" Now his response was a kind of "aha" experience. But later, as he had occasion to half-acknowledge/half-apologize for his failure since our last session to complete a job application, I felt that the enactment was being reinstated. Yet somehow it did not occur to me to ask him if concluding our conversation in this way might not reflect exactly what we had just been discussing.

Needless to say, enactments like this one have a rather extraordinary adhesiveness. Along with our patients, we can get stuck in them. Time and again, we need to muster the awareness and initiative to work our way through these enactments so that something unexpected and useful may occur.

Patients like Rodney generate patterns of interaction with their therapists that reflect a dynamic tension between the old and the new, security and risk, repetition and transformation. As therapists, we experience a similar tension between the pull to enact our side of the transference–countertransference configuration and the relative "objectivity" that can strengthen our impulse to understand rather than yield to this pull or reflexively defend against it. Steven Stern (1994) discusses these dialectics in terms of the "repeated relationship" and the "needed relationship," each of which has the potential to be enacted in psychotherapy.

Stern (1994) suggests that projective identification may be the means by which the patient "coaches" the therapist and thus brings these patterns to life in the relationship, either re-creating old experience or making new experience possible. Described by Karen Maroda (1999) as "body-to-body communication" (p. 72), projective identification is said to occur when the patient treats the therapist in such a way that the therapist comes to identify with what the patient is projecting.[4]

Stern's dialectical notion that the patient has conflicting impulses that activate at times the *repeated* relationship and at other times the *needed* relationship fits well with the conclusion of attachment researchers that among insecure individuals a dominant state of mind with respect to attachment is regularly accompanied by an opposing state of mind that tends to be dissociated. For example, dismissing patients may behave as though they have little interest in emotional closeness, yet that very disowned disposition can be discerned in their preoccupation with the prospect of pressure from the emotional demands of others. Patients like these who habitually evoke responses from the therapist that seem to re-create the problematic past can also be expected to pull implicitly for responses that fulfill unmet developmental needs. Against the potent forces that invite repetition are apparently arrayed the shared desires of patient and therapist for experiences that reveal new relational possibilities.

Self-Disclosure

If there is a single transformation of technique that distinguishes the new paradigm from the old, it is the opening up of the option of deliberate self-disclosure (see Ehrenberg, 1992; Maroda, 1999). Recall that from the relational perspective, preserving the therapist's anonymity is not only an impossible aim but also an undesirable one. In that light, the traditional rationales for proscribing self-disclosure start to evaporate. Surfacing in their place are a number of compelling reasons to add this intervention to the therapist's repertoire. Most important perhaps is the fact that explicitly disclosing our thoughts and feelings can help our patients to recognize and "own" experiences they have previously felt the need to disavow or dissociate.

Just as attachment theorists like Fonagy (2001) have insisted that in order for the child to know her own mind she needs the mind of another, relational clinicians (Bollas, 1987; Spezzano, 1995) have observed that in order for patients to integrate disowned thoughts, feelings, and desires, they need the psyche of the therapist to temporarily *contain* experience that they have been unable to bear on their own. In the setting of the therapeutic relationship, the patient's "unthought known" (in Bollas's phrase) can come to reside within the therapist.

Under these circumstances, the therapist's own subjective experience can remain an underutilized resource—unless and until it is disclosed to the patient. The underlying assumption here is that patients unconsciously but purposefully test their therapists to determine the truth of their belief that certain things are simply too dangerous to know, to feel, or to want. The therapist who contains, considers, and now gives voice to her own "personal" experience—say, the sadness she finds herself feeling in a given patient's presence—may disconfirm the patient's belief about the peril of knowing and showing what one feels. The therapist's self-disclosure here serves to demonstrate that more can safely be experienced and expressed than the patient had apparently assumed (Hoffman, 1992, 1994).

Clearly, intersubjectivity theory encourages us not only to make silent use of our subjective experience but also to discuss that experience with our patients when doing so seems likely to further the aims of treatment. Beyond its role in facilitating integration, how can deliberate self-disclosure enhance our therapeutic effectiveness?

It is a crucial resource in our efforts to deal with enactments. To turn these potential obstacles into opportunities for healing, we need at certain times to "work ourselves out of" enactments (otherwise there's raw experience without usable understanding) while we need at other times to "work ourselves into" them (lest there be "understanding" without the lived experience that makes emotional learning possible).

Enactments often signal their presence by straitjacketing the therapist. In other words, when we become aware that our range of motion has significantly narrowed with regard to how freely we can think, feel, or interact with the patient, then we may well be in the grip of an enactment. The more rigid, repetitive or hard to escape the enactment is, the more important it becomes to do what we can to loosen its hold. In such situations, taking the risk of putting our experience into words can often break the spell of the enactment, enabling us to relate to the patient with greater freedom, authenticity, and clarity.

On the other hand, when we feel remote from the patient—persistently bored, sleepy, or distant—or when the nature of the ongoing enactment is all too vague, then disclosing our experience to the patient can enliven a deadened interaction and help make the latent enactment manifest. For example, in a recent session, I said, "I find myself having a much harder than usual time feeling really involved in what you're saying. It feels harder for me to be present right now. This may have to do entirely with me or it may have to do with what's going on here between the two of us. Can you tell me what your experience has been like? And how is it for you to hear me say what I'm saying now?"

The patient sighed deeply and said she was relieved to hear me admit what she thought she had observed, namely, that I seemed to be somewhere else; she added that she hadn't felt present either, she'd been on autopilot, "just yakking." But after this exchange we were off to the races, so to speak. The therapist's expressive participation has the potential to resolve the empathic impasse, bring both parties more fully into the room, and facilitate understanding of their jointly created enactment.

The therapist's self-disclosure can also provide the patient with a model that embodies many of the capacities we hope to strengthen in the course of treatment, including both the reflective capacity that Main and Fonagy link to secure attachment and the capacity for mindfulness. The therapist who can thoughtfully consider her experience, who can question it rather than taking it at face value, and who can entertain various interpretations of it specifically models mentalizing—the ability to respond to experience in light of the shifting mental states that shape it. Similarly, the therapist who can discuss her here-and-now experience undefensively while encouraging the patient to do the same invites a quality of nonjudgmental, present-centered awareness that is the hallmark of a mindful stance.

Self-disclosure on the part of the therapist also models the capacity to put difficult feelings or reactions into words, and giving verbal expression to the kinds of experience the patient has found it necessary to suppress or dissociate fosters the work of integration.

Finally, self-disclosure can be of value in giving patients a view of their impact on the therapist, and thus possibly of their impact on others. I think here of the treatment in which I told a patient that I found myself taking

great care in choosing my words when I spoke to him, that I felt I needed to communicate a message that would be bulletproof, because he seemed so ready to find fault with what I had to say. He found this astonishing: Rather than imagine that *I* might feel threatened by him, he actually felt the need to be on guard in relation to *me*. As the therapy has gone on, we have repeatedly returned to this exchange, most recently when he was confused by a critical performance evaluation at work indicating that his communication with subordinates had put them on the defensive. Now recognizing a familiar pattern, he realized that he needed to deal with his fears of being judged not by relocating them in others but by understanding them and perhaps seeking reassurance.[5]

Relational theory makes deliberate self-disclosure an always available option; whether or not we choose to exercise it in a given moment should depend, like all sound clinical judgments, on what we believe will best serve the patient's interests. The risk that the subjective experience the therapist discloses may have nothing to do with, and/or may not be useful to, the patient is diminished when the therapist communicates it with "skillful tentativeness" (Safran & Muran, 2000) and a willingness to take the patient's reactions very much into account.

There are also risks in keeping our own counsel, of course. While it can be hard to acknowledge, much less disclose, the intense feelings—or indifference—patients stir up in us, our understandable reticence often has its costs. Concealing difficult feelings may do more damage than revealing them. In withholding what we feel, we may be able to offer only a pretense of being present with the patient when, in fact, we have withdrawn. Moreover, there is the risk that we may destructively act out when, in an unpredictable moment, our feelings become too strong for us to contain them. Maroda (1999) and Renik (1995) both suggest that our personal reluctance to reveal these feelings may be rooted in the fear that such disclosure will destroy our authoritatively beneficent image in the patient's eyes, leaving us flawed and vulnerable.

Consistent with my own character, perhaps, it seems to me that attempting to do effective psychotherapy without the benefit of the resource that is self-disclosure makes no more sense than attempting to play the piano with one hand. But while traditional theory proscribed self-disclosure, the new paradigm does not prescribe it—certainly not for every therapist with every patient. Self-disclosure is only an option. As we are about to see, it is the nature of the particular therapist and patient that should determine whether or not the choice of this option makes good clinical sense.

The "Interactive Matrix"

Jay Greenberg (1995) coined this term to describe the jointly created context within which specific events in therapy acquire their meanings. It is

made up of the concordant or discordant subjectivities of patient and therapist. Greenberg argues that it's the particular interactive matrix in treatment rather than any "Book of Standard Technique" that should determine
how a given therapy will be conducted. What is healing, in other words,
will depend entirely on what works for a particular patient working with a
particular therapist.

When the sensibilities of the two partners are in synch, they may mesh
so smoothly that the interaction between them seems a nonevent, in which
case the relational and attachment issues drift to the periphery. Discord, by
contrast, highlights interaction and makes these highly charged issues absolutely central. Now negotiation (mixing empathy, interpretation, and sometimes the therapist's self-disclosure) is required to restore the therapeutic
couple's equilibrium. This notion that discord between therapist and patient requires negotiation to restore equilibrium parallels the conclusion of
infant–parent researchers that a key factor in generating security is the repeated experience, not of perfectly smooth interaction but of (inevitable)
disruption followed by repair.

The issue of discord or harmony, congruence or conflict, is both an interpersonal issue and an internal one. At an interpersonal level, the therapist's way of working may or may not accord with the patient's needs or
desires and the patient may or may not be able to make good use of the
therapist's interventions. But what goes on at that interpersonal level—say,
the patient's response to the therapist's disclosure—will have a great deal to
do with the internal fit (congruence or conflict) between what the therapist
does (intervention) and who the therapist *is* (character).

For example, a given therapist might choose to practice in the most
traditional mode because he has been taught that maintaining anonymity is
good technique. If he finds that mode characterologically comfortable, then
his clinical persona may be accepted by the patient as a natural expression
of his efforts to help. If, on the other hand, the therapist is built psychologically in such a way that he feels as though attempting to function as a blank
screen means being withholding, and thus induces guilt, his efforts may be
experienced by the patient as destructive. Once again, therapists are inescapably subjective and patients pick up on cues that reveal our subjective
experience. Thus, it is not only what we do that matters, but—perhaps even
more important—how we feel about what we do (Wallin, 1997).

The "Analytic Third"

Thomas Ogden (1994) argues that the interactions of patient and therapist
generate an atmosphere rich with unconscious meanings. They are, so to
speak, in the air. This atmosphere of intersubjectively created meanings is
what Ogden calls the analytic third. He believes that this "third" penetrates
and shapes the experience of both parties to the interaction. Accordingly,

attending to the subtlest aspects of our own experience with the patient—including the physical sensations or stray thoughts that are usually dismissed as distractions or evidence of narcissistic preoccupation—may be a key to the patient's dangerous affects and dissociated states of mind. Such traces of the "analytic third" offer another window into the unconscious.

Further evidence of the "third" can be found in striking instances of overlap between the experiences of patient and therapist. Some years ago, I was working with a young man four times weekly. He was the last patient I saw on a Monday evening. The following morning I awoke early from a dream about a woman with three penises. When I saw my patient that afternoon, he began the session by telling me that the night before he had had the most peculiar dream. I knew immediately what he was going to tell me next. He said, "I had dream about a woman with three penises." Examples like this suggest the uncanny way in which an intense intersubjective relationship can generate shared experience that belongs neither to the patient nor the therapist alone but to a mysterious amalgam of the two.

WHAT THE INTERSUBJECTIVE PERSPECTIVE ADDS TO ATTACHMENT THEORY

Charles Spezzano (1998) has asked—doubtless with tongue planted firmly in cheek—what relational therapists do to kill time between enactments and self-disclosures. The question actually raises a crucial issue. If intersubjective and relational theory has got it right that authentic corrective emotional experience partly derives from falling into, and eventually extricating ourselves from, enactments that originate outside awareness, then what are we to attempt *consciously* to do with the patient until we recognize them?

Much of the power in integrating the theories of intersubjectivity and attachment is that the former so usefully frames this question while the latter with equal effectiveness helps us to answer it.

To recap: Attachment theory suggests that the therapist is potentially a new attachment figure in relation to whom the patient can develop fresh patterns of attachment. In identifying aspects of parenting that foster security in the child, attachment theory helps the therapist choose and deliberately manifest a stance geared to generate greater attachment security in the patient. Through its description of distinct attachment styles, the theory also helps the therapist identify the attachment pattern of the particular patient and develop specific approaches accordingly. Finally, in illuminating the centrality of the reflective function and the course of its normal development, attachment theory focuses the therapist's effort to strengthen the patient's mentalizing capacity by coupling efforts to provide a secure base with communication that reflects consistent awareness of the "intentional

stance" of the patient—however nascent that stance may be. As I will be elaborating in Part IV, attachment theory offers therapists a powerful framework for deciding what they might deliberately attempt to provide for their patients.

From an explicitly clinical perspective, intersubjective/relational theory addresses a number of crucial facts. First, as every therapist must know, much if not most of what occurs in psychotherapy is *not* the outcome of deliberate intention on the part of the therapist or the patient. Instead, what occurs is more often than not the product of an interaction of conscious intention with experiences in treatment that are unpremeditated, inadvertent, and unconsciously motivated. Second, patients are usually very conflicted about taking advantage of the new attachment relationship that the therapist is implicitly offering. And third, patients are frequently unwilling or simply unable to be articulate about important facets of their experience.

By providing tools to work with the unintended aspects of our own participation in the patient's world and tools to engage those crucially influential parts of the patient's experience that are not, and often cannot be, put into words, intersubjective theory makes vital contributions to an attachment-oriented approach to treatment.

To begin with, the relational perspective highlights the fact that in becoming part of the patient's world through *enactments,* the therapist is able to experience and know the patient in an emotionally direct way that is unmediated by language. This gives the therapist access to the "unverbalized and unverbalizable" realms of the patient's experience.

The relational perspective also expands attachment theory's understanding of "sensitive responsiveness." In addition to promoting empathy and attunement, there is the emphasis in relational theory on the deep feeling of being understood and held that can arise *not* out of our effort to provide what we presume the patient needs, but rather out of our immersion with the patient in the complex, difficult, sometimes painful interactions that occur unpredictably in spite of our conscious intentions. To the guidance attachment theory offers clinicians regarding deliberate provision, an intersubjective approach adds a focus on the advantages to be derived from working with our (initially) unconscious participation in the relationship with the patient.

Furthermore, an intersubjective approach highlights the opportunity to learn, through attention to enactments, about the *conflict* the patient experiences when it comes to making use of the empathy and containment— the *new* attachment—that the therapist is presumably attempting to provide.

Finally, intersubjectivity theory adds to attachment theory the emphasis on mutuality and dialogue that invites the patient to occupy multiple roles in the treatment relationship—including that of "consultant" to the therapist. Give that all of us have an unconscious, implicitly enlisting the

patient as an interpreter of the therapist's experience can be enormously helpful.

There is a potent synergy in the integration of the theories of attachment and intersubjectivity, which converge and, in this sense, confirm one another. Both identify close relationships as the crucibles in which human beings are originally shaped and in which—whether in love or psychotherapy—their early emotional injuries can potentially be healed. And both theories highlight relational experience that lies outside the strictly verbal realm. More importantly, each theory can be seen to complement and even, perhaps, complete the other. Intersubjectivity theory fills in the largely undeveloped clinical dimension of attachment theory. Attachment, in turn, immeasurably deepens the developmental and diagnostic dimensions of intersubjectivity. In terms of their yield for psychotherapy, then, the two theories when wed are a conceptual "marriage made in heaven."

NOTES

1. As Mitchell (1993), Stolorow et al. (1987), and Daniel Stern (2004) have all suggested, the "isolated mind" is a fiction, an oxymoron.

2. "I cannot recommend my colleagues emphatically enough to take as a model in psychoanalytic treatment the surgeon who puts aside all his own feelings, including that of human sympathy, and concentrates his mind on one single purpose, that of performing the operation as skillfully as possible" (Freud, 1912/1924a, p. 327).

3. Owen Renik, former editor-in-chief of the *Psychoanalytic Quarterly*, has said that whereas he used to believe the traditional approach was more effective for some patients than for others, he's now persuaded that it is not optimal for *any* patient and is more damaging for some than for others (personal communication, 2002).

4. To the "needed" and "repeated" dimensions correspond the patient's "Type One" and "Type Two" projective identifications (Stern, 1994) that evoke distinctive reactions from the therapist that, on the one hand, re-create old experience and, on the on the other, make new experience possible. Stolorow et al. (1987) cover related ground with their "bipolar" conception of transference—that alternately threatens the patient with traumatic refinding and nurtures the patient psychologically by fulfilling unmet selfobject needs. Similarly, Weiss and Sampson's (1986) control-mastery theory can be seen as a guide to the transformation of repeated into needed enactments through transference tests in which the therapist either confirms or disconfirms the patient's pathogenic beliefs.

5. In this connection, it is worth underlining that—given each therapist's uniqueness—we cannot assume that the patient's experience in the treatment relationship necessarily matches his or her experience in other relationships. I find it helpful to suggest to patients that, very likely, there are both similarities and differences between what they experience with me and what they experience elsewhere—but that paying attention to the overlap may turn out to be very illuminating.

PART IV

ATTACHMENT PATTERNS
IN PSYCHOTHERAPY

V*ery little of what we do as therapists can be scripted in advance. As the Change Process Study Group has observed, psychotherapy proceeds through the* improvisation *of relational moves. Yet such improvisation is likelier to be helpful if the therapist's moves are informed by an awareness of what a developmentally facilitative relationship actually looks like.*

Attachment research has identified the features of collaborative dialogue associated with the development of security, resilience, and flexibility later in the child's life. Given the overlap between the change processes of childhood and psychotherapy, this research gives us a framework for fostering correspondingly collaborative dialogue with our patients. The research can also enable us to identify our patients' dominant attachment pattern(s) and thus to "imagine" their early relationships, including in particular what those relationships likely could and could not accommodate.

Chapter 11 translates the empirical findings into clinical recommendations for facilitating coherent communication and for assessing the particular "incoherencies" of our insecure patients. In so doing, it sets the stage for the following three chapters that detail the treatment implications of recognizing that the patient's prevailing state of mind with respect to attachment is dismissing, preoccupied, or unresolved.

CHAPTER 11

Constructing the
Developmental Crucible

Whether in childhood or psychotherapy, the provision of a secure base is a defining feature of a "good enough" attachment relationship. Such a relationship strengthens the vital capacity for affect regulation by fostering the individual's expectation that a stronger and wiser other will be available to help restore emotional equilibrium in the face of threat. It also fosters the flexible balance between connection and exploration that Ainsworth regarded as the signature of secure attachment. To the extent that this kind of relational experience can become portable—an "internalized secure base"—it gives our children and patients a resource of inestimable value. For it reinforces confidence in the self, trust in others, and the sense that the world is a safe place within which to love and to grow. The question, of course, is how we can generate such a relational experience.

FOSTERING COLLABORATIVE COMMUNICATION IN PSYCHOTHERAPY

Noting the convergence across multiple studies and research traditions, Lyons-Ruth (1999) identifies four key features of parent–child communication that are linked to the most positive developmental outcomes. Such communication is collaborative and coherent, and requires the parent to: (1) structure interaction so as to learn as much as possible about the child's feelings, desires, needs, and views; (2) initiate interactive repair when disruptions occur; (3) upgrade the dialogue to keep up with the child's emerg-

193

ing potentials; and (4) actively engage and struggle with the child during periods when her sense of sense of self and others is in flux.

Correspondingly, in light of the symmetry between what we provide as sensitively responsive parents and empathically attuned therapists, we should be aiming for: (1) an affective as well as linguistic dialogue that accommodates as much of the patient's subjective experience—feelings, thoughts, desires—as possible; (2) a sensitivity to disruptions in the relationship and a readiness to initiate repair; (3) a stance of acceptance combined with an expectation of a little more from the patient than she currently believes herself capable of; and (4) a willingness to confront, set limits, and struggle with the patient—as is often appropriate during periods heralding change in the patient's identity and in the therapeutic relationship.

In explaining how we might implement this framework in clinical practice, I'll be describing the ingredients of our *deliberate* effort to provide for the patient an attachment relationship that is friendlier to his psychological development than the relationships that launched him.

Make the Dialogue Inclusive

Our patients need us to help them access and express the full range of their subjective experience, including in particular their emotional experience. As Bowlby (1988) writes, "It is the emotional communications between a patient and his therapist that play the crucial part" (p. 157). Such questions as *What do you feel? What do you want? What do you believe is going on here now between the two of us?* (whether posed explicitly or silently entertained in the therapist's mind) must be a consistent feature of our effort to generate an inclusive dialogue.

They are often unanswerable by the patient precisely because they involve experiences of the sort that the patient's first relationships excluded. Therefore, we have to tune in to what the patient can only convey nonverbally. As discussed earlier, such implicit communication of the "unthought known" can be expressed through the patient's face, tone of voice, posture, or gesture. It can register in us as a feeling, bodily sensation, image, or thought, and it can be enacted in the relationship. Apprehending these kinds of implicit signals requires an oscillating attention to the patient, on the one hand, and our own subjective experience on the other. "Self-reflective responsiveness" (Mitchell, 1997) and "empathic introspective inquiry" (Stolorow et al., 1987) are terms that describe the sort of binocular vision I have in mind.

In the interest of including what might otherwise be excluded, I sometimes find it useful to make explicit my experience of the patient, of myself, or of our interaction. Putting such experience clearly into words can help

the patient to access dissociated or disowned aspects of her own experience.

> Recently, for example, I found myself feeling surprisingly unmoved by a patient's account of her relationship troubles. Silently wondering why, I noticed that the patient concluded nearly every statement with a rising inflection as if asking a question; she also spoke very quickly as if doubting that I had much patience for her story. When I shared these observations with her and suggested that perhaps she was feeling uncomfortable with what she was saying, or dubious about my interest, she demurred: "Not really. Not with all those 'you're entitled to your experience' kind of looks on your face." Yet I persisted, telling her of a conversation I'd overheard between two little girls. One spoke as if she were certain the other was interested, while the other, seeming less confident of her friend's attention, sped through her words and ended each sentence on a questioning note. To which my patient replied: "I think you're probably onto something, because as you were speaking I felt myself settling in, whereas before that I was just buzzing." It soon became clear to both of us that, despite her words to the contrary, she actually felt quite unentitled to her experience and assumed it wouldn't count for much with others.

Our patients' words often represent a very partial, and sometimes misleading, account of what they actually feel. Consequently, our empathy for a patient's immediate experience can be both an important starting place and—if we stop there—an obstacle to a more inclusive conversation. Frequently, for example, patients can articulate either their desire to change or their fear of changing. To integrate the two—for both are usually present—it can be useful for the therapist to speak to that side of the experience about which the patient is currently silent. In order for such a response to be meaningful, however, the patient must be able to find a reflection of herself in the therapist's words. When she can, such an intervention can enable the patient to feel recognized by the therapist at a deeper level and accepted as more of a whole person.

To foster the inclusive dialogue that makes integration possible, we need not only to *recognize* the patient's experience, especially emotional experience, but also to *communicate* that recognition in such a way that the patient feels understood. Yet often this feeling of being understood by the therapist is itself insufficient. To feel fully recognized, at such times, the patient must also feel *felt* (Siegel, 1999). Susan Coates (1998) puts it this way: "rather than get the patient's feeling, what the therapist must do is let the patient's feeling *get* to him or her (i.e., take him or her over in a way that is recognizable to the patient)" (p. 127). When affect is "contagious" and the therapist's response matches the quality of the patient's communication, it

can represent an exceptionally powerful form of contingent responsiveness and intersubjective meeting. Certainly such a response ratifies that what the patient is experiencing—perhaps with considerable trepidation—can, in fact, be contained in the relationship with the therapist.

Beyond the responsiveness that allows our patients to feel recognized and felt, there are two further elements to the therapist's communication that further the goals of inclusiveness and integration. In this connection, Fonagy's suggestion that parents in response to their child's distress should provide empathy, a coping attitude, and attention to the child's "intentional stance" is entirely to the point. In psychotherapy, as in childhood, the individual certainly needs the empathic resonance, attunement, and mirroring of the other. But, as Fonagy's prescription implies, our patients need more than mirroring if they are to sense that their relationship with us is safe enough to risk fuller self-revelation.

First, our patients need to experience us as capable of helping them to cope with their difficult feelings—otherwise, why should they allow themselves to feel any more than they have to? Paraphrasing Schore (2003), attachment *is* the interactive regulation of emotion. Such regulation depends significantly on our own ability to tolerate and manage painful feelings. When this ability is well developed, we are generally able not only to recognize and resonate with the patient's difficult feelings, but also to communicate that they can indeed be coped with. Here an attitude of calm is useful (if we can muster it) as well as behavior that expresses our desire to understand and, through understanding, to help.

Second, we must respond to the underlying intentions, feelings, and beliefs that are the context within which our patients' words and behavior can be seen to make sense. Responding in this way, in light of the "intentional stance" of our patients, allows them to feel understood in depth—and this translates into a feeling of being accepted. Feeling understood and accepted fosters confidence that their experiences—even those they have had to bury—can be safely contained in the new attachment relationship.

Perhaps most important to encouraging an inclusive dialogue, we have to be emotionally present in order to be receptive enough, and involved enough, to sense what is emotionally alive in the patient, even (or especially) when it is not being expressed directly.

Actively Initiate Repair

Our empathy, deliberate self-disclosure, and/or interpretation can be enlisted to restore equilibrium in the therapeutic couple. Whatever the intervention, repairing a rupture usually involves some form of intersubjective negotiation. Resolving conflict through negotiation with the therapist rein-

forces the patient's trust that the secure base is, in fact, secure—that it can survive the strain of disappointment, difference, and protest.

Returning to therapy after a two-week vacation, Randall, a patient I had seen for several years, spoke in a familiarly "objective" way about his fear that he would never be able to have a lasting intimate relationship. He said he was afraid of being rejected, but lost interest whenever someone was seriously interested in him. He asked what I would suggest, after a preamble implying that what I'd offered to date had not done the trick. Rather too facetiously, I suggested that he try psychotherapy.

Randall looked a little startled; clearly he was not amused. Complaining that therapy of late had not been of much use to him, he alluded to an earlier period during which we had been looking closely at our relationship. Then, he said, our work together had been emotionally involving and valuable to him—but certainly not now.

I found myself thinking that recently (today being a case in point) he had seemed to me to be quite disengaged. For my part, I had noticed earlier in the hour that I was feeling less close to him than I would have expected. Possibly my "joke" reflected my frustration at his distance and deprecation. Then I recalled that the hour before his vacation, I had been feeling preoccupied. Consequently he might well have experienced *me* as distant, and perhaps rejecting.

In the course of several exchanges, I said to him that the wish he'd expressed for my help might have felt especially urgent in light of his intensifying desire for a romantic partner and his fear that we might be making no progress. Then I asked if he had retained any impression of our last session. He told me he'd found it very depressing, all our talk then about the dead ends in his quest for a mate. I said, "I'm not sure that what I'm about to say is related to your feeling depressed then, but I know that I had a lot on my mind during that hour. I suspect I was having a hard time being present and you might very well have picked up on that." I added that in this context, my rather flip remark might have been jarring, at the very least.

He became a little tearful telling me he was relieved to hear my words: He had thought I was withdrawn and had worried that perhaps I was angry at him for saying "no" to an earlier request of mine to change the time of our appointment. As the hour ended, he expressed his appreciation, saying that he felt connected to me again.

Such sequences of disruption and repair—particularly repair initiated by the therapist—strengthen the patient's confidence that the relationship can be relied on to contain difficult feelings and help resolve them. In the process, they build the patient's capacity to make use of interactive affect regulation which is a forerunner of self-regulation. Successive episodes of repair tend, in addition, to disconfirm the patient's preexisting transference

expectations—in my patient's case, the expectation, borne of experience with his astoundingly narcissistic mother, that no one would ever take responsibility for problems they caused and that he alone would be held liable.

Upgrade the Dialogue

Bromberg (1998b) describes psychotherapy as a process that allows patients to change while staying the same. Along the same lines, Friedman (1988) suggests that we as therapists need to accept our patients on their own terms while also refusing to settle for those terms. Striking this kind of balance requires us to assume that our patients are capable of somewhat more feeling, thoughtfulness, connection, or initiative than they believe they are. Expect too little and the patient may feel his hopes have been betrayed; expect too much and the patient may feel his vulnerabilities have gone unrecognized.

Upgrading the therapeutic dialogue to higher levels of awareness and complexity requires what developmentalists call "scaffolding." Parents, for example, scaffold their child's emerging capacity for language by speaking *for* her before she acquires the words to describe her own experience and later by asking her to "use your words."

Therapists can similarly scaffold their patients' emerging capacities for feeling, reflection, initiative, and so on. In practice this may sometimes require us to speak for the patient, say, by articulating her unarticulated or unrecognized feelings. At other times, our receptive silence is called for, in order to make room for the patient to feel, or feel more deeply. And at certain moments we may need to bridge the dialogue to a more openly emotional level by "going first" and expressing our own feelings.

To help kindle the reflective capacity we usually need to talk about the mental states that underlie the patient's experience and, sometimes, about how hard it is for the patient to consider her experience in this way. We may also want to let the patient in on our own efforts to make sense of experience: In the process, we "model" mentalization. To strengthen the capacity for agency or initiative, we may need to keep a focus both on what the patient wants for herself (inside and outside therapy) and on her difficulty knowing or acting on what she wants. We may also decide to share our quandary about how to actively foster the patient's initiative without implicitly usurping it through our activity.

One of the most effective ways to upgrade the dialogue is to make the dialogue itself the focus of discussion. Having a "conversation about the conversation" is an *inter*personal version of an *intra*personal development that we aim to promote in all our patients—namely, the development of

mentalizing. Remember that the medium here is the message: In fostering a metacommunicative dialogue—that is, communication about the communication—we may also be fostering metacognition, also known as thinking about thought. For patients who are all too embedded in their experience, this kind of dialogue helps open the door to deeper, more emotionally informed reflection.

Consider, by way of illustration, the patient just discussed to whom I made the offhand (but "overdetermined") suggestion that he "try psychotherapy." Having fairly successfully repaired the rupture occasioned by my remark, we found ourselves returning in the next session to the scene of the crime.

Randall is struck that he seems to "hunt for rejection" as if to confirm the mistrust that makes it so difficult for him to really be himself in his encounters with others. I say that he seems burdened by a similar mistrust here, and remind him of his initial reluctance to tell me of his disappointment, his sense that I had withdrawn from him, and his fear that I was angry. A little exasperated, he says, "So what am I supposed to do? Ask what's going on with you? Tell you you're not doing this right? You're the expert here. I'm sure you'd be upset." I say that, given this expectation, I can understand his relief and appreciation last week at my willingness to consider my role in the difficulties between us. He replies that this kind of openness has been one of the most meaningful features of his experience with me, virtually from the start. Each time I've been willing to admit my part, he says, he has been surprised and moved.

"Do you notice," I ask him, "that even though you've had the same emotionally telling experience with me a number of times, it still always comes as a surprise? It's as if you can connect with the experience and feel more trusting, but only for the moment. So the next time something is really bothering you, something you don't like or something you need from me that you're not getting, it's very hard for you to speak up."

After a longish silence, he says, "It never even occurs to me to speak up. The whole things is automatic, I don't question it. It's like I've got a moat around me. I'm not coming out from behind the walls because other people always feel like they could be dangerous. But maybe that's part of the hunt for rejection I was talking about before, like I don't want to take in your response, so it doesn't stick, it's always a big surprise. I'm thinking now that if you or anybody else really cared for me and seemed safe, it's like I wouldn't know what to do with it."

Conversations about the conversation—about what's ruled in and what's ruled out—facilitate change in the patient's internal rules and mod-

els by allowing him more than a single perspective on experience. (This is, of course, the essence of the reflective stance that makes possible greater freedom not only to reflect but also to feel and to connect.) By enabling the patient to stand, as it were, in two places at once—both inside the experience as a participant and outside it as an observer—such conversations upgrade the dialogue to new levels of awareness and complexity.

Be Willing to Engage and Struggle

At times, a child invariably requires a parent to come up against, a parent to provide the structure the child needs. And invariably, as the child grows up, the parent is required to loosen the structure and relinquish greater initiative to the child. Much the same can be said in relation to what the patient needs from the therapist.

It must be understood that our patients at times need confrontation more than they need empathy. To the extent that this understanding goes against the grain for many of us, it can be useful to remind ourselves that the therapeutic relationship is also a *real* relationship: Just as we would not knowingly countenance destructive behavior in our other relationships, we certainly would not want to do so in relation to our patients. Accepting the patient is in no way inconsistent with taking a stand against his self-defeating conduct, inside or outside therapy.

I had struggled for several years with a chronically, acutely suicidal male patient, simply to keep him alive. After too many harrowing close calls, multiple hospitalizations, and the achievement through arduous limit setting of a structure that finally seemed to make real progress possible, I listened to the patient tell me that, yes, the structure we had established was indeed important, and, yes, we might now be in a position to get somewhere, but that I needed to know one thing: He *was* eventually going to kill himself. Hearing the patient's words, I blew up. The expurgated version: "You can talk about suicide all you want, but I refuse to let you hold the threat of it over my head! You do *not* have a terminal disease and I'm not *ever* signing on to provide hospice care for you." Hearing my words, the patient settled down, seemed relieved, and actually appeared grateful for my anger. Then he told me again, as he had before, that he needed me to be "bigger" than he was. Needless to say, my enraged response to this patient was unpremeditated and I'm not recommending it as a technique. Nevertheless, it illustrates that our attuned responsiveness can take unexpected forms.

In the intimate partnership that is psychotherapy, our willingness to struggle serves not only to protect both partners but also to make room for the patient's protest and anger. Such active engagement helps avoid the pit-

fall to which one patient of mine delicately alluded: "How can I be shitty, when you're so nice?" The therapist who sets a limit or spontaneously expresses displeasure at the patient's conduct *may* give the patient a context within which to develop the sense that she can be separate in a relationship while also maintaining connection.

In the wake of such potentially unsettling moments, what will be decisive is the degree of "fittedness" or intersubjective understanding between the partners that can eventually be achieved. The event itself—say, the expression of anger by patient and/or therapist—is one thing, while the process through which its meaning gels is quite another. Usually, it is this follow-up that consolidates the therapeutic value of the event—particularly when the process involves negotiation that softens hard feelings and restores the sense of a bond or alliance between the two partners. Notice the synergy here among several key aspects of "collaborative communication": Active engagement is conducive to an inclusive dialogue as well as to sequences of disruption and repair.

The need to struggle and to actively provide structure may be particularly pronounced with patients who might be described as disorganized or unresolved with respect to trauma. Yet, early in treatment, as we are about to see, nearly every patient benefits from the provision by the therapist of a modicum of structure.

INITIATING THE PATIENT INTO PSYCHOTHERAPY

Lyons-Ruth (1999) suggests that collaborative dialogue involves "getting to know another's mind and taking it into account in structuring and regulating interactions" (p. 583). In taking the mind of our patients into account, we have to assume that most of them require an orientation to the unfamiliar rules and roles of psychotherapy. Initiating our patients involves a process of helping them to become actively engaged in a relationship that can't succeed without their collaboration. Much of this initiation occurs implicitly, of course. But keeping the structure of therapy a mystery does the patient a disservice. To foster collaboration we need to be explicit with our patients about what we expect of them and what they can expect of us. The therapeutic relationship is a unique one with no parallel in ordinary social interaction and, therefore, the therapist must assume responsibility for "training" the patient how to make the best possible use of the relationship.

In an initial hour, I generally begin by asking new patients what they are hoping for from this sort of ongoing conversation with a therapist. Later in the hour, if it appears that we may be going forward with treat-

ment, I usually add that it may take a few sessions for us to get clear about exactly what we're going to be working on together. As therapists, we often need to walk a fine line between accepting the patient's goals (or definition of the problem) as our own and imposing our goals (or definition of the problem) on the patient. For example, a dismissing patient may want us to help him become more self-sufficient, while we believe it would be better for him were he less compulsively self-reliant.

In subsequent sessions, particularly when patients seem uncertain about how to make the best use of their time with me, I may suggest that they say whatever comes to mind that seems relevant to the therapeutic goals we've identified. This communication and others like it are aimed at letting patients know what I expect from them and how I think we can most effectively work together. With regard to what patients can expect from me, my communication here is both implicit and explicit. Alongside what I express implicitly though the quality of my responsiveness, I usually make a point of being explicit about what I think I'm doing with them and why. Such explicitness may well be of use to most patients, but it is essential for those who are insecurely attached or unresolved with respect to trauma or loss, because they so often have difficulty accurately reading others' intentions on the basis of their nonverbal cues alone.

The rationale for exploring the therapeutic relationship is almost never self-evident to our patients. Yet the need to be explicit about how a focus on their interactions with the therapist can help them reach their goals in treatment is often ignored. For most of our patients, this vital way of working (formally described as transference–countertransference analysis) simply does not make sense, since, quite understandably, they are far more interested in looking at the relationships they have *outside* therapy. Thus if patients are to do more than simply comply with our lead, they must be given an explanation or, better still, a demonstration of the usefulness of this approach.

Most desirable is to link the patient's stated problems or goals with what is going on in the relationship with the therapist. Here's an example of what I have in mind:

A female patient told me in our first session that her relationships with men always fell apart because, as she put it, "I never met a man I couldn't find fault with." Previous therapy had begun to give her some insight into this pattern of defensive devaluation. Early in our work, not very surprisingly, she began to find fault with me. Her impression, she complained, was that I was cold and unsympathetic. She added that this was troubling to her, looking ahead, because "leopards don't change their spots." At this point, I said to her something like the fol-

lowing: "I'm sure you remember telling me you wanted to work with a male therapist to get some insight into how you relate to men. I'll bet if we take a look at what's going on now between the two of us *here* we might very well get some insight into what goes on in your relationships with men out there. I say this because it *may* be that you're on the verge of repeating with me the very pattern you say has doomed your relationships with other men." These words caught her attention, prompting an exploration of the possible parallels between her experiences inside therapy and out. They also helped her appreciate that focusing on our interaction might help her become aware of aspects of her interactions with men that she had not yet been able to articulate to herself or to me.

Conversations like this one generally have to occur more than once before patients can begin to fully collaborate with us in making use of the transference–countertransference enactments that arise in every therapeutic relationship. Usually, of course, it is the therapist who must take the lead in focusing attention on the here-and-now interaction. The point at which patients first take the initiative in exploring their here-and-now experience of the relationship, including their perceptions of, and feelings about, the therapist, is a marker of real collaboration.

When we initiate the patient in this way, we also set the stage for an effective approach to specific events in the therapeutic relationship that have particular salience within an attachment framework.

SEPARATIONS, INTERRUPTIONS, AND TERMINATION

Separation and loss are as central to Bowlby's theory as attachment is. It was in fact the need to understand the profound developmental impact of children's experiences of separation and loss that led to the original formulation of attachment theory. Considering that attachment is vital to the child's emotional and physical survival, the loss of the attachment figure—including the temporary loss that is separation—can be seen as the prototypical attachment trauma. Therefore, in the patient's new attachment relationship, events that involve the real or feared loss of the therapist, temporarily or permanently, will usually evoke feelings—or defenses against feelings—that are directly related to the patient's attachment history.

When development has been marred by loss or trauma that remains unresolved, the patient may react to the therapist's vacation, for example, as if it threatened catastrophe. A resourceful and energetic, but highly self-destructive patient became paranoid and briefly suicidal the first time my summer break interrupted our work. Like many patients with a history of

unresolved loss, he could not easily differentiate between a temporary separation and an irreversible abandonment. And as is frequently the case with such patients, progress in this man's therapy was signaled by a gradual toning down of his distress in response to our separations. Slowly he came to realize that a break in our relationship was not the same as the relationship being broken and that my wanting a break was not the same as my wanting to get away from *him*.

Progress of this kind hinges centrally on the therapist's ability to make room for the patient's responses to loss as they are evoked by separations, including at times even the separation occasioned by the ending of the session. A disciplined attention to the impact of separation fosters the sort of inclusive dialogue that makes integration possible. Working with separation is also a way to ensure that disruptions in the relationship are repaired. Finally, dealing effectively with reactions to separation contributes to the patient's confidence in the relationship as a secure base.

Not infrequently, a patient will react strongly to a separation without realizing that his reaction was actually triggered by the separation. Often, it is only through our persistent focus on the patient's characteristic responses to breaks that the meaning of these responses can be clarified. But, of course, it is not just a matter of meaning. When we make room for the patient's reactions and respond in an attuned way, we make a new experience possible. For note that it is not loss or trauma per se that eventuates in disorganized attachment, but rather loss or trauma that has never been resolved. When we work with the patient's reactions to the potential trauma of *new* loss—as represented, say, by the therapist's vacation—we heighten the probability that the patient, rather than being retraumatized, may have a healing experience of resolution.

Many of our patients, like the one whose experience I described a moment ago, have suffered in childhood precisely the sorts of severe loss that research associates with an unresolved state of mind with respect to attachment. Yet loss of a different, less disorganizing kind is a feature of the history of most of our patients, the majority of whom we might describe as insecurely attached.

To provide a context here, recall that young children who endure protracted separations from their parents exhibit a characteristic sequence of reactions (Bowlby, 1969/1982). First, there is *protest*—expressed actively, tearfully, angrily as if the sheer intensity of the child's distress might bring about the parent's return. Then there is *despair:* As hope seems to wane, the child though still tearful, becomes increasingly quiet and inactive, as if in a state of deep mourning. Finally, as hope fails, despair shades into *detachment:* The child, despite a superficial sociability and even cheerfulness, now seems remote, having apparently lost all interest in the parent whose absence was so recently and painfully mourned.

Protest, despair, and detachment are phases of response to dramatic losses that might be described as acute. The less dramatic losses that figure in the experience of many insecurely attached patients are chronic.

Often we find that adults with an anxiously preoccupied attachment style have grown up with parents who were unpredictably responsive— alternately present or absent, moderately attuned or immoderately mis-attuned. Thus, such adults experienced when they were children the repeated loss of the (available and attuned) attachment figure. Then and now, their behavior in attachment relationships—including that with the therapist—reflects their fear of such loss. Like the child in the phase of protest, they are intensely emotional, both as a reaction to the threat of loss and as a strategy to avert it. Patients like these need us neither to write off their emotionality as manipulation nor to be knocked off center by it. We have to make room for their protest—their tears and anger—without ratifying their sense that, on their own, they are helpless.

By contrast, dismissing adults behave like children in the detachment phase of Bowlby's sequence. Research suggests that adults like these have frequently had emotionally distant parents who rejected their early overtures for comfort and connection, such that as infants they were never allowed to be babies. The detachment of dismissing adults from others and from their own feelings is thus a response to their hopelessness about being cared for; it also provides protection both from further loss in the present and from the sadness that is the legacy of past loss. Dismissing patients need us to help them connect to the needs they minimize and the feelings they avoid.

In general, present losses evoke echoes of the losses of the past. For the patient in psychotherapy, every break in the continuity of the relationship is a potential trigger for old feelings and old defenses—and a potential opportunity to address unfinished business around separation and attachment. Depending on their predominant state of mind with respect to attachment, our patients tend to react to separation in different ways—as do we. Patients and therapists in a preoccupied state of mind often become anxious around separation, while those who are dismissing generally respond as if it were a nonevent. And, as I've mentioned, adults who are unresolved may become disorganized or disoriented when faced with separation. It is vital that we be aware of our own characteristic responses to separation, lest we risk repeating with our patients problematic scenarios with which they (and we) may already be far too familiar. A dismissing therapist, for example, may collude with a dismissing patient in treating separations as if they were insignificant—which is tantamount to affirming that attachment itself is insignificant.

The ultimate separation in psychotherapy comes, of course, with termination. While patients can (and sometimes do) return after therapy is

over, concluding treatment is invariably a process with enormous emotional significance and therapeutic potential. It can be deeply affecting—painful and bittersweet—to experience the prospect of ending the new attachment relationship that therapy has provided. As such, termination provides an extended opportunity to revisit and further resolve the patient's past and present issues around attachment and loss. Needless to say, termination involves not only an emotionally charged backward look, but also the possibility of saying goodbye in a way that is as complete and fully felt as possible.

I'll have more to say about the different attachment categories in the chapters that follow, but here are a few generalizations that bear directly upon termination: Preoccupied patients with their fear of abandonment and their overplayed helplessness may need the therapist to structure therapy's end when the time is appropriate—and to make room for the patient's resulting protest. Dismissing patients who avoid their feelings and minimize the importance of relationships may need the therapist to bar the door in order to make room for the emotional experience the patient both fears and desires. Unresolved patients who can be undone by loss, but are also terrified of being alone, may need the therapist to legitimize a staggered termination in which they may leave "prematurely" with the understanding that they can (and very probably will) return to treatment when it feels necessary and tolerable to do so.

ASSESSING THE PATIENT'S STATE OF MIND
WITH RESPECT TO ATTACHMENT

Recognizing the patient's prevailing state of mind with respect to attachment can enable the therapist to identify what may be the primary organizing principle(s) or guiding metaphor(s) that give a characteristic shape not only to the patient's relationships, but also to the various facets of the patient's self.

Consider, for example, a patient with an avoidant attachment style. Having grown up with emotionally distant parents who were rejecting and/or controlling, such a patient does to himself (and others) what was done to him. He tends in relationships to be the one who rejects, makes distance, and attempts to exert control. He rejects, distances from, and tries to control his feelings. Initially experiencing his goals and desires as his own, he can easily come to feel controlled by them and inclined, consequently, to reject them. He is, in short, as out of touch with himself and others as his parents were out of touch with him. The guiding metaphor here is self-isolation to avoid being rejected or controlled.

Identifying the patient's state of mind with respect to attachment also enables the therapist (in a tentative and provisional way) to envision the patient's childhood and make informed guesses about the patient's formative relationships. What kinds of feelings, desires, thoughts, and behavior could these relationships accommodate? What did the patient need to deny or suppress? What relational and affect-regulating strategies was the patient required to adopt in order to maintain the attachment bond? Answering such questions helps us determine what the patient may need from us. Recognizing the feelings, desires, and abilities that the patient has had to deny or inhibit helps to clarify the kinds of responsiveness we might most usefully attempt to provide.

There are a variety of ways to identify the patient's predominant attachment pattern(s). Patients generally have a different "feel" depending on their state of mind with respect to attachment—and we may tend, correspondingly, to feel differently when we are with them. In addition, familiar and easily recognizable diagnostic categories (obsessive, hysteric, borderline, etc.) tend to map pretty well onto the attachment classifications. However, the most valuable clues for identifying our patients' attachment patterns come from the Adult Attachment Interview.

Clinical Assessment and the AAI

Although the AAI is a research instrument, it is structured very much like a clinical interview. In drawing conclusions from a research subject's AAI narrative, the emphasis is on process and form rather than content—just as it should be in an initial session with a patient. Spoken content is by no means irrelevant, but the ultimate aim of assessment in AAI research and therapy alike is to grasp aspects of the person that *cannot* be spoken about directly. For the "state of mind with respect to attachment" (Main, 1995, p. 437) is the product of internal working models and the rules they encode, which are largely nonconscious and implicit. Hence, what turns out to be most revealing is not what someone can explicitly *tell* us but what he implicitly *shows* us through his mode of discourse (Main, 2000).

Through AAI research that has been replicated many times, Main demonstrated that coherent and collaborative discourse reflects secure working models, and that, conversely, discourse marred by incoherence, irrelevance, and/or lapses in reasoning reflects working models that are insecure or disorganized. The discovery that an individual's *discourse* about attachment reflects that individual's internal working model(s) of attachment is directly applicable to clinical assessment in the therapeutic setting. Along with what patients evoke in us, enact with us, and embody, the *way*

patients use words reveals, paradoxically, aspects of experience that cannot be put into words.

The patient is, by definition, someone whose distress has brought him for help to someone else who is presumed to be stronger and wiser. Thus, the initial hour or two of psychotherapy (like the Strange Situation and the AAI itself) is a context geared to activate attachment behavior, or defenses against such behavior. Probably from the first phone call and certainly on crossing the threshold to the therapist's office, the patient begins to show us his characteristic ways of attaching. It is particularly revealing to listen to the way the patient talks to us, for research using the AAI has codified the distinctive ways in which secure, dismissing, preoccupied, or unresolved adults tend to communicate about attachment.

How coherent is the patient's communication? And how collaborative is it? To identify the patient's state of mind with respect to attachment, these are the key questions to keep in mind as we listen. Taking our cues from the AAI, we need to attend to four aspects of the patient's discourse that Main—following the philosopher Paul Grice (1989)—calls quality, quantity, relation, and manner.

With regard to *quality*, the issue is the patient's truthfulness: Does he have evidence for what he says? Or, are we left with the impression that the patient's assertions are unsupported or contradicted by what he says later?

With regard to *quantity*, can the patient be succinct, yet complete, in his communication? Or, do we feel either swamped by extraneous detail or left clueless by the brevity of the patient's responses to our questions?

As for *relation*, can the patient remain relevant to the topic at hand? This is another way of asking if the patient can tune in to his own experience while also keeping our questions in mind.

Finally, with regard to *manner*, can the patient communicate in a clear and orderly way? Or, is the patient vague, confused or confusing, and/or illogical?

In general, patients who are secure can communicate truthfully and succinctly, while remaining relevant and clear. They can talk thoughtfully and with vivid affect about emotionally evocative experiences. They seem capable, even when absorbed in strong feeling, of staying connected to the therapist and mindful of the purpose of the conversation.

Dismissing patients, by contrast, have a hard time being coherent and collaborative. In particular, they have trouble being truthful: They often fail to support, and sometimes contradict, what they assert. They are also overly succinct and have very little to say about attachment-related experiences, often explaining that they simply don't remember. Very likely, the insistence on lack of recall is tied to the relational context in which their habits of representation developed: To maintain the best possible attachment, it

served them not to be aware of, and not to remember desires, feelings, or experiences related to the need for connection.

Correspondingly, dismissing patients may have little to say about the difficulties that bring them to therapy; communicating about such difficulties risks activating the attachment system. In keeping with the finding that the AAI transcripts of dismissing adults tend to be the shortest, dismissing patients often fall silent, leaving the therapist to fill the airtime.

The communication of preoccupied patients presents very much of a contrast: They may be truthful, but they are rarely succinct, relevant, or clear. Their intense and troubling feelings, especially about past attachments, often contribute to a narrative that can be tangential, vague, and hard to follow. As if the pressure of their distress overwhelms their ability to collaborate, these patients seem to have an impossible time staying with the topics about which we've asked. As a result, the session may be over before such patients can get to the apparent point of their story. Asked about childhood relationships, they may discuss current ones—and vice versa. Old feelings of anger, fear, or helplessness in relation to parents seem to spill into their present relationships, including that with the therapist.

Not long ago, I received from a preoccupied patient a nearly interminable phone message that ended only when the recording time on my answering machine ran out. The patient began speaking in a very adult tone, but gradually shifted into what sounded like the voice of a desperately unhappy little girl. So preoccupied is this patient with the unresolved attachments of her past that she can drift in the present into a mode of relating akin to that of a small child forlornly beseeching her unresponsive father for help.

As this example suggests, preoccupied states of mind sometimes overlap with unresolved ones, particularly in the way in which absorption in the disturbing events of the past can color communication in the present. The communication of unresolved patients is marked by what Main (1995) calls "lapses in the monitoring of reasoning or discourse" (p. 442). When touching on attachment and themes of trauma or loss, the discourse of these patients can briefly depart from ordinary reasoning about space, time, and causality. The patient I've just described worried that her mother had died because the patient had stopped thinking about her; another patient talked about her long dead father as if he were still alive.

Lapses in discourse may be reflected in rather striking shifts in the patient's tone of voice or bearing, of a kind that suggest the patient has entered a different and dissociated state of consciousness. And, indeed, dissociation is a frequent feature of the experience of unresolved patients. The patient may seem suddenly dreamy, or begin to speak in a whispery tone of voice. Or, having begun to talk about a disturbing experience, a patient

who had been sitting might now lie on his side on the couch, facing toward the therapist, or even facing away.

In the pages that follow I'll focus on the therapeutic implications that flow from a recognition that the patient's predominant state of mind with respect to attachment is dismissing, preoccupied, or unresolved. In particular, I'll be considering the kind of relationship we might deliberately attempt to foster so as to integrate aspects of the patient's experience that have previously been disowned or dissociated.

CHAPTER 12

The Dismissing Patient
From Isolation to Intimacy

In conventional diagnostic terms, dismissing patients can be seen to fall on a continuum with obsessives at one end and narcissists and schizoids at the other. Such patients all have enormous difficulty trusting others enough to be genuinely intimate with them, even though they may have stable long-term relationships. And they are no more intimate with themselves. Their "compulsive self-reliance" (Bowlby, 1969/1982) and defensive overestimation of their own value require that they remain remote from whatever feelings, thoughts, or desires might provoke them to seek support, connection, or care from others.

They cannot extinguish their biologically driven attachment needs, however. Dismissing adults may claim in the AAI context to feel that "all is well," but physiological measurement indicates otherwise—just as avoidant infants display little distress in the Strange Situation while elevations in their heart rate and stress hormones tell a different story (Fox & Card, 1999). Clearly our dismissing patients are reluctant to feel emotions that might spur them to connect deeply to others, and even more reluctant to express such emotions. Yet only through making an emotional connection with these patients can we actually engage them in the kind of relationship that makes change possible. The key here is to follow the affect.

We have to be keenly attuned to the dismissing patient's subtle affective cues, usually as these are communicated through the body. What do we see in the patient's eyes? (Is his gaze averted, possibly in shame, or directed

downward, as in sadness? Do his eyes appear moist, as if he might be moved? Are his upper eyelids raised, as in an angry glare?) What do we observe in the set of the patient's jaw, mouth, or brow? What might be expressed in his posture? And what can we infer from his tone of voice?

Perhaps even more important, we need to tune in to subtle shifts in our own psychobiological state as we sit with the patient. For what patients are reluctant to feel, they will often inadvertently evoke in their therapist. Shifts in our internal experience are rarely unrelated to the emotional experience of the patient. Attention to our internal experience tends to be most fruitful when we can be at once quite deliberate about allowing ourselves to feel and not overly concerned with concealing our feelings. (Recall Ekman's research showing that adopting a poker face flattens not only the expression but also the *experience* of emotion.) Bringing our own feelings to the treatment of dismissing patients can help them to begin to integrate their own dissociated feelings.

But for psychotherapy to provide the secure base that makes such integration possible, the therapist has to matter to the patient—and allowing the therapist to matter is, of course, at odds with the deactivating strategy of the dismissing patient, which depends on diminishing the importance of others. Thus the central challenge is to enable the patient to allow the therapist to matter.

More often than not, such a patient begins treatment behaving as if the therapist either has little to offer or represents a threat that must be kept at bay. The Catch-22 here is that the patient's barriers against feeling make it impossible for him to feel much for the therapist, while the therapist's relative insignificance to the patient reinforces the barriers against feeling. Of course, this is the essence of the dismissing adult's defensive strategy in the face of his broader life problem. The patient's self-protective constriction of feeling and avoidance of closeness generate the emotional and relational difficulties that typically bring the patient to therapy.

Finding our way through that Catch-22 requires that we balance empathic attunement with confrontation. Usually patients need the former in order to feel that we understand them. Often the dismissing patient, in particular, needs the latter in order to feel that we exist—that we can have an impact upon him and that he can have an impact upon us. To really get to the dismissing patient, we may need to let the patient know how he gets to us.

EMPATHY AND CONFRONTATION

Both empathic attunement and confrontation are geared to the essential aim of opening the patient to more of his emotional experience. For with

regard to feeling, the dismissing patient is very much a closed system, having learned that the acknowledgement and expression of distress would likely result in frustration, or worse.

Putting our empathy for the patient's experience into words may diminish the patient's fear that we are controlling or rejecting, in which case such a response will be reassuring. But it can also backfire. Dismissing patients, we may assume, knew little in the way of empathy from attachment figures when they were growing up. As a result, our empathic communication may be Greek to them; they may experience it as a lame substitute for "real" help ("Is that all you have to offer?"); or—because empathy can evoke the multiple threats associated with closeness and dependency—they may be unconsciously compelled to reject it.

While I almost invariably lead with empathy, believing it provides an essential ongoing background of safety, I find with dismissing patients that in order to connect with them early in treatment something more than empathic mirroring is necessary and, for that matter, something more than interpretation. The "something more" here is the deliberate or spontaneous expression of our subjective experience of what it's like to be on the receiving end of the patient's communication. This is what I'm calling confrontation.

Letting the patient in on our experience of the relationship usually means disclosing something of what we're feeling, and our showing some emotion may be particularly important with patients who feel so little of their own. Their self-awareness is severely constricted by what they can't allow themselves to feel, think, or remember. Their preverbal experiences are lost to explicit memory and their later recollections may never have been encoded because of the deactivating in these patients of the strong emotions that ordinarily "tag" experience as worth remembering.

But what such patients lack access to in themselves may nonetheless be evoked in others, including the therapist. Thus, our subjective experience may provide a key route to their otherwise inaccessible feelings, thoughts, and memories. Moreover, since the defensive strategy of dismissing patients compromises their ability to empathize and, in turn, blocks their awareness of their impact on others, our subjective experience can be an exceptionally vital resource when it is divulged to them.

Recall the patient I discussed in Chapter 8—a forceful, rather intellectual executive—with whom I found myself anxiously "bulletproofing" my words as if I were facing the threat of prosecution. When I disclosed this experience to "Gordon," he was astonished. It seemed to him that I was giving voice to *his* experience of feeling somehow endangered—an experience for which he had previously lacked the words, but which had driven him to "goldplate" his performance at work lest he be judged or attacked. He recalled his mother, a Holocaust survivor, making the assumption that

he was anxious at work ("You must be the only Jew there"). His feeling of being under threat seemed to be the legacy of his mother's history, the probable result of the intergenerational transmission of trauma. Confronting patients like Gordon with the therapist's experience of the relationship with them has the potential both to connect them to their own emotional experience and to illuminate something of their impact on others.

Sometimes, but by no means always, confrontation has the kind of "edge" the word brings to mind. Previously I mentioned a somewhat reluctant patient who in an early session made it clear that she was finding my every word and gesture of attuned understanding completely useless. To my empathic overtures, she responded as if I were actually an adversary toward whom she was becoming increasingly contemptuous. After 20 minutes or so of this futile and frustrating exchange, I told the patient (with a bit of an edge) that I was beginning to feel quite exasperated with her, that this was not my customary response to her, and that we needed to understand exactly what was going on here. A little taken aback, the patient collected herself, then admitted that her relationships at home and at work were regularly marred by her tendency to be contentious and, sometimes, bullying.

Such patients, especially (though not exclusively) early in treatment, have one foot in (if that) and one foot out. They can appear to be "resistant" in the old problematic sense of the term—that is, they can seem to be functioning in opposition to the therapist or the aims of therapy. But understanding the dismissing patient's apparent resistance as a *communication* is far more useful and true to the patient's experience. In being reluctant, unengaged, or controlling, these patients are conveying their fears of closeness and dependency. And as attachment research makes clear, dismissing patients have come by these fears honestly: In the context of their attachment history, acknowledging the need for help may feel like an invitation to rejection or a humiliating admission of insufficiency.

Needing help and not finding it is always a risk, but *getting* it may represent an even greater risk. To feel helped in a significant relationship is to risk destabilizing a dominant conscious working model in which the self is valued as strong and complete while the other is devalued as weak and dependent. What is likely to surface in its place is the feared unconscious model in which the self is helpless and vulnerable while the other is rejecting, controlling, or punitive; under the sway of this model, the patient is liable to feel angry as well as anxious. Moreover, experiencing the therapist as someone who is willing and able to help may evoke a terrible sadness in relation to earlier attachment figures who were unable or unwilling to do so.

Psychotherapy places dismissing patients in a bind by implicitly invit-

ing their dependency upon a new attachment figure whose help cannot be expected to be helpful. As therapists, we may begin to disconfirm this expectation when we shift between efforts to attune to the patient's experience, on the one hand, and to recognize—and sometimes disclose—our own experience, on the other. Perhaps it should be clarified here that what can appear to be two opposing modes of responsiveness nearly always interact.

After all, I am able to understand and empathize with the patient largely through, and on the basis of, my own experience. In this connection, I'll occasionally preface my words to the patient by saying that my understanding of him derives from experiences of mine that may (or may not) turn out to be relevant to his. Additionally, in the process of deliberate self-disclosure, I usually find myself feeling more attuned, as well as closer, to the patient. Conversely, the experience of empathizing with the patient, and sometimes expressing that empathy directly, often leads me to feel more self-knowledgeable and more connected to myself.

THERAPEUTIC INTERACTION AND THE DISMISSING PATIENT

An authentic expression of the therapist's subjectivity may be necessary in order for the dismissing patient to *feel* the therapist's presence as a separate person. This is especially true when the patient has experienced his parents as rejecting or emotionally absent, in which case the therapist's affective responses may be bracing, but also reassuring. Even when the patient has felt overly controlled by his parents and has consequently drawn inward, it may be important to hear from the therapist, as a sometimes vulnerable human being with the ability to feel and express feelings.

Particularly when dismissing patients are more remote, they may need the stimulus or encouragement to be present that an affectively substantial expression of the therapist's subjectivity can provide; when patients are more emotionally engaged and available, on the other hand, they may simply need the therapist to stand beside them, as it were, to help them feel more deeply and understand their experience. The risks of the therapist's self-disclosure are real, but so are the risks of his appearing overly controlled or reserved—a blank screen. Stereotypically neutral or "objective" therapists (especially those with a dismissing attachment style) may wind up colluding with the defenses of the dismissing patient, inadvertently reinforcing the emotional isolation that has hobbled the patient's development.

The point, of course, is not to deliver a barrage of honesty but, rather, to communicate our experience in a form the patient can make use of. Nat-

urally, this can be quite challenging at times. While the dismissing patient may succeed in remaining out of touch with many feelings, anger is not inaccessible: Unlike sadness, say, anger helps make for distance. And, as expressed through the overt (or covert) devaluation intrinsic to the patient's deactivating strategy, that anger often winds up provoking strong feelings in the therapist.

Exactly what feelings and how they are expressed will depend largely on our own attachment pattern(s). Therapists who lean in the dismissing direction may become cold or withdrawn. Or, they may become controlling. Or, they may interpret, adding insight to injury, so to speak. Preoccupied therapists with powerful fears of abandonment may find it impossible not to show how crushed they feel or they may fly into a rage.

Ideally, we are secure enough to convey something of our feeling, with just enough affect to reach the patient at an emotional level. Obviously, we are not (nor should we be) entirely in charge of the emotions that unfold in our interaction with the patient. Sometimes we overshoot and sometimes our responses mirror the patient's withdrawal or overcontrol. To be able to recognize and understand the characteristic patterns of transference/countertransference that are likely to arise with our dismissing patients is no guarantee of optimal responsiveness, but it can help.

Three such patterns stand out, and each seems to be associated with a somewhat different history of avoidant attachment. One pattern is played out with patients whose first line of defense is devaluation, a second with patients who (initially) idealize, and a third for whom control is the watchword. Usually we experience more than a single pattern with the same patient, but early in treatment one tends to predominate; because it represent the patient's first line of defense, it often reemerges during times of difficulty both inside and outside therapy. And because the therapeutic relationship is co-created, our own attachment characteristics inevitably have an impact on the patient. If we have a need to be idealized, for example, the patient may be more likely to lead by idealizing us.

The Devaluing Pattern

Dismissing adults in couples have been described (Goldbart & Wallin, 1996) as "merger wary," and those among them who devalue as "the merger wary who sabotage love" (p. 93). In conventional diagnostic terms, these patients tend to be labeled "narcissists." Frequently the children of deprived and narcissistically devaluing parents, they have grown up in an emotional desert. Borrowing their parents' defenses, they have learned to shield themselves from their unmet needs and angry frustration by thinking too well of themselves and too badly of others.

Over time, however, the illusions of specialness that protect and comfort these patients can prove an increasingly hollow substitute for love. Yet genuine intimacy risks exposing the feelings of dependent longing and anger which their parents could not tolerate. Consequently, their response to a potentially intimate relationship is akin to that of a starving man at a banquet who tells himself the food just isn't good enough and therefore refuses to eat.

What we need to keep in mind about our dismissing patients is that the self-generated propaganda about *their* perfection and—still more so—*our* imperfection provides them with (a very prickly kind of) protection from shame. As vital as this protection may feel at an unconscious level, it is also self-defeating and, as such, requires therapeutic attention.

More effective than a direct focus on the patients' protective hostility, however, are comments that highlight their difficulty in letting others matter. In therapy, that difficulty is reflected in the patient's (often unconscious) efforts to make sure the therapist does not become too important to him. Faced with an impending interruption in the treatment, for example, the patient may cancel sessions or comment on the money he'll save in the therapist's absence, as if to reassure himself about how little the therapist will be missed.

A year or more into the relationship with one such patient, I finally commented on his rather striking way of beginning and ending our sessions. Upon entering the office, he would stride by me, handing me his check without a look in my direction, and often, in fact, briefly shutting his eyes. When parting, he would stride out, silently showing me his back in response to my usual "take care" or "see you next time."

Without mentioning that I often felt shut out and slighted by his behavior, I simply described it to him and suggested that it probably had some meaning. On hearing what I had to say, he initially seemed to try to normalize his behavior, observing that a kind of "military crispness" marked most of his professional relationships. As we explored his experience, however, it became clear that he was uncomfortable with the "personal" dimension of these relationships.

Therapy, for example, was bound to end, he pointed out, so why would he allow himself to get too personal or close here? He admitted that trust was an issue and went on to elaborate that his mother probably provided the model for his behavior as well as the reason for it. She would regularly withdraw into her bedroom without the slightest gesture or word of parting. Nor would there be any sign of acknowledgment, much less welcome, from her when he arrived home from school: She would remain sequestered in her bedroom, silent; it felt, he said, like coming home to an empty house.

With patients who are defensively devaluing, either implicitly (like this one) or explicitly, we may find ourselves enacting a couple of different responses. In a dismissing state of mind, we may respond to the patient's devaluing transference with a devaluing or angry countertransference. When in a preoccupied state of mind, by contrast, we may feel all too vulnerable and respond as if the patient's devaluation were warranted by our insufficiency: If the patient won't let us matter, maybe that's because we have nothing of importance to offer him. In either case, if we are able to bear both our own discomfort at the potential for further devaluation and the patient's discomfort at feeling "exposed," we have the opportunity to explore an important *relationship* pattern (as well as a defensive one) that may shape the patient's interactions not only with the therapist but also with others.

The Idealizing Pattern

Dismissing patients who idealize, like those who devalue, have often grown up with overtly self-absorbed, covertly insecure parents. Sensing that their parents' narcissistic needs would always come first, such patients as children came to realize that they could find an oasis in the emotional desert by satisfying these needs. Through helping their parents to feel special, they could feel special themselves—while avoiding the risk of being dependent or angry.

Knowing this pattern of childhood adaptation gives us a way to understand the tendency of some of our dismissing patients to idealize us. What is crucial to keep in mind is that the admiration of these patients is overdone because it is overdetermined. No matter how terrific we are, patients at some level usually feel that their admiration for us is obligatory. They "know" that in order to maintain the relationship they must prop up what they imagine—or perceive—to be our shaky narcissistic equilibrium. Generally such patients keep to themselves (and sometimes from themselves) the implicit assumption that the therapist has feet of clay and requires reassurance. Unspoken, this assumption gives their relationship with the therapist an "as if" quality and preserves distance. Seen from this angle, idealizing patients, while *appearing* significantly more engaged than their devaluing counterparts, may actually be no less avoidant.

Probably we need to be as respectful of such a patient's need for idealization as we are of another's need to devalue—and just as committed, ultimately, to addressing the defense in a way that will be helpful to the patient. Many years ago, I had a powerful and regrettable lesson about the perils of failing to do so:

After a long, seemingly successful therapy, a patient I'll call Andrew experienced a profound and embittering awareness that his relationship with me had reproduced his compulsorily idealizing relationship to his narcissistic mother—a formidable, and only superficially available, woman who seemed to have required and received the admiration of all around her.

This patient abruptly and angrily concluded treatment, accusing me of being blind to this dimension of our relationship (presumably on account of my own need to be idealized) and the limitations it had imposed on his treatment. Years later, I crossed paths with Andrew, and told him what I had been thinking for quite some time, namely, that he was right: I had been blind to the enactment and deaf to his earlier words entreating me to be more emotionally involved with him, more self-revealing, and more self-reflective.[1]

Like devaluation, idealization can be driven by a more or less unconscious sense of necessity. But whereas devaluation is mainly motivated by the need to avoid dependency, idealization may largely serve the patient's need to maintain the two-person mutual admiration society that he has learned to use to reinforce his sense of specialness. This understanding suggests that rather than challenge the patient's idealization, we ought to focus on the patient's worry about our vulnerability and his conclusion that we need to be propped up and shielded from his doubts that we are really so "idealizable" after all.

Preoccupied therapists may be uncomfortable with their patients' idealization and, consequently, they may feel compelled to puncture the balloon the patient has inflated to keep them both aloft. Dismissing therapists, in contrast, may take their patients' idealization of them too much at face value or enjoy it too much to recognize its role as part of a defensive pattern of relating. Noticing either our discomfort or pleasure at the patient's admiration can often be a clue to the presence of idealization.

The Pattern of Control

Some dismissing patients can be counted on to turn their relationship with the therapist (and others) into a power struggle. Often labeled "obsessive personalities," these patients seem obsessed with control and the fear of being controlled. Unsurprisingly, such patients often grew up with controlling, brusque, and fastidious parents who suppressed their own anger and appeared uncomfortable with close physical contact. Probably these were parents with little tolerance for their children's distress, messiness, or temper tantrums. But unlike the parents of devaluing and idealizing patients,

these responded less with angry rejection or withdrawal than with intrusive control. As children, these future patients coped in two ways. First, like all who adopt dismissing defenses, they became as remote from their feelings as possible. Second, they (often covertly) resisted their parents' control as if turning away from the hazardous pursuit of comfort and connection to a preoccupation with the struggle against powerlessness.

In the psychotherapy of such patients, issues of power and control may seem to pop up with exasperating frequency. We may be drawn into struggles around the fee, the schedule, or the way we choose to work with the patient. Meanwhile, the patient often sees the therapist (who may actually be feeling quite beleaguered) as a controlling figure intent on imposing her will. The key is to identify the meaning to the patient of all these struggles. Frequently, they turn out to represent a rematch with the parents, so to speak, as well as an avoidance of the underlying attachment issues: People generally don't wish to be close to those with whom they feel embattled.

The challenge with these patients is neither to avoid the control struggles through submission nor to attempt simply to dominate them. Enacting the first is likely to leave us feeling resentful. Enacting the second may lead us to feel guilty. Neither alternative looks particularly therapeutic on its face—yet, assuming we're aware of our role in the enactment, both may open up meaningful exploration of the control struggle, as the following clinical summary illustrates:

"Selena" was a patient for whom the fee was a very contentious issue. A businesswoman fallen on lean times, she was determined, as she put it, not to be screwed. Wanting to make therapy possible and having arrived at a sense of what she could actually afford, I proposed a reduced fee. From her side, it wasn't reduced enough. She made a counteroffer. I agreed to it.

Some time later, however, I learned of some rather considerable financial assets the patient had not disclosed. In this context, I suggested that we probably ought to revisit the issue of the reduced fee. My suggestion left the patient feeling betrayed, exploited, and vulnerable. Complaining bitterly that I was taking advantage of her candor, she added that she should have known better than to trust a therapist who had already evidenced an overinterest in money. Shortly thereafter she interrupted treatment. A couple of years later, however, she returned, and though her personal economy was somewhat improved, I nonetheless agreed to a reduced fee (though not so reduced as before). Then her business took off spectacularly.

For more than year, I said nothing about the fee, nor did she. It seemed to me that her acute vulnerability to feeling exploited was reason enough to set the issue aside. Finally, I realized that my reticence

was also driven by my fear of reigniting her anger and suspiciousness—and that in keeping silent I was experiencing a toned-down version of Selena's own feelings of anger, distance, and vulnerability at being taken advantage of. It took me another month to brace myself and tell her that I was raising her fee.

With a slightly guilty smile, she said she'd been wondering when I was going to do so. She asked if I was raising her fee only, or that of my other patients as well. I answered that I'd raised my fees with other patients some time ago, but that I'd hesitated to hike hers because of how deeply troubling it had been for her when I had brought up the issue of the fee in the first round of our therapy. She said she was moved that I was taking her feelings so much into account.

Tempted to leave my newly burnished image intact, I nonetheless pushed on, telling her that, in fact, what had kept me quiet was my fear of arousing her feelings of anger and betrayal—feelings so intense that they had previously made it impossible for her to stay in therapy. However, I added, keeping quiet also kept me more distant from her than I wanted to be.

I asked what it was like for her to hear what I was saying. She said she was still grateful that I hadn't brought the fee up earlier, before she felt as trusting as she did now. But she was also both intrigued and disturbed to learn that her anger and potential for suspicion could have such a problematic impact on me, and, by extension, on her relationships with others. Interestingly, she had completely forgotten that her flight from therapy had been precipitated by the issue of the fee.

The struggle for control has different meaning to different patients. The loss of control can be equated with a threat to the patient's identity, or self-sufficiency, or autonomy. Giving up (or even sharing) control can feel like surrender or submission. For Selena—especially early in therapy—feeling subject to the perceived control of the other in a relationship was to feel endangered. As the treatment progressed, she could begin to consider that her sense of danger was less real than her worry about being close, vulnerable, and dependent. In short, while the issue of control here has importance in its own right as it does with many dismissing patients, it is at the same time also a refuge from the risks associated with intimacy and attachment. Often as psychotherapy proceeds and our relationship with the patient deepens, the focus shifts from aggression to love—from the risks of being controlled or controlling to the risks of loving and being loved.

Concluding on a Neurobiological Note

The right hemisphere has been described as *the social–emotional brain.* Ideally, the therapist's relationship with the dismissing patient nurtures the

development and integration of the "right mind" (Ornstein, 1997) in ways that the patient's original attachment relationships did not.

The *relational* connections that normally nurture the *neural* connections of thinking with feeling, language with experience, and the sense of the self in relation to others may have been largely absent for such a patient, growing up as an avoidant child with dismissing parents. Remember that attachment and caregiving behavior, face recognition, and the reading of nonverbal, bodily cues in oneself and others are all functions of the right hemisphere. In avoiding closeness and feeling—activities largely mediated by the right brain—the dismissing patient may have learned to dwell mainly in a left-hemisphere world organized by linear logic and language.

Coaxing the patient's "right mind" into the relationship with the therapist depends on *right-brain-to-right-brain communication* (Schore, 2003) that is largely nonverbal and implicit but can also arise through the exchange of words that embody and evoke emotion. Certainly a (dismissing) therapist who deals exclusively from the left hemisphere is unlikely to activate the patient's undeveloped capacities to relate intimately and to feel. On the other hand, a (preoccupied) therapist who has trouble harnessing the left brain's linguistic and interpretive resources may be unable to speak in a language to which the patient can respond. Depending on our own psychological organization, we may need to still our mind enough either to inform our thoughts with feeling or to let our feelings be effectively translated into thoughts.

The ability to enter a mindful state may be particularly helpful when working with dismissing patients because mindfulness fosters in the therapist the sort of open and integrated experience we are hoping to encourage in our patients. A mindful stance enhances our capacity to both sense and articulate the nonverbal and emotional undercurrents in our relationship with the patient. Not unimportantly, facilitating the development of the *patient's* capacity for mindfulness may also be very helpful. Dismissing patients (as one of them said in describing himself) often hover over their lives, never really landing in their own bodies. As therapists, we need to be as fully present and grounded as possible with these patients, if we are ever to enable them to connect—as deeply as they are entitled to—with themselves, and with those they might love and be loved by.

NOTE

1. When my patient attributed my reserve to my need to hide the chinks in my armor, and so maintain his idealization of me, his interpretation may have been correct, but it was incomplete. For my reserve also reflected my thoroughly misguided adherence to what I now

regard as a very problematic, if not downright destructive, view of the therapeutic relationship. In that traditional view, of course, it is rarely if ever to the patient's advantage to be informed about what is going on inside the therapist. I now believe, to the contrary, that this kind of knowledge can often serve the patient well—while the refusal to disclose it often does damage, as exemplified in my work with Andrew.

CHAPTER 13

The Preoccupied Patient

Making Room for a Mind of One's Own

Patients with a predominantly preoccupied state of mind with respect to attachment are in many ways the polar opposite of dismissing patients. The latter often appear low on life, cut off from their feelings, and uncomfortable being close to others. The former often seem lively and vivid—but also overwhelmed by their feelings and absorbed in avoiding distance from others. Superficially, at least, dismissing patients have little problem with their own self-esteem or autonomy, while those who are preoccupied are filled with self-doubt and fearful of being too independent. Dismissing patients almost always have trouble relying on others; preoccupied patients have trouble believing they can sometimes rely on themselves. And if the dismissing appear cut off from the resources of the social–emotional right brain, the preoccupied appear to have trouble harnessing the linguistically oriented left brain's ability to make orderly sense of disorderly experience. Paraphrasing Diana Fosha (2003), those who are dismissing can *deal*, but they can't *feel*, while in contrast, those who are preoccupied can *feel* (and *reel*), but they can't *deal*.

Preoccupied patients can be seen to fall on a diagnostic continuum with hysterics at one end and borderlines at the other. The former appear overwhelmed and helpless, but superficially cooperative and sometimes seductive. The latter appear angry, demanding, and chaotic. Both variations

on the preoccupied theme involve patients whose lives are shaped most fundamentally by the fear of abandonment.

Such patients have been characterized as "merger hungry" (Goldbart & Wallin, 1996): "Because [their] greatest threats are separation, loss, and being alone, closeness is experienced as the greatest good: it is the solution, never the problem" (p. 90). As it happens, however, the way in which these patients pursue closeness usually winds up turning the solution into a problem. The hyperactivating strategy of preoccupied patients buys a modicum of security, but at an exorbitant cost.

Early experience with unpredictably responsive attachment figures has taught these patients that their best hope for securing the attention and support of others is to make their own distress too conspicuous to ignore. The problem with this solution is that it requires them continuously to scan for internal and external cues to amplify their distress. Thus, they tend to be all too aware of threat-related thoughts, feelings, and bodily sensations, and prone to exaggerate their significance; similarly, they are hypervigilant for actual or imagined signs that a relationship partner might be disapproving, withdrawn, or rejecting. The need to keep the attachment system chronically activated undermines the preoccupied patient's potential not only for emotional balance but also for self-esteem and trust in others.

In psychotherapy, therefore, if we are to help such patients to strengthen their capacities for emotional balance, self-esteem, and trust, we must offer them a relationship that presents an alternative to their hyperactivating strategy. Effectively, this means a relationship in which patients can come to count on the therapist's emotional availability and acceptance rather than feeling that they can obtain this quality of responsiveness only by defensively amplifying their affect, helplessness, and/or superficial cooperation. In other words, we need to provide preoccupied patients with a relationship that renders the hyperactivating strategy increasingly unnecessary.

This is far more difficult than it might seem. Conspicuous insecurity has become the most reliable means for gaining the attention of unreliable others. Thus it is hard to relinquish. In addition, these patients experience their overwhelming feelings, insecurity, and mistrust not as a "strategy" that they might be (at least consciously) willing to change, but rather as facets of their reality that anchor their sense of who they are. Unconsciously (and sometimes consciously), the preoccupied patient embraces these burdensome aspects of her approach to herself and others because they support both a strategy *and* an identity.

In dealing with the patient's felt need to embrace an approach that is self-defeating, it may be helpful to keep in mind that a therapeutic process is generally one that heals by allowing the patient to stay the same while changing (Bromberg, 1998b). Far from denying the importance of the strong feelings and the pursuit of closeness around which the preoccupied

patient's sense of self is organized, we need to make room for *more* in the way of feelings and closeness. Specifically, we need to respond to the deeper feelings that underlie the patient's displays of distress. And we need to foster a more expansive version of closeness in which the patient can be more fully and authentically present rather than disappear into her preoccupation with the availability of others.

In working with the feelings—fear, anger, and desire—that underlie the drama, we bring the patient's once adaptive, now self-defeating strategy of hyperactivation into focus. In working with the patient's narrow sense of what is required for closeness, we illuminate aspects of her identity that the patient has previously had to deny—in particular, the strengths, ambitions, and needs for which her fears of abandonment have left so little room.

Exactly how we can work most effectively using this double focus on emotions and intimacy depends to some extent on our assessment of the patient—specifically in terms of their position on the continuum anchored by hysterics at one end and borderlines at the other. (Note that for didactic purposes I describe the "subtypes" here as if preoccupied patients could always be clearly differentiated along these lines; it's my clinical impression that often they can, but not invariably.) The different behaviors of ambivalent infants upon reunion with their parents in the Strange Situation may presage the different behaviors of the preoccupied patients we see as adults—the apparently helpless infant developing the more hysteric style, the infant who oscillates between clinging and angry rejection becoming someone who looks more borderline.

Regardless, there are preoccupied patients who clearly "lead" with helplessness while others all too quickly reveal their anger and their desperate demands. (The latter frequently have histories marked by trauma and loss and, thus, they may also be well described as unresolved.) Each of these two variations on the preoccupied theme requires a somewhat different therapeutic approach.

THE PATTERN OF HELPLESSNESS

Patients described with the term "hysteric" are so labeled because they appear hyperemotional and even melodramatic, just as most preoccupied patients do. What differentiates these hysteric-like patients from their more troubled cousins is that their dependency needs are less extreme, as are their reactions when these needs are frustrated. Because such patients are less apt to feel as if their lives are one long emergency, their approach to satisfying their relationship needs can be relatively more appealing and more successful.

Generally, they connect with others more through their helplessness

than their anger. But while making no secret of their neediness, they do a poor job of satisfying their own needs—or even really knowing them. Their center of gravity seems to lie outside themselves, as if they lived less inside their own mind than in the mind of others. Desperate to avoid being abandoned, they are too fearful to assert themselves and too willing to please.

When they enter therapy, they often present us with a contradiction. They may appear to have considerable psychological resources and may be quite accomplished. But in the treatment setting they conduct themselves as though they were powerless, both to manage their distress and to try to understand it. Early on, hoping for our help, they may strike us as eager patients, fully prepared to commit themselves, and very much in touch with emotions that evoke our desire to help. Quickly, we may develop with patients like these the expectation that they will be easy to work with. But first impressions can mislead. There's both more—and less—here than meets the eye.

Often these patients have more ability to manage and make sense of their feelings than they believe they do, know more about their experience than they are willing to grant, and have more assets as people than they are prepared to acknowledge. On the other hand, their apparent readiness to engage in a therapeutic relationship is less an indication of their ability to collaborate than a sign of their desire to comply and to please. To secure the comfort they hope that closeness to the therapist will bring, these patients "know" they must maintain the appearance of helplessness while also helping the therapist to feel good.

The challenge for us here is not to confuse the surface with the reality that lies beneath it, not to mistake the patient's defensive strategy for the difficulties it was designed to deal with. If we take the helplessness at face value, we may try to be helpful in ways that ratify the patient's sense that she is helpless. And if we are charmed or seduced into playing the great therapist, we may lose sight of her need to be the perfect patient. In so doing, we may deny our patient the opportunity to grapple with the fear and distrust that make her compliance and pleasing feel so necessary.

With such patients, we need to be alert to our overeagerness to rescue or to be idealized. But when, as so often happens, we find ourselves enacting such impulses, we have an opening both to do things differently and to illuminate key facets of the patient's experience. Once again, as the clinical material that follows makes vivid, the therapist can constrain as well as contribute to the patient's progress in treatment.

An extremely competent academic whom I'll call Elaine sought my help after a series of panic attacks. Early in therapy, she told me that whenever there was a silence in our conversation, it made her acutely anxious. Apparently the last thing I wanted to do was to make this

anxiety-ridden patient more anxious. Rather than take up the issue, I got into the habit of filling every silence. It took me several months to realize that in so doing I was doing her no favor. With some trepidation, I decided that when next a silence arose, I would let it be.

Unsurprisingly, in the quiet that came Elaine began to feel very anxious. But we were able to talk about it. It emerged that her anxiety bloomed in the silence because she felt helpless on her own to make sense of her experience—and feeling helpless, she said, scared her. I suggested that it was a bit of a puzzle that someone who made her living by making sense of experience should feel helpless to make sense of her own. In the conversation that ensued, she became aware of what she called a "surplus helplessness" that she had learned to cultivate as a child. Then and now, being overwhelmed was her best bet, she realized, when it came to connecting with her unpredictably available mother. Similarly, she connected with her father mainly around problems she was unable to solve by herself—homework when she was young, and later academic or work problems.

Farther into therapy, as Elaine became more comfortable with silence, she realized that, previously, she had felt threateningly alone when we were not in verbal contact, as if without words she would be unable to keep me with her. Now, in a way that was altogether new, she was capable of experiencing in the silence a more certain and ongoing connection between us. This was for her a cherished experience of being able to be alone with me, but alone together.

My fear of triggering Elaine's anxiety resulted for a time in my colluding with her defenses instead of grappling with the underlying experience that made them necessary. In the process, I inadvertently confirmed her sense that she was helpless to deal with her feelings—most important, her anxiety about abandonment. On the other hand, once I realized what I was doing, and found a way to tolerate my own anxiety enough to change my behavior, her "surplus helplessness"—a version of the hyperactivating strategy—could begin to be understood. Later, when she was able to relax into being "alone together," I read her achievement as reflecting her gradual internalization of the experience of a secure base: She no longer needed to coerce me (through helplessness or distress) into being with her, because now, for the most part, she trusted that I was.

For patients like Elaine, a diminished reliance on the hyperactivating strategy goes hand in hand with a growing ability to experience the therapist as a secure base. Initially, of course, such patients bring their fears of abandonment to the therapeutic relationship. They cannot rely on the therapist's emotional availability or good intentions. Like ambivalent infants whose preoccupation with mother's availability leaves little room for exploration, their energies are absorbed in maintaining their connection to the therapist.

Yet it is only to the extent that preoccupied patients feel less compelled to monitor or manage the therapist's responses that they can turn their attention more fully to their own experience. We make ourselves a secure base rather than a source of all-too-contingent support when we generate a relationship that offers more to the patient—and asks more *of* the patient—than the relationships that launched her.

Among the key features of developmentally facilitative relationships cited earlier (Lyons-Ruth, 1999), two are particularly salient here: inclusiveness and the necessity for a "developmental gradient." Specifically, we must aim for a relationship that encourages the patient to connect with as much of her experience as possible—especially that experience for which her original attachments made no room. And we must expect more of the patient than she may initially feel capable of. That is, we have to recognize and enlist resources in the patient that she may be unwilling or unable to recognize in herself.

Inclusiveness

The emotionality of the preoccupied patient often has an "other-directed" quality. When preoccupied patients express their feelings, the purpose is usually less to express themselves than to get the attention or help of others who, they believe, would otherwise be unavailable. This is, of course, the essence of the hyperactivating strategy.

Rather than collude with that strategy by being oversolicitous or overprotective (a seductive possibility), the trick is to be no more or less available when the patient expresses such "public" emotions than when she does not. Just as important, we need to deploy a kind of empathic Geiger counter that cues us with regard to the "private" emotions the patient can only express indirectly.

Here, once again, attention to the nonverbal language of the patient's body—as well as a focus on our own subjective experience—provides the best access to what the patient has learned to exclude. Obviously, the details here will vary depending on the particulars of the patient's history. However, in my own clinical experience, I've found that what frequently emerge, often in sequence, and are gradually integrated into the patient's sense of self are: mistrust and fears of abandonment; then anger and the allied ability to say "no"; and finally, sadness and authentic need, as well as the ability to say "yes"—and really mean it.

The Developmental Gradient

After getting off the phone with a patient who had just scheduled an initial hour with me, I realized that in the course of our conversation I had been

inhibiting myself, verbally and intellectually, so as not to "hurt" her by exposing a contrast with her own apparent deficits in this area. Yet when we actually met, I became aware that she had the capacity (though she didn't typically exercise it) to be much more forceful and articulate than she had appeared to be over the phone. Clearly, she led with her vulnerability, and I initially responded by being conspicuously and unhelpfully overprotective.

With this patient (and others like her) it has proven essential to expect more, rather than less. Of course, we have to meet the patient where she is. Yet we usually fail the patient when we're too ready to assume that's as far as she can go. Far more helpful is the assumption that the patient is actually capable of feeling and thinking in greater depth than she appears to be. Across the board, in fact, there tends to be in preoccupied patients an underestimate of their strengths and resources—and it can be very problematic if we seem to take the patient's negative self-appraisal at face value.

On occasion, I have spontaneously confronted a patient's overmodest self-appraisal: "You say no one could possibly be interested in you. But I'm thinking: What's not to like?" In the moment, such an intervention can seem quite unproductive; over the long haul, however, it has sometimes provided a sort of touchstone—a vivid image of the patient's defensive denial of her own strengths. Though offered in a supportive spirit, this kind of confrontation is rarely welcomed because it is incongruent with the patient's sense of herself and presents a challenge to the patient's adaptive strategy. Probably more useful as a rule is simply to explore the patient's view of her own capabilities and how that view developed; in addition, it is vital to intervene in ways that implicitly communicate our conviction that the patient is capable of more than she believes.

For example, after one patient began a session angry and distraught about several recent interactions with her husband by whom she felt unheard, unseen, and gratuitously criticized, we deconstructed the episodes that troubled her and she recognized—almost in passing—that her husband had not actually ignored or attacked her at all: "It wasn't that he really didn't hear me or recognize me, it was just that I felt that way. The same for the criticism. I know he respects and loves me, he's not attacking me, he just has another opinion. But that's not how it *feels*."

When I asked how it did feel ("What's your sense of how it happens that you feel he's ignoring or attacking you, when with some other part of you, you think that he's not?"), she replied, "I honestly don't know"—as if that were clearly the end of her exploring. "But just because you don't know, does that mean you can't think about it?" Which she then, in fact, proceeded quite productively to do.

Because strong displays of emotion may have helped these patients make the best of a bad situation, they tend to let their feelings drown out their thoughts. We have to make room for their feelings, to be sure, but we

must also encourage them to think about what they feel. A balancing act is required from us as therapists if we are to help activate the reflective self of the preoccupied patient. We have to do some thinking for the patient, but not too much. We need to model mentalizing—say, by articulating our thoughts about the feelings evoked in us as we relate to the patient. But rather than take sole responsibility for making sense of the patient's experience, we would do better to invite her to join us in the effort, or ask her to think aloud about her own experience.

As therapists, we must keep in mind that the patient is actually fearful of developing a sense of confidence and independence, because autonomy and self-initiative have been discouraged early on and so are inconsistent with the patient's beliefs about how best to secure the attention of others. Therefore, we will want to convey our awareness of how difficult it is for the patient to trust in her own resources.

Further, it may be particularly important—given the constraints on the patient's autonomy—to notice and make room for the surfacing of anger, criticism, or disappointment in relation to the therapist. When both partners can get through such protests relatively unscathed, it reinforces the patient's dawning awareness that autonomy and separateness can in fact coexist with closeness, contrary to the lessons of the patient's original attachment experience. But whether these early lessons are, or are not, updated will largely depend on what occurs between patient and therapist in the context of the new attachment relationship.

The Relationship: Patterns and Pitfalls

While it is true that the patient–therapist relationship, like all attachment relationships, is co-created, it is true in a particular way in the case of preoccupied patients, who tend to adapt, chameleon-like, to the expectations of others. Their desire to merge, driven by their fear of our unavailability, leaves them all too ready to submerge themselves—with the result that what we get is often what they think we want. The shape of the therapeutic relationship is, thus, very much a function of the preoccupied patient's attachment strategy in interaction with that of the therapist.

Of course, every such relationship is unique and unpredictable. Regardless of the clarity of our therapeutic intentions (attune to what lies beneath the affective surface, don't collude, don't reinforce helplessness) we are bound to be surprised. If we're not, we're probably treating a theoretical rather than a real patient, or conducting ourselves as though we were therapy machines, rather than spontaneous, emotional, and vulnerable human beings. Yet the surprises notwithstanding, there are characteristic patterns and countertransference pitfalls that mark the treatment of many preoccupied patients. Knowledge of these patterns won't stop us from fall-

ing into them—nor should it. For recognizing the nature of our interaction with our patients may be the most significant part of how we get to know them and how they get to know us. At the same time, general knowledge of this kind can help us identify the character of our own unwitting participation in the relationship, which allows us, in turn, somewhat greater flexibility.

The patient's abiding fear of the therapist's unavailability results in (but is also sometimes hidden behind) the patient's zeal to connect. Her need for the reassurance and comfort of closeness may be expressed in a number of ways. Whatever else they may represent, the patient's apparent helplessness, displays of distress, compliance, seductiveness, and/or efforts to be a "good patient" are also implicit attempts to diminish distance and win the therapist's support. The earlier in treatment these overtures emerge—and the more intensely or inflexibly they are enacted—the deeper, I presume, is the patient's distrust and her anxiety about abandonment. As therapists, our responses to such overtures will be shaped, to some extent, by our own attachment style.

If we are more secure, rather than less, it will be easier to resonate with the deeper feelings that underlie the patient's indirect appeals for connection: the fear of not being taken care of and the anger at having to lose herself in order to secure the attention of others, as well as profound need and sadness. In a secure state of mind, we will be able not only to interact relatively freely, but also to help the patient make sense of her role in the interactions we co-create.

When our state of mind is more dismissing, we will probably need to be cautious about a number of possible pitfalls having to do with the fact that the patient's attachment strategy is the opposite of our own. Fearful to one degree or another of feeling and of closeness, we may find ourselves uncomfortable, or even put off, by the patient's intense affect and hunger for merging. To feel more comfortable, we may choose to help by trying to "corral" the patient's intense emotion with intellectual understanding. Rather than resonate with the patient's deeper feelings—or notice the lack of fit between what is being said and what seems to be felt—we may prematurely aim to provide the reassuring (for us) structure of words and interpretation. To which the patient may well respond by feeling alone and misunderstood, or by joining us compliantly in a "pretend" version of meaningful therapeutic exploration—or both.

Alternatively, we might be unconsciously relieved to be able to find our disavowed affect and dependency in the patient rather than in ourselves. In this case, we may be inclined to collude with the patient's defensive strategy. For example, we may take her emotional neediness too much at face value, while feeling implicitly reassured that we have no such needs of our own. Similarly, to buttress our self-esteem, we may take on too readily the

role of the brilliant therapist idealized by the overtly helpless (but covertly controlling) patient. In this enactment, we may remain unconsciously, but purposefully, ignorant of the patient's mistrust and anger, while for her part, the patient is self-protectively manipulating our narcissistic needs.

When we are in a more preoccupied state of mind with respect to attachment, the issues we confront in the relationship with the preoccupied patient will be different. On the one hand, we will likely be more capable of empathy with the patient's experience because of its overlap with ours; on the other hand, our own fears of abandonment can make it difficult for us to do much more than empathize. Should we wish to address the partly defensive nature of the patient's helplessness, for instance, we would need to convey a perspective that differs from hers. But doing so requires a degree of separateness that we may easily confuse with aggression or experience as threatening to our ongoing relationship with the patient. Thus, our own preoccupation with attachment may incline us to "join" the patient in her distress, but without intervening in the ways that might ultimately help her cope with it better. By the same token, we may yield to the impulse to "rescue" the patient rather than help her to recognize her own resources. In addition, our own bias toward feeling rather than thinking can interfere with our ability to mobilize (both in ourselves and in the patient) the "left brain interpreter" that makes sense of emotional experience so that it can be used as a signal, rather than experienced as a burden, a symptom, or merely a fact.

The Erotic Transference

Beyond the foregoing interactions that commonly occur in the treatment of preoccupied patients, we frequently encounter what I would describe as "intimate transferences" along with their countertransference complements. Ordinarily discussed under the heading of erotic transference, these interactions have a dimension of sexuality, romance, and/or unappeasable longing that is often significant in its own right, but may also obscure underlying attachment issues.

As a number of writers have pointed out, the nature of the erotic transference–countertransference situation that develops depends largely on the gender of the patient and therapist involved (Person, 1988; Wrye & Welles, 1994; Kernberg, 1995). I would add that a second influential factor here is attachment style.

Very briefly, intimate and (especially) sexualized transferences are overall most likely to arise when the patient is a woman and the therapist a man—at least to the extent women in general tend to fear separateness, while men, again in general, are more likely to fear closeness. Hence, for women, particularly those who are preoccupied, the pursuit of a romantic or sexual connection to the therapist often represents not only a defense

against distance, but also a defense against more fundamental attachment issues. For men, by contrast, the *avoidance* of romantic or sexual feelings for the therapist often represents a defense against deeper involvement as well as the characteristic masculine solution of segregating sexuality and attachment. When men, especially dismissing men, *do* develop sexual feelings for the therapist, those feelings are still apt to reflect avoidance of closeness and dependency, because sexualizing the therapist can be, for a man, a way of devaluing him or her as an attachment figure on whom the patient might be tempted to depend.

The emotional impact upon us as therapists of the patient's erotic transference may differ according to our state of mind with respect to attachment. If our style is more dismissing, we may welcome the patient's romantic or sexual longing because it bolsters our self-regard. Alternatively, we may be put off because we experience such longing as a challenge to our customary distance from others. But if our style tends to be preoccupied, we may welcome the patient's desire as a signal of closeness. On the other hand, the same desire may be experienced as deeply discomfiting because it represents an overture we must reject—and we assume the patient will feel that it is she herself, not just her desire, that we are rejecting.

Ideally, we can allow ourselves to be the object of the patient's longing, without either encouraging it unduly or feeling compelled to shut it down. To the extent that we can make a place for this longing, we have an opportunity to explore its role in the therapeutic relationship—and, by extension, its role in the patient's other close relationships. Is sexuality used as a surrogate for attachment, an indirect route to it, or an avoidance of it? Central in the treatment context is the fact that the patient's longing for the therapist is one that can never be fully gratified. As such, it may represent the living out of the pattern of frustrated desire that characterized the patient's original attachment(s) as well, perhaps, as her contemporary ones. Sometimes the erotic transference is an important waystation for the preoccupied patient en route to the development of a deeper capacity to trust and to love. But if the therapist is either too pleased or too discomfited by the patient's desire that welcome development may be thwarted.

As I mentioned at the outset, preoccupied patients can be understood to fall on a diagnostic continuum. Thus far, I have focused on that end of the continuum occupied by those patients whose hysteric-like features include helplessness, the amplification of affect, and seductive compliance. It is the opposite end of the continuum to which I turn next.

THE PATTERN OF ANGER AND CHAOS

Research suggests that many, if not most, borderline patients have a preoccupied state of mind with respect to attachment. These patients are found

with great frequency to fall into a particular subclassification: fearful pre-occupation with traumatic events (Patrick, Hobson, Castle, Howard, & Maughan, 1994; Fonagy et al., 1996). It appears that patients at the more troubled end of the preoccupied continuum have often experienced histories marked by recurrent trauma or losses that remain incompletely resolved. In AAI terms, such patients are both preoccupied *and* unresolved. Therefore, much of what I'm about to say may well apply not only to patients at the more troubled end of the preoccupied continuum, but also to patients who are unresolved.

Preoccupied borderline patients often experience life as an ongoing crisis. Their emotions are not merely painful but overwhelming in their intensity. Rather than sensing a stable sense of self, these patients feel chaotic inside, and empty. Their relationships are frequently stormy, ending often in what feels like betrayal. Torn between their terror of dependency and their bottomless need, they may appear desperate for help, but tyrannized by their conviction that their needs will drive help away. In desperation, they may approach, but in fear and anger they withdraw. As a therapist with such patients, I have often felt like someone trying to save a drowning man who fights off aid as if it were an attack. The challenge with such patients is not to let ourselves be pushed away.

Margaret Mahler uses the term "hatching" in writing of the psychological birth of the human infant (Mahler et al., 1975). As the therapist of a borderline preoccupied patient, it's very much as if we're called upon to sit on a chick or an egg that seems to be doing its best, or worst, to knock us off our maternal perch. To provide (and preserve) the new attachment relationship the patient needs, we must be able to offer a combination of empathy and limit setting. Neither is sufficient on its own to "contain" overwhelmed and overwhelming patients like these or the fear, anger, and hopelessness they are all too capable of evoking in us. When the therapeutic relationship *can* become sufficiently containing, the patient has the opportunity to develop the kind of internal and interpersonal stability for which her first attachments provided no models.

Empathy

Unless we can understand and, to some extent, resonate with the patient's internal experience, we will be unable to help. Without the therapist's empathic attunement, the patient is likely to feel unrecognized and alone, or worse, threatened and betrayed. Yet such attunement is usually hard won. It depends on at least three things: our ability to draw on relevant theory and research, our openness to the full spectrum of our own experience, and our capacity to interact with the patient in ways that neutralize, at least temporarily, the mutually generated obstacles to empathy and connection.

Fearfully preoccupied with trauma, these patients are often quite ex-

plicit about experiences with their parents—or experiences of being abandoned by their parents—that left them overwhelmed and sometimes terrified. Their parents, like parents of preoccupied patients generally, were unpredictable, to be sure, but they could also be angry or unavailable in ways that were scary.

A patient told me that his father, an alcoholic police officer, could be unpredictably brutal. The patient's job had been to somehow keep this explosive man entertained or distracted when he appeared on the verge of violence. Sometimes the patient was successful. When he wasn't, he could become the target of his father's rage. Once, his father drew his pistol and pointed it at the patient's head.

Part of the tragedy for patients like this one is that such scenes of childhood victimization continue to be enacted in the patient's subsequent relationships, including, most importantly, the patient's relationship with himself. Fonagy (2000) theorizes that In place of the "constitutional" or true self, these patients have internalized the representation of an "alien" self that embodies the responses of the abusive attachment figure. But because this alien self is both persecutory and at odds with the true self, it must be expelled. The resulting projection of this dangerous internal presence ensures that others will be experienced as persecutory. When others are not available, the patient may feel compelled to persecute himself, through vicious self-attack, including, sometimes, self-mutilation. Fonagy's theory can help us make sense of disturbing behavior that might otherwise function as an obstacle to empathy. Such understanding may be especially vital when our interaction with the patient threatens to mimic the interactions of his past—as was the case with the son of the policeman whose traumatic history I touched on a moment ago.

Following an unusually collaborative session, this patient arrived twenty minutes after the hour was to have begun, making no comment about his lateness. He was to have paid me, but told me he didn't have his checkbook. He said that he was sick of therapy, and that all this talk was just getting in his way; without it, he'd probably feel much better.

Around the lateness and the missing check, I found myself feeing irritated, but when he began to attack our work together, I started to feel quite angry. Then it occurred to me that I was being invited to play his angry persecutor, because if I were instead a collaborator, then he would be left alone with the persecutor inside him. Moreover, he might experience me as inviting him to take the foolish (perhaps unconsciously life-threatening) risk of trusting me.

I wondered aloud if perhaps he were trying to pick a fight rather than feel close. I added that my guess was that a session like the last one in which we had been able to work so closely together might very well have made him anxious. I should not have been surprised when he

angrily took issue with my suggestion. My interpretation, however, served both of us well. It enabled me to stay with him, rather than feel pushed away. It was also an interpretation he could eventually make increasing use of as we re-experienced, many times, scenarios very much like this one.

Obviously, there's a lot more theory and research to draw on in our efforts to grasp the experience of our more troubled preoccupied patients. Splitting, embeddedness in experience, failures of mentalizing, and the overarching metaphor of the self overwhelmed by a powerful, malevolent other are all useful constructs to which we will shortly return. But beyond theory, personal experience is a resource that can enhance our compassion for patients whose blatantly self-destructive and frequently offputting behavior can be hard to tolerate, much less feel empathy for.

In this connection, I have found it valuable to be able to locate within myself echoes of the patient's experience. For example, when feeling exasperated with a patient whose tenacious resentment over past injustices seemed to hurt only herself, I helpfully recalled how extraordinarily difficult forgiveness has been, on occasion, for me. We understand others most deeply, I'm quite certain, on the basis of shared experience. Sometimes, of course, the commonalities can be difficult to recognize, or too uncomfortable to acknowledge, even to ourselves.

Making empathy possible—our empathy for the patient and our patient's empathy for herself—often necessitates interventions that have the potential to dissolve barriers to it. The primary barrier to empathy is the therapist's negative countertransference. When we feel frightened, angry, diminished, or dominated by the patient, it can be difficult to put ourselves in the patient's place enough to grasp the emotional logic of her experience. And without the therapist's doing so, the patient has no basis upon which to extend empathy to herself.

Feeling the negative countertranference is probably inevitable. Perhaps it is even desirable, as a way of getting to know the patient and the reactions she may evoke. On the other hand, drowning in the negative countertransference is not inevitable, nor is it desirable. Sometimes, finding a way to put our troubling experience into words, either silently or with the patient, is sufficient to modulate our feelings. But sometimes it is not. This is where limit setting comes in.

Limit Setting

When we communicate a limit, we are not attempting to control the patient. It's unwise to attempt the impossible. Our capacity for self-control, however, allows us the option of telling the patient what we will or will not do, given a particular set of circumstances. The formula here is: If you do

X, I will do Y. If you throw something at me, the session is over. If you allow me to speak to your physician and your psychiatrist, then I will continue to meet with you. If you call me to talk about your suicidal feelings, the only thing I will talk to you about is whether or not I need to call the police to get you to the hospital. Obviously, different limits are called for with different patients with different therapists in different situations. But with the kinds of patients I've been describing, some limits are almost invariably necessary in order to protect both parties and the treatment. They guard all concerned against too intense a negative countertransference, which can make empathy impossible and in the process eliminate the potential for the patient to experience the therapeutic relationship as a secure base.

Acting on a limit we have set is often initially disruptive, as when I called the police to the home of a patient after he was unable to tell me that he would not commit suicide, and he became enraged. But such disruptions are also occasions for repair. The patient was eventually able to recognize my action as springing from a desire to protect him rather than a wish to cause him harm or exert my control. With a patient like this one, the therapist's willingness to engage and struggle is absolutely essential; in its absence, the patient may feel we have given up on him—and the feeling may be justified. Of course, the engagement and struggle that are so necessary also take a toll. Yet when our efforts result in a deeper, closer, more productive relationship—and particularly when the patient gets better—such a patient can come to be among those who matter to us most.

The Relationship: Patterns and Pitfalls

In some ways these more tormented patients who lead with anger can be seen to present the same psychology as the preoccupied patients who lead with helplessness—but everything about that shared psychology is amplified. The affects are more extreme as is the sense of embeddedness in experience, the limitations on mentalizing, and the associated impulsivity. And although both kinds of preoccupied patients live in a mental space that has been colonized, so to speak, by their original attachment figures, the nature of those figures is different.

In the helpless patient, the subjective experience is of the internalized other looming so large as to take up most of the mental space, leaving little room for self-definition. In the internal conversation here, the voices are largely those of others responding loudly and clearly to the self, whose voice is indistinct. In relationships, the patient is correspondingly preoccupied with the other and vague about her own needs, views, and ambitions.

For the angry patient, it's as if the internalized other not only looms large but also is malevolent and seems regularly to threaten the self. In rela-

tionships, this malevolent other is frequently projected onto (or into) those upon whom the patient might be inclined to depend, including the therapist. The result is that the patient is mainly absorbed in fending off perceived danger rather than recognizing and trying to satisfy her own desires.

In framing a stance with such patients, it is helpful to recall Fonagy's account of the responses of secure parents to their children. These responses convey the parents' empathy for the child's distress; their appreciation of the wishes, feelings, and beliefs that are the context for the child's behavior; and, finally, their ability to cope with experience the child finds overwhelming. As therapists, we need to aim for a similar kind of responsiveness with patients whose internal and interpersonal experience is so threatening, specifically because they have so little capacity for compassionate understanding of themselves, so little awareness of their own intentionality, and so little confidence that their experience can be managed.

Largely lacking a reflective or mentalizing self, these patients live in a subjective world whose character is defined by physical rather than psychological realities, actions rather than words or thoughts, bodies rather than minds. Consequently, we need to demonstrate that we are on the patient's side, that we understand, and that we can cope. With such patients, in a variety of ways, it is initially more what we *do* than what we say, more what we *show* them than what we tell them, that has impact.

When their behavior regularly pushes us away, seems incomprehensible, and leaves us feeling that we'll be lucky to muddle through, it can be helpful to keep in mind that patients like these are struggling internally with titanic emotional forces. Externalizing or *interpersonalizing* this excruciating struggle—handing it off to us or "sharing" it—can be a way for the patient both to manage overwhelming feelings and to communicate them.

In one memorable session, the patient whose father had threatened him with a gun told me that he was comforted by the knowledge that he could always blow his brains out with his own pistol, recently purchased, that he kept in a drawer near his bed. Just taking it out and holding it, his finger round the trigger, helped him feel more at ease. He had no intention of killing himself now, he assured me, but he felt suicide was his ultimate destiny.

Hearing about this gun for the first time, I felt myself becoming extremely anxious, not to mention angry, at being placed in the position of dealing with a threat over which I had such limited control. (I also had a sickening recollection of a man whom I had seen in therapy just once as part of a couple: Before we could meet for a second session, I learned in a message from his wife that he had shot himself.)

I asked the patient how it felt to have told me about the gun. He

said he was relieved, both to have the gun and to know that I knew about it—this way there was no secret. Great, I thought, I'm glad you're being so honest with me: Now I'm going to have to punish you for trusting me by taking away your security blanket. I felt as if he were pointing his gun at my head. I told him that guns scared me, that suicidal patients with guns really scared me, and that I couldn't be any help to him if I were to continue to feel this scared. If he wanted me to keep on working with him, I said, he was going to have to bring me the gun.

There is a great deal that could be said about this episode. For now, let it illustrate several points about patients like this one. First, the patient's subjective world is a world of physical actions and the therapeutic dialogue here is, above all, an action dialogue. Second, the patient communicated the nature of his world to me through behavior that evoked it in my own experience: In some sense, I felt *his* fear, powerlessness, and anger, along with my own. Third, the knowledge that his behavior was communicative and that my behavior also needed to be, helped me to intervene firmly but without being punitive or threatening—in other words, it helped me to cope. Fourth, we were able over the course of subsequent sessions to situate the patient's superficially calm, but deeply desperate behavior in the context of his unbearable feelings and his conflict about hoping for my help. These were experiences that allowed the patient (paraphrasing Fonagy, 2000) to find himself in the mind of a benevolent other as a thinking and feeling being. And, yes, he did bring me the gun.

Of course, we are "tested" repeatedly by such patients. It is to be hoped that we succeed more often than we fail. But even when we fail—say, by becoming punitive or withholding—there is the opportunity for repair. Moreover, we can show the patient in this context and others that there is room for failure, that some failure is inevitable, and that it can be tolerated to the extent that we don't confuse the part with the whole. In other words, we can show the patient a relational and affective world that is not all or nothing, black or white, now or never. Beyond the world of splitting that the patient generally inhabits, there is also one that is more integrated.

Again, however, it must be stressed that in dealing with patients who split and who, rather than articulate their feelings, act them out with dangerous and sometimes life-threatening consequences, our ability to maintain a thoughtful and integrated perspective can sometimes simply evaporate. In the face of the stress and the demands of the work, we will inevitably, at times, feel overwhelmed, frightened, helpless, and/or enraged—very much as these patients must have felt with parents whose own difficulties placed impossible burdens on their children. As the therapist of such patients, our saving grace may be the support we are able to find, after the

fact, in others, in ourselves, and, to some extent, in our theories. There is, moreover, the reality that many, if not all, of these patients can effectively make use of their relationship with us to get better, to heal.

The Place of Mindfulness and Meditation

The "hyper-hyperactivating" strategy of the patients I've been discussing appears to be associated with a highly reactive autonomic nervous system. Literally, as well as figuratively, these patients have an exaggerated startle reflex and are slow to regain equilibrium. They are vulnerable to intense and rapid reactions to perceived threats, as though the responses of the amygdala were unmodulated by the hippocampus. When the sympathetic branch of the autonomic nervous system is activated, they can become extremely agitated as if in the mode of fight or flight. When the parasympathetic branch is triggered, they can become drowsy, can appear dissociated, or may "freeze."

Because meditation seems to have the potential to calm the body (as well as to strengthen mentalizing) it can play an especially useful role in the treatment of this subgroup of preoccupied patients, some of whom I have consequently taught to meditate. With some of these patients, I begin each session with a brief period of meditation. Such patients have not infrequently entered my office in a state of apparent agitation. Typically, we have exchanged a few words in acknowledgment of their feelings before beginning to meditate. Emerging from a five- or ten-minute meditation, these patients usually appear calmer and seem more capable of considering their experience without feeling emotionally and physiologically overwhelmed by it.

The background for their autonomic overreactivity may well be early attachment experiences that were either acutely or chronically traumatic (Schore, 2002). As I've suggested, the more troubled patients with a preoccupied state of mind with respect to attachment often bring with them to therapy a history of unresolved trauma or loss.

CHAPTER 14

The Unresolved Patient

Healing the Wounds of Trauma and Loss

The AAI identifies as unresolved not only some adults who are preoccupied, like those described in the preceding chapter, but also others who are dismissing or even secure. This finding may be in keeping with the fact that most of us have "islands" of trauma and dissociation in our history (Bromberg, 1998a). More often than not, however, there does appear to be a link between an unresolved state of mind, on the one hand, and severe psychological problems, on the other. Borderline, dissociative, and posttraumatic stress disorders are all apparently associated with lack of resolution of trauma, as is a childhood history of disorganized attachment (Dozier et al., 1999; Hesse, 1999; Solomon & George, 1999; Liotti, 1995; Solomon & Siegel, 2003; van IJzendorn, Schuenzel, & Bakermans-Kranenburg, 1999).

To identify patients who are unresolved, we need to be alert to lapses in reasoning or discourse when our patients touch on personal experiences of trauma and/or loss. For remember, it is not overwhelmingly painful experience per se that has a persistently disorganizing impact on the personality. Instead what is decisive is the patient's *lack of resolution* with regard to such experience, specifically as revealed through the sorts of lapses Main and Hesse describe (Main, 1995; Hesse, 1999). To the extent that we become aware of such lapses, we know that trauma and/or loss will figure significantly in the patient's therapy. But importantly, working with the im-

pact of trauma is not *sui generis*. As in all attachment-oriented treatment, the relationship is where the therapeutic action is.

Some years ago I met with a couple who were ostensibly seeking only to upgrade their communication. In the second session, the husband exchanged glances with his wife, Sarah, along with words I could barely make out, the gist of which seemed to be a pitch for her okay to discuss . . . something. As I recall, he wound up giving the headline and she took up the story from there. It turned out that when she was a teenager, she had come home from school one day to find that her mother had been murdered by her father.

Hearing the disclosure of this horrifically traumatic loss left me stunned, nearly into speechlessness. Sarah, for her part, made the calm, but transparently desperate, assertion that the event and its aftermath had nothing to do with who she was today. When I encouraged her to open up a little about her experience if she felt safe enough to do so, her response was very striking.

Whereas earlier in hour she had seemed engaged and emotionally available, she now spoke about her discovery of the murder in flat tones that conveyed an eerie detachment. Her account was interrupted several times by extremely long silences, during which she seemed to be turning inward and turning off, as if she were becoming lost to herself. Each time, it appeared that she needed to be brought back into the room with a word or a question from me or from her husband. Intermittently, in discussing her catastrophic past, she lapsed into the present tense.

All these markers of unresolved trauma—the apparent shift in Sarah's state of consciousness, her eerily detached tone of voice, the present-tense description of the past, and the lengthy pauses—can be understood to reflect the disorganizing and disorienting "return of the dissociated." Clearly this patient was unable to discuss her experience of trauma without feeling, in some sense, retraumatized.

At my urging she initiated her own individual psychotherapy in which, over time, I learned, she was gradually able to integrate and resolve the trauma she had originally had to dissociate. Further into our couples treatment she said that, while she had long tried to think about her past as little as possible, it had always been with her: "It's like a sharp pebble in my shoe, and when you've got a pebble in your shoe it can't help but deform your stride."

Extraordinarily difficult, but potentially extraordinarily rewarding, the therapy of unresolved patients resembles that with other patients—but writ large. With most of our patients, promoting integration is a significant part of our work. With unresolved patients for whom dissociation is so central and defining a feature, promoting integration of various kinds is the very heart of the work. Similarly, while with most patients the relationship with

the therapist is a significant part of therapy, for patients who are unresolved the therapeutic relationship *is* the therapy. And, finally, there is the matter of memory, which is more problematic for unresolved patients than for others.

All our patients are influenced by preverbal attachment experiences that are imprinted and stored as implicit procedural memories—building blocks of the right-brain working models that shape the patients' original patterns of relating, feeling, and thinking. Such implicit memories have registered prior to the development not only of language but also of those brain structures—in particular, the hippocampus—that place memories in a context within which their meaning can be grasped.

But recall: the developing hippocampus is temporarily deactivated by trauma. For unresolved patients, therefore, it is not only implicit memories of preverbal experience—often of a disorganized nature—but also of later *traumatic* experience that may remain wordless, timeless, and without context. Unable to consciously retrieve such experiences from memory, traumatized patients tend simply to relive them, with no sense of recollection.

Often these patients have grown up in disorganizing attachment relationships that were traumatic in at least two senses: They were overwhelmingly painful *and* they provided the child no safe context whatever within which to cope with this pain. The experience here was of regular and devastating disruption without repair. Such experience generated in these patients multiple incoherent models of the self, the other, and the relationship between them. These are the profoundly dispiriting models that unresolved patients bring with them to psychotherapy.

As practitioners of what Freud called an impossible profession, our mission with such patients is to provide them with a different experience and a different model of relationship. That is, we need to generate a new attachment relationship that is safe, reliable, and inclusive—and in which disruptions can be repaired. This relationship should also promote the development of the patient's resources, including those necessary to resolve past trauma. The problem here is that the patient who may consciously wish to have his suffering relieved is unconsciously compelled to recreate with us the old, profoundly unsafe relationship in which neither help nor hope was possible. And in the context of a therapeutic relationship that is felt to be unsafe, resolving the patient's trauma is, of course, impossible.

OVERCOMING THE PATIENT'S FEAR OF SECURITY

That the unresolved patient has trouble tolerating a secure relationship with an empathically attuned therapist is a paradox that defines much of the treatment. Creating a relationship in which the patient *can* actually feel

safe is essential and difficult. It should be seen as both the ultimate goal of therapy and a precondition for beginning to resolve the patient's trauma. This way of putting it will probably sound contradictory until it is grasped that creating a secure relationship and confronting trauma are intertwining processes. As I will explain, the incremental achievement of a sense of safety in relation to the therapist *does* resolve trauma, while the incremental resolution of trauma gradually obviates the necessity in the patient to reexperience the therapeutic relationship (and others) as a rendezvous with old threats.

The distinction has been drawn between "large-T trauma," like 9/11 or my patient's discovery of her mother's murder, and "small-T trauma"—the child's repeated experiences of fear, helplessness, humiliation, shame, and/or abandonment in relation to attachment figures who provided no repair (Shapiro & Maxfield, 2003). Small-T trauma has also been called "relational trauma" (Schore, 2002) and "cumulative trauma" (Kahn, 1963). Such trauma requires the child—and later predisposes the adult—to resort to primitive mechanisms of self-protection including dissociation and projective identification. It is these defenses that are largely responsible for bringing the patient's dangerous internal world alive in the relationship with the therapist.

Working with these defenses—through the kind of empathic attunement and limit setting described earlier—can gradually modify the patient's experience of the therapeutic relationship. As this relationship comes to feel progressively safer, it establishes a new working model that "competes" with those models that arose in response to the trauma of the patient's childhood. In this sense, the experience of an increasingly secure relationship indirectly modulates the impact of the original trauma while setting the stage for the patient's trauma to be confronted more directly.

Keep in mind again, however, that working with the therapeutic relationship and confronting trauma are processes that interweave. Dealing with the relationship often leads to feelings associated with trauma, while discussing traumatic experience often raises issues in the relationship. It is only for purposes of clarity that I discuss these ways of working as if they were strictly separate and sequential. To the extent that there is a sequence—security in the relationship, then dealing with trauma—it is one that is repeated over and over again.

The road to an increasingly secure relationship is usually an exceedingly rocky one precisely because the defenses the patient uses to avoid the painful past often wind up provoking its re-creation in the present. The therapeutic challenge, then, is to respond to this evocation of the past in a firm but empathic fashion that establishes by degrees a wedge between the old attachments that enrage and terrify the patient and the new attachment relationship whose promising possibilities the patient can initially barely imagine.

Put differently, our aim is to enable patients who are thoroughly embedded in experience—and thus inclined to simply equate their every feeling and belief with reality—to catch glimpses of a world that may be at odds with those feelings and beliefs. Over time, the combination of seeing themselves through our eyes and participating in interactions that disconfirm their rigidly held expectations can begin to kindle their capacity to consider more than one perspective on their experience—that is, to mentalize. How do these ideas about the interaction of past trauma, defenses, and the patients' relationship with the therapist play out in practice?

Toward the opening of the initial session of a very long psychotherapy, the patient—an emergency room physician whom I'll call Casey—told me that both his parents had killed themselves. Probably observing the expression on my face, he quickly clarified that they had "killed themselves slowly" through alcoholism and related forms of self-neglect. Confronted with a series of losses several months into the treatment, Casey himself became suicidal. He was now visibly desperate for help but unable to seek or make use of it, for reasons that fast became apparent—if only, at first, to me.

From early childhood on, Casey had been required to play the caregiving parent to his frail mother and violent father as well as to his younger siblings. While clearly he felt abandoned and neglected in this role, it enabled him to avoid some (though not all), of the explosions of rage and abuse that regularly tore his world apart. Taking care of others became for him a source of identity, as well as insurance against attack, yet it was a role, particularly in relation to his parents, that he had played out of fear.

Long angry at having to assume responsibilities that should never have been his, Casey had "chosen" not to impose on others the burdens his parents had imposed upon him—with the result that he had been regarded as a Rock of Gibraltar. But this counterdependent defense was apparently not only rigid but also brittle. He became suicidally depressed when faced with real and threatened losses that, I suspect, raised the specter of past abandonment and trauma. Even feeling overwhelmed, however, he had an extraordinarily difficult time acknowledging his need directly or accepting my help.

For more than a year, our therapy felt like a series of back-to-back emergencies that often seemed to have as much impact on me as they did on my patient. There were innumerable late night phone calls, suicide threats, gestures, and attempts, as well as multiple hospitalizations. Feeling that I had to battle the patient to keep him alive, I was nearly overwhelmed at times by anger, anxiety, confusion, and a sense of compulsive involvement—as if a single lapse in my caregiving might lead to a death or some other catastrophe.

Stepping back from the fray (as I was capable of doing only intermittently) I recognized that these feelings were probably related to

those Casey had experienced as a child with two parents who were not only threatening but also quite likely already "killing themselves." He had never before gotten close to integrating these overwhelming feelings, and he was certainly in no position to do so now. Instead he dissociated, and managed (largely unconsciously) to evoke his own unbearable experiences in me.

By virtue of my own history, I was all-too-ready to identify with them—not in the sense that I had literally known the same trauma but rather that my own experiences had primed me to resonate deeply with Casey and, at times, to enact with him dissociated aspects of his traumatic relationship with his parents.

DISSOCIATION, PROJECTIVE IDENTIFICATION, AND COUNTERTRANSFERENCE

Before returning to the account of my work with this patient, I need to situate it in the context of the defenses that protect patients like this one from the impact of trauma, while also unfortunately ensuring that elements of their trauma will repeatedly be relived. Such defenses play a role in evoking the therapist's countertransference—and, because that which is evoked in the therapist is often enacted with the patient, these defenses exert considerable influence in shaping the therapeutic relationship.

Let's start with "dissociation," a term that has two distinct meanings. It refers to "disintegration" of various kinds, including the self-protective splitting off of an unbearable state of mind (in which, for example, one's father has murdered one's mother) from other states of mind that are more tolerable and readily integrated with one's ongoing sense of self. Dissociation also refers to a defensively altered, trance-like state of consciousness, like that into which my patient in couple therapy fell when the trauma of her mother's murder resurfaced. Both kinds of dissociation play a central role in the experience and the psychotherapy of unresolved patients.

Failures of integration, to begin with, are pervasive in the psychology of many of these patients. Splitting—also known as "primitive dissociation" (Kernberg, 1984)—is the defensive hallmark of patients with a borderline personality disorder. It involves all-or-nothing, black-or-white, either-or forms of feeling, thinking, and relating that produce experiences of self and other that are compartmentalized, oversimplified, unrealistic, and unstable. In the subjective world of many unresolved patients, human beings are heroes or villains, persecutors or victims, those who rescue or those who are helpless. And given the tendency of such patients to confuse the part with the whole, they and the figures with whom they interact can easily slide from the valued category to its opposite. This makes for relationships

with others—including the therapist—that are unstable, stormy, and extraordinarily difficult for these patients to count on.

From a slightly different angle, the internal world of unresolved patients is built to a greater or lesser degree on working models and states of mind that have had to be defensively dissociated from one another. For example, in order for a maltreated child to avoid living in a state of perpetual terror, the models derived from the child's fear-filled experiences of abuse may have needed to be dissociated from other models arising from interactions that were less threatening. Such a history leaves radical discontinuities in the internal world of the adult, resulting in a vulnerability to sudden shifts from ordinary to overwhelming states of mind.

From a neurobiological standpoint, part of the price of early relationships that necessitate dissociation is that the child for whom attachment figures are frightening may fail to fully develop those integrative neural structures (such as the hippocampus, orbitofrontal cortex, and corpus callosum) that help modulate the brain's emergency response system, the amygdala. Without such integration and modulation, the overreactivity of the amygdala makes it likely that relatively innocuous triggers will provoke extremely intense autonomic responses in many unresolved patients.

In addition to shaping the psychobiological structure of these patients, dissociation also functions as a first-line defense. Frequently described as "the escape when there is no escape" (Putnam, 1992, p. 173), dissociation is not only a matter of failed integration, but also a hypnoid state in which the relation of the self to reality is altered for defensive purposes. Like all defenses, it provides self-protection at a price. Unresolved patients, by making reality less real, by spacing out, by becoming drowsy, and so on, have been able to blunt the impact of experiences they feared would overwhelm them. But the same altered state that keeps painful realities at bay also makes it impossible for those realities to be confronted effectively. The result is that unresolved patients live as if refusing to identify the smell of smoke rising from a fire smoldering in the basement. They remain always on the edge of being overwhelmed, as if (to mix metaphors) endlessly waiting for the other shoe to drop without realizing that it has dropped already.

Moreover, dissociation as an altered state usually entails experiences of "leaving the body" which can have a number of very problematic consequences. The body that is psychically abandoned in order to avoid painful experience is in some sense lost; it is no longer the person's own body. In the process, the somatic markers of emotion become inaccessible or difficult to read for many unresolved patients. Bessel van der Kolk puts it this way in writing about survivors of trauma: "Their failure to translate somatic states into words and symbols causes them to experience emotions simply as physical problems. . . . [They] experience distress in terms of physical organs, rather than as psychological states" (van der Kolk,

McFarlane, & Weisaeth, 1996, p. 423). The body of patients who dissociate can thus become a battleground on which psychological issues are fought out. Partly as a result, such patients often have many physical problems. A further complication: Because they are overly capable of disconnecting from their bodies, they often have a hard time taking good care of them. Finally, patients who dissociate may wind up in a panic when they begin to feel too cut off from themselves and from their bodies—necessitating drastic measures to reconnect. Self-mutilation in the form of cutting, burning, or beating themselves enables such patients to feel more embodied again, when dissociation has left them feeling disturbingly disembodied and unreal. Working with the body—a key feature of the psychotherapy of unresolved patients—is a matter I address in Chapter 16.

Dissociation that splits off what Sullivan (1953) calls the "bad-me" and "not-me" parts of the self enables unresolved patients to "disidentify" with a range of subjectively unbearable experiences, past and present. Yet that which is defensively dissociated does not disappear, although it may be relegated to the very periphery of awareness. Experiences, memories, representations, and feelings that are unintegrated and denied seem, figuratively speaking, to seek a home.

If they can't be psychologically accommodated within the patient, they must be relocated in the other. This is defensive projective identification, and in the treatment setting, the "other" is of course the therapist. In the process of relocating dissociated experience in us, the patient treats us in such a way as to evoke in us what he cannot bear in himself and we come to identify with it.

Countertransference, broadly conceived, arises out of the interplay between the patient's projective identifications and our own psychology. It is probably inevitable that as the therapist of an unresolved patient, we will enact in some form that which the patient projectively invites us to. For countertransference until it is recognized and dealt with tends simply to be enacted. Thus, if we are to succeed in generating a relationship with the patient that is better than those of his traumatic past, it is imperative that we try to recognize the unfolding transference–countertransference situation.

Awareness of countertransference has the potential to put the brakes on destructive enactments. This may be the most important rationale for attending to what we do, feel, and want in relation to our unresolved patients. For to the extent that we recognize the nature of our participation in the therapeutic relationship, we are likely to be able to conduct ourselves in such a way that our difficult, so-called "negative" countertransference reactions can eventually be contained, rather than simply acted out and/or denied.

In this connection, I have found it enormously helpful in relating to unresolved patients to think in terms of their working models of self and other. It has been theorized (Liotti, 1995, 1999) that traumatized patients

who dissociate—like Casey, discussed earlier, the physician son of a violent father—may have as many as four distinct experiences of themselves in relation to others. Having experienced abuse, neglect, loss, or cumulative relational trauma at the hands of attachment figures, they have a model of themselves as victims. Having experienced themselves as both responsible for the trauma and angry in response to it—and also, perhaps, identifying with the aggressor—they have a model of themselves as persecutors. Having experienced with attachment figures the role reversal involved in being "parentified"—recall that disorganized infants often become caregiving (i.e., controlling) children—they have a model of themselves as rescuers. And finally, because they have had frequent recourse to dissociation, they have a model of themselves as cognitively incompetent or confused.

Keep in mind that what is actualized in the interaction of transference and countertransference interaction is a *relationship*. For example, I continually found myself feeling compelled to rescue Casey, probably very much as he had felt compelled—by fear—to rescue his parents. Meanwhile, Casey appeared in our interactions to be as uninvolved in his own care as he felt his parents had been in theirs. In this mode, my countertransference identification was with the "self" component of the patient's working model, while he seemed identified with his mother or father. As will become apparent in a moment, on the other hand, I could as easily occupy the countertransference role of his angry or abandoning parent, while Casey—understandably distrustful of such a figure—approached me warily, if at all, and then invariably withdrew.

OVERCOMING THE PATIENT'S FEAR OF SECURITY (CONTINUED)

During the period in which Casey was most dangerous to himself, I was meeting with him three times weekly and talking to him briefly on a nearly daily basis. It was very clear to me, to his physician, and to his psychopharmacologist that we were fighting to save his life. The patient, however, buffered by dissociation and self-medication, repeatedly cycled out of crisis into denial. While in crisis, he desperately and angrily flailed about for help; while in denial, he stubbornly claimed not to need it. In the latter mode, he frequently threatened to quit therapy—having told me that if indeed he were to quit, I would know for certain that he was going to kill himself. I found myself variously enraged, scared, and confused in relation to this patient but almost always consumed by the need to protect him.

Sometimes it was possible for me to grasp that all these feelings were, in part, the outcome of Casey's nonverbal, projective, enactive communications about his internal world. When I was thoroughly embedded (read, "stuck") in my experience of our relationship, these communications had

me by the throat such that I was by turns Casey's persecutor, victim, incompetent helper, or rescuer. When I was able to free myself from their grip, they enabled me to empathize with my patient's dissociated experience. They also gave me clues with regard to how I might need to intervene.

At one point, as Casey began regularly to arrive for his appointments late, I began to feel increasingly angry. His chaotic and self-destructive behavior was self-evidently a cry for help, yet he seemed to be doing virtually nothing to help himself. I felt that he was generating a relationship in which I alone was supposed to be responsible for him, much as I guessed he had felt angrily alone with the responsibility his parents had foisted on him as a child.

Then during a session to which he arrived late, without a word about why, he threatened once again to quit therapy. Initially exasperated, I then felt stunned by the rather excruciating sensation that I was being dropped. But along with this sensation, an image crystallized, and with it came a shift in my feeling about, and understanding of, Casey's behavior.

Prompted by that as well as by some much-needed consultation, I told Casey that it made sense to me that he might wish to stop. I said I had the image of him in my mind as a baby who had been held—then suddenly dropped. Our relationship, I guessed, must feel like an invitation to be held again and then—inevitably—dropped.

Now apparently it was his turn to be stunned. Gazing at me wordlessly, but as though he were for the first time in a long time actually present, he then said he was "awed" by the depth of my feeling for his experience, and, yes, it was impossible for him to believe that I wouldn't drop him. It was only a matter of time. Yet he averred that he also yearned to be able to assume otherwise. I sensed a shared recognition during the brief silence that followed that we had found the emotional equivalent of a calm in the storm.

After a few moments, I told him that if I were to be able to really hold him and not drop him, then I needed to insist that he try to allow himself to be held. I wasn't at all sure he could do this, I added, but for my part, I was going to try to help: Specifically, I was not going to agree that it was okay for him to stop therapy or, for that matter, to keep coming so late that we had sometimes less than half hour an hour to be together. In the future, if he were more than 20 minutes late, I said, I wouldn't meet with him, but I would charge him. He didn't protest and he began to show up for our sessions more punctually. Importantly, I had established a limit that enabled me to feel less angry, less like dropping him. I suspect the same limit helped Casey to feel less "bad," less unmanageable, and more effectively held.

What I hope I am communicating here is the therapeutic synergy between empathic attunement, on the one hand, and the setting of appropri-

ate limits, on the other. With patients like this one, both are necessary and neither on its own is sufficient. Without our empathic attunement, the patient can feel neither understood nor felt. Without setting the limits necessary to protect patient and therapist, we will likely feel too overwhelmed and angry to offer empathy or any other kind of meaningful help. I also hope I am conveying the necessity for, and the power of, enlisting our own subjective experience—our feelings, images, impulses—as well as our theories to help us sense what our unresolved patients might actually need from us.

Probably the most immediate, though also ongoing, need of patients like Casey is for our assistance in managing their overwhelming affects. Our attuned resonance and empathy, the limits we set, our reliable availability, and our concern are all elements of the interactive regulation of affect that we hope to supply in ways the patients' original attachment figures could not. The words we use to name the patients' feelings and give them a context are also key to this mutual regulation of affect. When we succeed in providing such help, we disconfirm the patients' transferential expectations and strengthen the sense of the therapeutic relationship as a secure base.

Effective provision of this kind of help can be difficult. Round after round of attunement, misattunement, and interactive repair are usually necessary before the unresolved patient can begin to trust in the emotion-regulating potential of the new relationship. Repeated sequences of disruption and repair are essential because our help in bearing painful feelings is so frequently felt by the patient to be unhelpful. It may be experienced as controlling, intrusive, and/or misattuned. Or it may register as a dangerous invitation to the patient to risk being "dropped" once again.

Such responses often reflect the absence of adequate affect-regulating interactions with the patient's original attachment figures—as well as the presence of interactions that were traumatic. Implicit memories of these interactions are relived in relation to the therapist, while the unresolved patient is, much of the time, unaware that he may be living out a memory. However, after repeated emotion-drenched sequences of disruption and repair that seem to disconfirm the patient's trauma-driven expectations, things may change. As the patient slowly comes to sense that the therapeutic relationship can be relied on as a source of security and safety, he may gradually grow more capable of recognizing his burdensome tendency to experience the present as if it were no different from the past.

PUTTING THE TRAUMA INTO WORDS

Yassir, a Palestinian contractor, had been in an on-and-off therapy with me for several years. Toward the middle of a recent session, he

began to seem uncomfortable. He was sweaty and looked anxious. It turned out that he was feeling claustrophobic and scared, without understanding why. As we explored his feeling of claustrophobia, he suddenly recalled an experience he'd had as an eight-year-old boy in Jericho at the start of the 1967 war.

He narrates the memory in the present tense. There are the sounds of air raid sirens and jet planes. Outside, looking up from the street, he sees jet planes, dogfights in the sky. He runs for the safety of what turns out to be a dangerously overcrowded bomb shelter. Having descended the steps, he feels he's suffocating. He's trying to claw his way out, but he's dragged back down. He feels terror.

Then he talks some about the months that followed: his family's flight to Jordan—the burning cars, the bodies of the dead and wounded en route—and the family's subsequent return via a clandestine night crossing of the Jordan river where the water was shoulder deep and the babies were held overhead. At this point, he goes quiet and I ask him what he's experiencing. He says he knows I'll find this hard to believe, but the answer is, absolutely nothing.

Then he says, "It's awfully stuffy in here."

I'll return to this session in a moment, but first I want to highlight the importance with most unresolved patients of recalling experiences of traumatic events and putting them into words, rather than simply reexperiencing trauma-related feelings in the relationship with the therapist, without the appropriate "time signature." Intrusive memories of unresolved trauma as well as the defenses against such memories produce a sense of helplessness. Naming the feelings associated with trauma confers a growing sense of mastery. Moreover, the memories of unprocessed trauma are "frozen" in time, with the result that the historical past is experienced as subjectively present. When old traumatic experiences can be revisited without the patient feeling retraumatized, the memories of trauma are changed. Paraphrasing Stern (2004), they now have a "new remembering context" that can be transformative as overwhelming events are recalled with feeling and their meaning elaborated in the (relative) safety of the relationship with a stronger or wiser other. Within such a context, the trauma of the unresolved patient can begin to be confined to its own time and place, rather than remaining a ubiquitously disturbing presence.

In establishing a new context for past trauma, we also need to make links between the disquieting past and its consequences in the moment. Thus:

When Yassir said the room was stuffy, I asked him if he were feeling claustrophobic here now. As he replied, "A little," I was already opening the windows of the office and pulling aside the curtains. He took a few deep breaths and immediately appeared relieved. We explored

why he couldn't ask me earlier for what he knew he wanted and needed, namely, more air in the room. That exploration led to a consideration of his survivor guilt.

A year before the war began, his mother had given birth to a profoundly disabled son, while his father, who had once been a "bigshot," had a heart attack and was reduced to selling lottery tickets in the street. It was during this time that Yassir decided that his needs ("for shoes, for an education") must take a back seat to the needs of others. Hence, his inhibition when it came to articulating his desires. We also touched on his everyday experience of nearly pervasive fear, which he seemed all too ready to rationalize. Clearly, making the connections between his history of trauma and his current apprehensiveness was going to be a work in process.

Like many unresolved patients, he was extremely reluctant to let his guard down. Braced for the next catastrophe, he was as yet quite unconvinced that the catastrophe he feared had already occurred.

MENTALIZING AND MINDFULNESS

Recalling trauma without being retraumatized, naming trauma-related feelings and bodily sensations, making implicit memories explicit—all within the context of an increasingly secure and effectively affect-regulating therapeutic relationship—are among the essential ingredients in the treatment of unresolved patients. So are mentalizing and mindfulness.

When we respond to the patient in light of the feelings, needs, and beliefs that underlie his behavior, we begin to kindle his biologically based capacity to mentalize. With this capacity, the patient can increasingly step back from his immediate experience—say, the experience of fear—in order to understand it. Such reflection confers a greater sense of control over feelings and behavior and makes both more meaningful and predictable. This helps generate, in turn, a quality of security that is usually in very short supply for unresolved patients in particular.

Mindfulness, finally, has a role to play both for the therapist of the unresolved patient and for the patient himself. For the therapist, the ability to enter a mindful state can diminish the countertransference pressures that arise in the treatment of patients who have been traumatized. For the unresolved patient, mindfulness meditation has the potential, emotionally speaking, to provide shelter from the storm (Linehan, 1993). As will be discussed in Chapter 16, mindful attention to the body (and especially the breath) can serve as an antidote to panic and dissociation, as well as a means to gradually toning down the patient's autonomic overreactivity. Lastly, the mindful practice of observing and labeling thoughts, feelings,

and bodily sensations (rather than avoiding them or being swept away by them) can support the patient's nascent mentalizing capacity (Allen & Fonagy, 2002). For the unresolved patient in whom the pull of emotions, sensations, and beliefs is nearly irresistible, this can be a very useful kind of support.

PART V

SHARPENING THE
CLINICAL FOCUS

I*n providing the patient with a secure base, we are offering a corrective relational experience that may be healing in its own right. From this perspective, the attachment bond the patient develops in relation to the therapist may be the key therapeutic intervention. Yet the attachment relationship can also serve as an exceptionally effective context in which to integrate dissociated facets of the patient's experience and nurture the patient's potential both to reflect and to live mindfully. How the therapist can make the best possible use of this new developmental context is the subject matter of the next three chapters.*

Chapter 15 spells out in detail the ways in which we can utilize our subjective experience and our awareness of co-created enactments as gateways to the nonverbal realm, which is often also the domain of the dissociated.

Chapter 16 concentrates on the body. The patient's somatic sensations, expressions, movement, and posture speak without words—as do the therapist's. Through working with the body, we can reach, and help to regulate, the patient's emotions. And because prelinguistic experience and trauma both register in the soma as well as the psyche, focusing on the body can bring inarticulate and dissociated experience to light.

Chapter 17 describes mentalizing and mindfulness as complementary paths of psychological liberation. The first frees us through understanding, the second through acceptance, presence, and awareness. As therapists, we can attempt in many different ways to help shift our patients' stance toward experience in a more reflective and mindful direction. How helpful we are here will ultimately depend on how effectively we're able to cultivate our own capacities for mentalizing and mindfulness.

CHAPTER 15

The Nonverbal Realm I

Working with the Evoked and the Enacted

In an attachment-oriented psychotherapy, our aim is to generate with the patient a new relationship that is more attuned, inclusive, and collaborative than those that originally shaped him. For many reasons, creating such a relationship with the patient requires a concentrated focus on the emotionally based nonverbal subtext of the therapeutic dialogue. The patient's preverbal attachment experience, trauma for which he has no words, feelings and needs that he has had to dissociate—all these are mainly made accessible, *not* as they are directly articulated by the patient, but rather as he evokes them in us, enacts them with us, or embodies them.

Therefore, while we listen to the patient's words and respond with words of our own, we need to pay as much, if not more attention to the emotional, relational, and visceral/somatic undercurrents that shape the verbal exchange. The words, in their own right, may or may not convey significant meaning. The implicit, nonverbal subtext almost always does. It is the *feeling* of what happens *here*—the sense of what is actually going on in the therapeutic relationship—that can lead us to what is most immediately salient both in the patient's experience and in the interactions we co-create.

To minimize the risk that our attention will be monopolized by the patient's words, we need to remind ourselves to "read" the language of the patient's body: the expressions of the face, the rhythm and tone of the

voice, the pace and locale of the patient's breathing, as well as the nuances of posture, gesture, and the like. Just as important, we need to remember to pause and take a deep breath, as it were, in order to be able to sense what is going on inside *us*—not our discursive thoughts primarily, but rather our bodily and emotional experience. Do we feel fully present, alive to our emotions, and engaged with the patient? If not, what *is* the nature of our experience? And how might it relate to the patient's experience? Here we are looking into ourselves in order to know more both about the patient and about the quality and meaning of our responsiveness to the patient.

Attachment research leaves no doubt that the parent's state of mind exerts a crucial influence on the developing infant. Clinical experience (both on and off the couch, so to speak) suggests that the therapist's state of mind with respect to attachment exerts a similarly crucial, though perhaps less powerful, influence on the development of the patient in psychotherapy.

To become aware of the impact of our own state(s) of mind upon the patient, we need to be keenly attentive to the patient's reactions to what we say and do, or fail to say and do. Recognizing these affective reactions requires attention to the patient's words, of course, but also to his nonverbal communication. Here we are focusing on the patient's experience both in its own right and as a way of recognizing the nature of our own participation in the relationship.

Of course, this brings us directly to the issue of transference–countertransference enactments—that is, the behavioral expression of the interacting subjectivities of patient and therapist. Given that enactments are ongoing and unavoidable, the question is not *whether* we are participating in an enactment but *how*. What are we really *doing* with the patient? What roles are we inclined to assume? What are we choosing to focus on? What are we avoiding? And what unconscious motivations might be driving our side of the enactment?

Because enactments arise from the *interlocking* influences of transference and countertransference, becoming aware of our own contribution to the interaction is often a preliminary to illuminating the contributions of the patient.

This kind of self-awareness often prompts intuitive interventions that foster an increasing sense of attunement and collaboration between patient and therapist in their pursuit of shared goals. Progressively deepening this sense of "fittedness" is among the most important ways in which the therapeutic couple generates a new attachment relationship that can transform the patient's insecure working models into "earned" secure ones.

As explained in Chapter 8, therapists and patients are involved together in a trial-and-error process of feeling their way toward such

fittedness through the "improvisation of relational moves" (Lyons-Ruth & Boston Change Process Study Group, 2001; Change Process Study Group, 2005). On the one hand, this process unfolds implicitly (and initially nonverbally) as both partners sense, and respond accordingly, to what is going on inside themselves, inside the other, and between the two of them. On the other hand, making such implicit experience *explicit* can be a key part of the recognition processes that heighten the probability that "moving along" in psychotherapy will also be "moving forward."

To help clinicians to work effectively with the implicit, nonverbal dimension of the therapeutic interaction, I have offered the shorthand that what our patients cannot articulate will tend to be evoked, enacted, or embodied. While the discussion that follows in this chapter and the next is organized accordingly, these categories are never as distinct in practice as they are in theory. What patients evoke in us, we often enact. What patients embody, they often evoke in us. And so on.

Moreover, as I've suggested already, the undercurrents in the therapeutic relationship rarely, if ever, flow exclusively in one direction. We can be as evocative a presence for our patients as they are for us. We can be as responsible for initiating enactments as the patient is. And we can be as prone as the patient to unwittingly express our feelings through the body.

Yet the therapeutic relationship is characterized not only by this kind of mutuality but also by asymmetry. While patient and therapist are inescapably mutually influential and share many of the same vulnerabilities, the therapist's training, clinical experience, and personal therapy (if not personal history) often confer advantages the patient may lack. These include— most importantly—a well-developed capacity to tolerate, recognize, and make sense of our own feelings and those of others, as well as an experientially derived recognition of the power of the unconscious.

In addition, the roles of therapist and patient are very different: One is there to help, the other to receive help. After all, it is the patient's vulnerability, discontent, and hope, rather than ours, which are the primary focus of, and *raison d'être* for, the therapeutic relationship. This asymmetry creates a context in which we may well feel both more secure than the patient and more secure than we ordinarily do. As a consequence, we are often more capable than we might otherwise be of providing the flexibility and empathic attunement (including attunement to nonverbal affective experience) that make a relationship of secure attachment possible.

As discussed in Chapter 10, intersubjective and relational theory is a uniquely powerful resource when it comes to working with the nonverbal experience that attachment research identifies as so central. Specifically, this body of theory illuminates how we might most effectively deal with what is evoked and enacted in the therapeutic relationship. In other words,

the theory helps us to recognize, understand, and intervene in transference–countertransference interactions that are implicit and unverbalized. These initially unconscious interactions can be an invaluable resource as well as a most challenging obstacle.

But before discussing them in detail, I want to touch on some research and clinical theory concerning individual differences in the perception and expression of experience in the nonverbal realm. For how therapists and patients communicate and interpret the nonverbal messages they exchange has enormous impact on the extent to which they wind up feeling that they are in synch and getting somewhere together. Because those of us with different attachment styles tend to communicate nonverbally in different ways, knowing something about these differences may be of use in understanding ourselves as well as our patients.

NONVERBAL COMMUNICATION

The "sensitive responsiveness" that helps to foster security in first relationships depends largely on the attachment figure's ability to accurately read the infant's nonverbal signals and to nonverbally communicate responses that are contingent—that is, attuned, matched, or fitted to the signals of the infant. Similarly, our empathic attunement to the patient depends largely on our ability to accurately read the patient's nonverbal cues and to respond nonverbally (as well as verbally) in ways that allow patients to sense that their own internal states are not only understood but also somehow *felt* by the therapist (Schore, 2003; Siegel, 1999).

While we might all wish to be fluent in the language of nonverbal communication, the capacity to understand and convey nonverbal messages varies from person to person. Social psychological research suggests that people who are secure may be more adept at communicating nonverbally than those who are not (Schachner, Shaver, & Mikulincer, 2005). Their readings of the nonverbal messages of others tend to be more accurate, while their nonverbal messages tend to be clearer and more direct.

The nonverbal communication of insecure individuals can be problematic in ways that are partly dependent on their attachment style. Let's start with the expressive dimension. When compared to that of secure individuals, the nonverbal behavior of those described by social psychologists as "avoidant" (that is, dismissing) tends to be quite restricted. Their facial expressions reveal less, they gaze at and touch others less, and their tone of voice may convey less positive feeling. In attachment-related contexts, they show less nonverbal support seeking, and more turning away and gazing elsewhere. By contrast, the nonverbal behavior of individuals described as

"anxious" (preoccupied) tends to be highly expressive, particularly when they are seeking support and/or when their emotions are negative.

As for their sensitivity to nonverbal cues, particularly cues signaling need or distress, avoidant individuals seem to ignore or be blind to them, while those who are anxious tend to overrespond, reacting sometimes to signals they imagine rather than accurately perceive. In general, insecure individuals appear to make appraisals of others that are biased, but in particular ways. Research suggests that avoidant adults are prone to assume that they are different and distinct from others—and they tend to see in others (projected) evidence of their own *unwanted* traits. Anxious adults, in contrast, are prone to assume that others are similar to them—and they tend to see (projected) evidence of *actual* traits of their own in others (Mikulincer & Shaver, 2003). These patterns of bias (false distinctiveness or false consensus) and projection (of unwanted or actual traits) may play a role in our patient's transference reactions. They may also be a factor in our countertransference responses. And, of course, the two interact.

For example, a dismissing patient who was guiltily inclined to deny his own aggression often read (or misread) anger in my tone of voice or the look on my face. From one angle, I could understand his tendentious interpretation as the result of projection and false distinctiveness: According to his reading of my nonverbal cues, I was angry and he was not. On the other hand, this patient's transference was unquestionably "ratified" at times by my countertransference. His eagle eye for hostility and my own tendency to assume that we *shared* a sense of vulnerability (false consensus) combined to evoke from me an overly protective, overly controlled response. And feeling straitjacketed by having to be so careful about what I revealed to the patient nonverbally, I gradually became irritated with him.

In much the same vein, a preoccupied patient who was often in distress didn't know what to make of it when she saw (or thought she saw) nonverbal signs that others were upset, only to be told in response to her solicitude that they actually felt fine. As for our relationship, she told me she thought we wouldn't make a good couple because we were both too moody. Was this a matter of false consensus? Needless to say, we had a very interesting conversation about her sense of our shared psychology.

Alongside the research on bias and projection, related findings suggest that avoidant and anxious individuals alike have a tendency to read hostile intent into their partners' behavior, even when cues suggesting such intent are absent (Schacter, Shaver, & Mikulincer, 2005). In general, it appears that patients with problematic attachment histories have difficulty accurately decoding nonverbal cues, such as facial expressions, and are consequently vulnerable to misinterpreting the emotions and intentions of others (Schore, 2003).

With such patients, in particular, it may be important for therapists to be more, rather than less, transparent. When we keep ourselves a riddle to patients like these we may inadvertently consolidate a surplus of negative transference. When such a patient seems to be misattributing feelings to me, I have often made a point of deliberately disclosing my emotional experience. When that disclosure has been met with skepticism, then I have asked the patient to *look at my face* while listening to me. *What does he see there? What does he hear me saying? Do the two channels match up, or not?* Of course, I explicitly keep open the possibility that the patient may be noting some aspect of my experience of which I'm unaware. Within such a respectful context, I'm aiming to strengthen the patient's ability to deliberately attend to nonverbal cues so as to be able to read them with greater accuracy. For patients, the first step here—often a disconcerting one—is to allow themselves to begin to at least question their automatic interpretation of such cues.

The nonverbal transmission and reception of emotion that we've been discussing is, according to the evidence of neuroscience research, a specialty of the right brain. In this connection, Schore (2005) makes the suggestion that clinicians might do well to focus on the left side of their patient's face, because it is the left side that is dominated by the nonverbal social–emotional right brain. Indeed, studies have shown that the left side of the face is more emotionally expressive than the right (Mandal & Ambady, 2004). Schore's suggestion may seem a trifle mechanical, but I have found it an extremely helpful one. That we should "tune in with the right brain" to the left side of the patient's face is, of course, a very specific recommendation that exemplifies the broader necessity that we focus attention on the patient's nonverbal cues.

Much that is communicated nonverbally remains implicit—an affective substrate of rapid cuing and response that shapes and reshapes the spoken dialogue moment by moment. Much of the time, one hopes, this ongoing exchange of visual and auditory cues between patient and therapist generates an atmosphere of safety in which the two partners feel emotionally in synch. On the other hand, there may be disturbing undercurrents in the shared implicit relationship that are only expressed nonverbally—and that the patient, for one, may be unable or unwilling to name.

Whether either of these two very different kinds of experience will be addressed explicitly often depends on the therapist. We can choose to make the implicit interaction explicit or we can choose not to. If we choose to make the implicit explicit, then we have a further question to answer: Should we directly disclose our experience of the interaction to the patient? Or, should we instead use that experience indirectly, say, in the form of an empathic comment or an interpretation? Questions like these are particu-

larly pressing when we feel that patients have succeeded in evoking aspects of their own experience inside us.

WHAT IS TO BE DONE WITH WHAT IS EVOKED?

What we think we *should* do with the experience the patient evokes in us and what we actually *will* do may turn out to be two different things. The first usually depends on our conscious sense of what is likely to be most useful for the patient. The second depends on a host of other factors, most of which are not initially conscious. These factors—including our own psychology, mood, and preoccupations of the moment as well as the influence of the patient—interact with our deliberate intentions to generate responses that are unpredictable and to some extent outside our conscious control. Often these unpremeditated responses turn out to be productive. Sometimes they are problematic.

> A divorced, hippie-ish attorney in his early 50s—"Neil"—sought my help in overcoming his anxiety. Over the course of several months together, we came to understand that anxiety, though the most overtly distressing of his feelings, was actually only one among many that were difficult for him to bear. One day our session began with a lengthy silence that I eventually broke, asking Neil what was going on inside him. As he was driving over, he told me, he'd heard on the radio about Jerry Garcia's death and just now he had experienced "a little twinge of sadness." He added that he had a number of friends, though, for whom the Grateful Dead's guitarist had been iconic, a real Sixties hero. They must really be feeling something.
> There was another brief silence during which I found myself thinking about how hard it was for *him* to feel. I considered inviting Neil to say more about his little twinge of sadness. At which point I became aware of my own sadness. I, too, had heard that morning about Garcia's death, but my reaction then had been muted. Now the feelings were stronger, sharper. Sensing that Neil was aware of my emotions, but not, of course, my earlier reaction to them, and guessing that communicating my experience might make more room for his, I said, "I'm not sure how this fits in with something that might be important for you, but I found myself remembering just now hearing about Garcia's death myself as I was driving over here. I think I stopped myself from feeling much with the worry that I needed to keep it together because I was about to be at work. I guess it can be a real question sometimes, how much any of us allow ourselves to feel." Saying these words, I felt my eyes well up. Then I saw that he, too, had become tearful. After a few moments, he briefly acknowledged that perhaps he

had felt "more than a little sad." And then he became intensely anxious.

As sketched so far, my interaction with Neil can be seen to illustrate several points about the usefulness of working with experience the patient evokes in the therapist—as well as experience the therapist evokes in the patient.

First, this way of working may contribute to a therapeutic relationship that is inclusive and that asks for a little more from patients than they may expect of themselves—two of the features of developmental relationships that researchers have found to be associated with secure attachment (Lyons-Ruth, 1999). Attending to the sadness Neil evoked in me—and disclosing my earlier reluctance to fully feel my own sadness—brought Neil's emotions and his anxiety about them directly into the room. Feelings from which he had learned to dissociate came alive in our interaction where they could be experienced, understood, and potentially integrated. Working in this way with Neil also led to an "upgrading of the dialogue" (Lyons-Ruth, 1999) that began to make a place for what might be described as the "unfelt known." Ensuring that the therapeutic conversation engages not only the thinking mind but the "feeling body" may be especially crucial with patients like Neil whose attachment orientation appears to be predominantly dismissing.

Second, our interaction illustrates the importance of keeping in mind that the evocative influence in the relationship of patient and therapist flows in both directions. When Neil discussed his (defensively minimized) experience of sadness he evoked my own (previously minimized) sadness. In turn, I believe, the sadness I communicated to Neil through my words and welling eyes evoked tears of his own and, moments later, his anxiety.

How much this sort of emotional "contagion" marks the experience of any given therapeutic couple may depend on a number of factors. From one angle, it's probably always built in. Having been equipped by evolution with mirror neurons, we're all hard-wired to participate in the subjective experience of other people. From another angle, it may depend on the degree of our willingness and ability as therapists to make ourselves emotionally available to the patient's influence. Finally, it may be that whatever the patient successfully evokes must be "evocable" in the particular therapist involved. That is, there may need to be an internal "hook" on which the patient can hang his hat. I'm referring here, broadly speaking, to the particulars of the therapist's character, but also more narrowly to the details of the therapist's lived experience. For example, I suspect I might not have been able to resonate so deeply with Neil's (largely) unfelt feelings had the musician who died been entirely unimportant to me.

Now let's briefly return to the session.

Shortly after he became tearful, Neil began to look very uncomfortable. When I asked him what was going on, he told me that he was starting to get increasingly anxious, and worried that the feeling might get out of control. I said it seemed to me that, for him, becoming tearful was very scary. He said he knew it made no sense, but he was sure that if he were to cry he'd wind up feeling small and weak, and that scared him. I found myself thinking that earlier I'd felt it necessary to contain my own impulse to cry: I was about to be at work. Then I remembered recently reading an article by Stephen Mitchell in which another analyst is quoted by a patient as having said to him: "Men work and fuck women."

Recall here Ogden's (1994) concept of the "analytic third"—the idea that our subjective experiences in the clinical hour (including apparently stray thoughts like the one immediately above) arise out of the unconscious psychic intermingling of both partners, and thus may reflect aspects of the patient's experience as well as the therapist's.

I asked Neil if perhaps he felt that it wasn't masculine to cry. He responded with a memory recounted in the present tense: He's at his mother's funeral. She has died of heart failure. He's struggling to contain his tears, and then with astonishment he sees—for the first and last time in his life—his father crying. He thinks, "What a wimp." This memory opened a discussion of Neil's need to keep an iron grip on his "negative" feelings, as well as his concern that I could apparently be so easily overcome by feelings of my own. It also brought into the therapy Neil's loss, and unfinished mourning, of his mother.

I think you can see here how the unfolding relationship of patient and therapist evolves unpredictably through a spiral of reciprocal reverberating influence. Neil evoked responses in me that evoked responses in him that elicited further responses from me, and so on. Most of this ricocheting influence has an impact that remains implicit and unspoken. When patient and therapist are emotionally in synch, neither may experience the necessity to be explicit about the (harmonious) nature of their interaction. However, what is required may be very different when the therapeutic relationship has come to feel uncomfortable, mechanical, adversarial, or disconnected. Then, to the degree that the implicit can be made explicit, we usually enhance the likelihood that the patient's relationship with the therapist may ultimately be experienced as safe, attuned, collaborative, and inclusive. What is key here—just as it is in our first attachment relationships (Koback, 1999)—is that the lines of communication between the two partners be kept open. In early development, such open communication largely depends on the caregiver's sensitivity to the infant's nonverbal signals. In

the context of therapeutic development, it depends on the therapist's sensitivity to the patient's nonverbal signals, including those that are conveyed by evoking experience in the therapist.

The precise meaning of our subjective experience as we relate to the patient is often hard to pin down. How much of this experience of ours is actually evoked by the patient? How much of it is, so to speak, ours alone? In this connection, I find it useful to assume that what I'm experiencing when I'm with the patient is almost always a matter of both/and, rather than either/or. With Neil, for example, my sadness was already there in me to be evoked. At the same time, his own sadness was hard for him to bear, and so, I believe, he "shared" it with me.

In clarifying the meaning of what the patient evokes, it may be helpful to consider the distinction between countertransference responses that are concordant (empathic) and those that are complementary (Racker, 1968). The first are thought to result when the patient evokes in the therapist an identification with a disowned aspect of the patient's *self* experience (Neil's partially unfelt sadness, for example, which I found myself feeling quite intensely). The second can be seen to result when the patient evokes in the therapist an identification with an aspect of the patient's internalized experience of an other. I recall, as an instance of this kind of complementary identification, that later in my work with Neil I found myself feeling angry at what appeared to be his lack of involvement with me. Exploring this experience, it seemed likely that I was identifying with his image of his mother as someone who became angry with him whenever he was, in his own words, "too independent."

Yet this useful framing of countertransference notwithstanding, we should never assume that the influence in the therapeutic relationship flows in only one direction. As I mentioned earlier, what we actually manage to do with what is evoked in us will depend, for better or worse, on more than our sense of what will be most useful for the patient. There is also the not insignificant matter of own relatively abiding patterns of feeling, thinking, and relating—our internal working model(s)—as well as the transient shifts in state of mind provoked by circumstances external to the treatment:

One morning I arrived in an unusually compromised frame of mind to see my first patient of the day. Virtually as soon as we sat down, the patient announced that while it was difficult for him to do so, he needed to tell me how far short I'd recently fallen in dealing empathically with his needs. This was not an unfamiliar conversation. On several previous occasions, he had communicated his unhappiness with me very directly and I had not felt unduly discomfited, partly because I sensed that his complaints, whatever their merit might be, were also part of a "transference test." Early in the therapy I had become clear

that this patient—whose father had killed himself—would need responses from me that might help disconfirm his fear that his own anger and power were lethal. Thus, my willingness to listen respectfully to his criticisms and to take responsibility for my role in them (when I saw that I had one) was extremely reassuring to him.

During this particular session, however, as he began to detail his discontents, I felt myself becoming increasingly cold and unsympathetic. I listened, but without empathy. It was as if I lacked the internal resources necessary to stretch far enough emotionally to put myself in his place, even for a moment. After a while I simply couldn't hear more. In a tense, strained, and vaguely angry tone of voice, I told my patient that I simply didn't know what I could say about his complaints: They were simply *his* complaints.

Not surprisingly, he was visibly taken aback, if not shocked, by my response. Appearing very confused and uneasy, he began to backtrack: Perhaps he'd been unfair to me and had been coming on too strong, maybe he'd been expecting too much, and so on. Jarred awake, so to speak, by his nearly palpable pain, I got enough of a grip on myself to explain that before I'd seen him that morning I'd had an extremely stressful time: Nothing serious, I reassured him, but the result of it was that I wasn't in a position now to respond in the ways I was ordinarily able to. He was relieved to hear my explanation, contrasting it with the failure of his previous therapists as well as his parents ever to acknowledge that, when there was a problem, it might be their own difficulties that were getting in the way. Yet he clearly had difficulty feeling entirely reassured. Near the close of this hour, and again in the next, we revisited his worry that perhaps I was unwilling or unable to deal with his anger.

This emotionally freighted encounter is a particularly obvious example of what is often a much more subtle reality—namely, that our experience of the patient's evocative influence is always in part a function of our own irreducible subjectivity (Renik, 1993). In previous sessions, the expression of my patient's discontent had evoked only the merest traces of anxiety in me, while in the session I just described it left me feeling angry and thwarted.

Thinking of these two very different reactions as opposite poles of a continuum suggests that the therapist's experience will vary at times in response to what is virtually the same aspect of the patient—and that reactions at either extreme (being unaffected or overly affected) usually leave something out. For example, wanting to hear no more of my patient's complaints in the hour in which I felt resourceless raised the possibility that my equanimity in response to his earlier criticisms reflected some denial: Probably I was reluctant to experience my own reactions to his "destructiveness" in relation to my efforts to help.

Just we as are never be a blank screen onto which patients project their

transference images, we can never be a pristine container of that which patients evoke in us. Our best hope is to become as knowledgeable as possible about the characteristics of the not-so-pristine container—our own subjectivity—that shapes our responsiveness to our patients' evocative influence. For in spite of what we may believe we're consciously *choosing* to do with the patient, it is often our *unconscious* needs, feelings, and intentions that are decisive. It is these that come through to the patient via the channels of nonverbal communication.

The mutuality of the nonverbal influence patients and therapists exert upon one another, as well as the internal influence exerted by the unconscious of each, ensures that making good use of what the patient seems to evoke in us will be an extremely complex matter. Like the complexity of the caregiver's task in responding to the young child's nonverbal cues, the complexity of the therapist's task here is real and inescapable. Ignoring it does the patient a disservice. Taking it into account, on the other hand, helps us both to know what as yet we *can't* "know" about the patient and to focus our attention where we need to—that is, on the separate subjective experiences of patient and therapist, and the relationship between the two.

The same mutual and unconscious influence that at once complicates and facilitates our efforts to take advantage of that which our patients evoke in us is at the very center of the work we do with enactments.

WHAT IS TO BE DONE WITH WHAT WE ENACT?

In the therapeutic relationship, as in others, words are not just words. They are also acts: "speech acts." McDougall (1978) makes this point in discussing the *patient's* words, but it applies no less to the words of the clinician: "Rather than seeking to communicate moods, ideas, and free associations, the patient seems to aim at making the analyst *feel* something or stimulating him to *do* something" (p. 179). "Enactments," as the term suggests, translate internal experience into action. By definition, enactments involve *behavior*—including verbal as well as nonverbal behavior. But even when enactments are played out in speech (as they often are in therapy) their essential meaning lies not in the words that are spoken but, rather, in the nonverbal subtext generated by what the words actually *do*. For example, the patient's words may pull us in or push us away, open us up or shut us down, make us comfortable or heighten our anxiety. And, of course, our words to the patient have the same kind of impact.

In an enactment of transference–countertransference, what is enacted, verbally and nonverbally, is a particular kind of relationship. It could be a parent–child relationship or a romantic relationship, a relationship of allies or of adversaries, a relationship that feels safe or one that feels perilous.

The variations are probably limitless, depending as they do upon the inter-action of two unique individuals—patient and therapist—both of whom bring to the relationship their own family of multiple selves.

Enactments are the scenarios that arise at the intersection, so to speak, of the unconscious needs and vulnerabilities of the patient, on the one hand, and the therapist, on the other. At this intersection, for better or worse, the relational patterns of patient and therapist meet and interlock. If we think of transference and countertransference as represented by two circles, enactments can be seen as emerging in the shared space where these circles partially overlap.

In an enactment, aspects of the therapist's representational world—the legacy of her original attachment experiences—are unconsciously activated and lived out. Exactly the same is true of the patient. For as long as the en-actment goes unrecognized, therapist and patient alike are simply embed-ded in their experience together. As such, each is acting automatically and unreflectively in relation to the other. Without being aware of it, both are responding not only to the actualities of the interpersonal encounter, but as much or more to internal pressures of which neither is presently aware.

To the extent that enactments continue to unfold outside awareness, they usually impose limits on what can be experienced and understood; in this way they make the therapeutic dialogue less inclusive and less collabo-rative. To the extent that they can be made conscious, however, enactments have the potential to provide access to highly significant, as-yet-unrecognized facets of the patient, the therapist, and the relationship they share. More-over, the very process of exploring these jointly created scenarios, rather than blindly playing them out, can itself constitute a corrective relational experience of inclusiveness, collaboration, and mentalizing. In this sense, enactments are (to paraphrase Renik, 1993b) the ever-present raw material of productive therapeutic technique. As such, avoiding them is not only im-possible—it is also downright undesirable.

Enactments are a particularly vivid expression of the fact that, like all relationships of attachment, the therapeutic relationship is co-constructed. What occurs in this relationship is necessarily a composite of the influences of patient and therapist. From the perspective of a two-person psychology, these influences are both internal and interpersonal. The experience and be-havior of patient and therapist alike will unavoidably be shaped uncon-sciously both by who they are independent of their relationship and who they are in response to that relationship.

Now what I've written in the previous paragraph may seem unarguable, if not literally self-evident. Yes, of course, therapists are no less vulnera-ble to the influence of the unconscious than their patients are. And yes, patients and therapists are equally subject to the inescapable reciprocal influence they constantly exert upon one another. These symmetries may

seem indisputably real once we acknowledge the clinical facts as described by two-person psychology. Yet the ways in which we practice frequently fail to take this theory sufficiently into account. What we actually do and think as therapists often seems to flow more from a one-and-a-half than a two-person psychology: It is the patient alone, in other words, whom we are inclined to view through the lens of two-person psychology. Let me be more specific.

Sometimes by virtue of our outdated training and almost invariably as a function of our own needs and defenses, we tend to work with our patients as if they were far more subject to the influence of the unconscious than we are. Almost automatically we reflect on the unconscious meaning of their behavior and communication, while the unconscious motivations that underlie our own words and actions attract no such automatic scrutiny.

Similarly skewed is the way we tend to work with the reciprocal mutual influence the theory describes. Think here about the concept of projective identification. Within this conceptual framework we're entirely prepared to consider that our experience may be evoked by the patient's unconsciously motivated behavior. We're generally much less inclined to consider that the patient's experience may be affected in just the same way by our unconsciously motivated behavior.

These asymmetries in the ways we habitually think about our patients and ourselves—while they seem to come all too naturally—make it far more difficult than it need be to recognize and work effectively with enactments. If there is to be a skew at all, then perhaps it should be in a direction opposite from the one that may come naturally. Rather than concentrate initially on the meaning of the *patient's* behavior, we would often do better to begin by focusing our own.

Just as is true of our patients, our own unthought and unfelt known is *enacted*. Noticing what *we* say and do, and what *we* avoid saying and doing, can therefore open a window onto the nature of our own unconscious participation in enactments. And because enactments are co-created, the product of mutual reciprocal influence, our conduct as therapists is, more often than not, meaningfully—rather than adventitiously—related to the patient's experience. Thus, becoming aware of the nature of our own unconscious involvement in an enactment almost always helps to illuminate the nature and meaning of the patient's involvement.

In this connection, we need to keep in mind that our behavior as therapists is shaped as much, if not more, by our unconscious motivations as by our conscious intentions. At one level, then, we may deliberately be attempting to generate with our patients a new and better attachment relationship. To this end, we may endeavor to be attuned and responsive listeners, trying to resonate empathically with our patients' emotions, to help

them make sense of their experience, and so on. At another level, however, we are always unwittingly enacting scenarios with our patients that stem from our own unconscious needs, internal working models, defenses, and so on.

Such enactments may, at least from one angle, be consistent with our patients' needs as well as our own. For example, the empathy we deliberately provide may be healing for the patient even though it is partly energized by our unconscious need to be seen as beneficent, rather than critical or controlling. Similarly, a confrontation may be exactly what the patient most requires, even though the confrontation is partly motivated by our unconscious need to feel powerful, rather than helpless or out of control. In instances like these, we usually feel that we're behaving as we do because our empathy or confrontation, say, is ultimately in the patient's best interest. Yet our efforts to be helpful—however conscientious—are always undergirded by motivations of which we are unaware.

Usually such motivations shape our behavior with patients in ways that have unintended consequences. Our consistent provision of empathy, for example, may dovetail too well with the patient's need to ignore her own distrust and anger. Similarly our confrontation, while useful as intended, may also be unhelpfully consistent with the patient's need to feel that, on her own, she is helpless to control herself. Obviously, what I'm describing here are enactments that arise from the overlap between the unconscious needs of patient and therapist.

Enactments like these can be difficult to recognize because they are so utterly embedded in what we ordinarily and un-self-consciously do as therapists. The trick here is to remember that we can never get away from ourselves. Our subjectivity penetrates every facet of our involvement with the patient from our most thoughtful interventions to our most obvious countertransference-based missteps. We should assume, therefore, that we are *continually* involved in enactments, just as the patient is. As I mentioned earlier, the essential question to ask ourselves here is not *whether* we're participating in an enactment, but *how*.

Recognizing Enactments

Like countertransference feelings that we recognize only when they become uncomfortably intense, some enactments eventually become too obvious or disturbing to ignore. But these are exceptions. Enactments are, by definition, initially unconscious, and they often remain that way for a considerable period of time.

Becoming aware of our role in enactments can be a considerable challenge because we're never completely transparent to ourselves. Much of what we do we remain ignorant of because it is simply an automatic, im-

plicit expression of who we are. In addition, our self-knowledge remains unavoidably incomplete precisely because we're motivated to keep it that way. We're inclined, in other words, to ignore or suppress awareness of that which is likely to trouble or unsettle us (Maroda, 1999; Renik, 1995).

To whatever extent we're short of the self-acceptance that facilitates self-awareness, it may be useful to keep in mind that in searching out our role in enactments we're not aiming to identify our shortcomings or psychopathology. Instead, we're trying simply to become aware of what we're actually doing. To further this sort of self-inquiry, we would do well to adopt a stance of mindfulness—that is, awareness of the present moment with acceptance. With such a stance, we may be more capable of regarding what we're doing as we relate to the patient as a "matter of fact" to be observed and noted, rather than judged as good or bad, right or wrong.

Having identified the distinctive features of our behavior with a particular patient, we need to try to be as objective as we can in answering two questions: What might be the roots of our behavior in our own psychology? And how might our behavior be affecting the patient? To the degree that we can become aware of the meaning of what we're doing in an enactment and can bring such awareness to the dialogue with the patient, that dialogue often becomes more inclusive and our role in the enactment less confining.

Patterns of Enactment

As I've mentioned, enactments can take a multitude of forms. Very broadly speaking, however, two patterns characterize these coauthored scripts: collusion and collision (Goldbart & Wallin, 1996).

The therapeutic couple who collude have made an unconscious "deal" that serves the self-protective needs of both partners. In such a deal, the individual defenses of one partner either mirror or mesh with the defenses of the other.

For example, a therapist and patient whose predominantly dismissing styles mirror each other may collude to steer clear of strong feelings. In so doing, they may enact an emotionally distant relationship that is familiar to both. In such a relationship—until the enactment is recognized—vital, but anxiety-provoking issues will continue to be avoided. Shared fears and defenses can thus make for collusive enactments that are all too stable, in part because they seamlessly mirror ways of being that are habitual—and therefore hard to recognize—for therapist and patient alike.

Less stable collusions may result when the defenses of therapist and patient differ, but nonetheless mesh, at least for the time being. For example, the therapist who is preoccupied with attachment may contain, or even

express, all the feeling that her dismissing patient disavows. This enactment may be psychologically convenient for the patient, who is spared the anxiety of dealing directly with his own relational and emotional issues so long as the therapist appears willing to take them on, almost as though they were her own. Meanwhile the therapist, in trying rather desperately to get the patient's attention, may be reenacting a role that is safely familiar, if also familiarly distressing.

Such a collusion, in which the partners' defenses differ, always has the potential to become a collision. The patient here may come to feel increasingly controlled or burdened by the therapist's apparent need for emotional contact, while the therapist may become increasingly exasperated at the patient's unyielding remoteness. Now the therapeutic couple may find themselves at odds.

This isn't necessarily a bad thing. So long as therapist and patient collude, the real fears and needs underlying their co-created enactment are likely to remain hidden. When the collusion breaks down, however, and a collision results, then some difficult but potentially liberating realities may come into focus, perhaps for the first time.

Such a propitious outcome depends on the ability of the therapist to reengage her capacity to mentalize sufficiently to recognize and begin to make sense of the enactments in which she has been embedded. Just like collusions, collisions can be the stuff of which enactments—and therapeutic impasses—are made. Transforming enactments, collusive or contentious, into opportunities for collaborative exploration and corrective experience requires a therapist capable, at least intermittently, of adopting a mentalizing stance.

For several years I saw in treatment a very brilliant physicist (I'll call him Jackson) whose dismissing attachment style kept him remote from his feelings and hobbled his ability to express them. One day he began the session by telling me that he wished that when he'd been a youngster someone had talked to him about himself as truthfully as he'd just talked to his teenage son. Then he wondered aloud if he would have been as resistant then as his son was now to hearing the difficult truth. He added that even as an adult he probably still wished for an authoritative someone to "tell it like it is." But the idea scares him because he knows he might not be told what he wants to hear.

Several days before this session, I had been thinking about my relationship with him. It had occurred to me then that emotionally speaking we were continuing to play in the shallow end of the pool despite my conscious intention to help him go deeper. Knowing something about the therapeutic needs of dismissing patients, I had avoided an overly intellectual approach (or so I thought) and tried to keep the focus on Jackson's feelings and the defenses against them. I was quite

unclear why it had been so difficult for me to help us break out of the mode of talking heads.

Now I thought I was hearing an allusion to this problem of ours as Jackson expressed his conflicted wish for someone to authoritatively "tell it like it is." But when I floated the possibility that his words might be a way of talking indirectly about me and about him, he demurred with a question: Hadn't we concluded together that he needed to become his own authority, rather than rely on mine?

Then in my mind's ear, I heard myself saying that I didn't like the idea of getting into a colloquy with him about this matter. *Colloquy?* The word I had silently spoken caught my attention because it was the sort of word I'd probably never use in conversation—except, perhaps, in conversation with this particular patient.

I realized then that, very likely, my unconscious need to bolster my intellectual standing in relation to his had resulted in my talking to him in a deliberately highly articulate and overly careful way. When I voiced this thought about the history of our communication—and how my own psychology might have inhibited the kind of direct talk he seemed to both want and fear—Jackson said he had no idea that anything of the kind had been going on. He couldn't imagine that I might see myself as someone at an intellectual disadvantage, while his confidence in his own intellect pretty much immunized him from any worries of his own on that score.

Then I remembered being both pleased and more than a little astonished when, a couple of years before, he had told me he thought I was a "genius." Now I suggested that my insecurity in comparing the two of us intellectually might have been *my* issue, while perhaps for him the comparison that provoked insecurity might concern a different kind of intelligence—namely, emotional intelligence.

Here he said that since early childhood he had derived his self-confidence exclusively from how bright and articulate he was, but that he had also felt compelled to hold himself back to avoid being picked on. I answered that today I was becoming aware of how *I* had been holding back, partly in the way I used language with him, but also in my reluctance to intervene more directly when he seemed, for example, to be dwelling on minutiae. What emerged then was the meaning of his hyper-detailed tangents: For him, these were safely oblique ways of communicating his emotional experience without actually feeling his feelings. In so doing, he said, he was guarding against the risk of being seen—or seeing himself—as "an emotional retard."

For both of us from this encounter, there came a sense of relief and renewed promise once we recognized the nature of our unwitting collusion. In avoiding our separate but related insecurities, in order to keep things safe and under control, we had unconsciously enacted an emotionally constrained relationship. But it was also a relationship that was feeling to both

of us increasingly—and unnecessarily—incomplete. The patient's words (a metaphorical message about the shortcomings of our communication) along with my observation of my own behavior (my competitively overliterate way of speaking) helped me to identify and begin to understand my role in the co-created enactment. Sharing this awareness led to a dialogue that illuminated the patient's role. In the process, we deepened our relationship and expanded our sense of what each of us could safely feel, know, and communicate in the presence of the other.

Often a careful scrutiny or sudden awareness of the nature of our own behavior with the patient—repetitive or strikingly out of character—is sufficient to lift the scales from our eyes. Sometimes, however, enactments are only recognized with the help of a consultant or in personal psychotherapy. When still in graduate school, I presented a case to my supervisor and another student. I was troubled by the conflicts that seemed to erupt all too regularly in my relationship with a particularly contentious female patient. Listening to an audiotaped session, my consultants exchanged amused and knowing glances before one of them finally let me in on the joke: "Doesn't it strike you that the two of you aren't so much fighting with each other as flirting with each other?" Eventually in dialogue with the patient it was borne out that the contentiousness—the collision—my patient and I were enacting was indeed a defense against our troubling feelings of attraction to one another.

Sometimes the patient functions as a kind of consultant—an interpreter of the therapist's experience—whose "intervention" helps make visible the invisible straitjacket in which an enactment can confine both partners in the therapeutic couple. In the following example, my patient enabled me to become aware of my impulse to be close that was enacted in a rather problematic way.

Just before I was to leave for a vacation, I met with a patient I'll refer to as Daniel who confessed to some anxiety about the impending interruption of our work together. He was dating someone new and was worried about confronting independently the sexual issues we had recently begun to discuss. As we spoke, I noticed that he was becoming increasingly uneasy. I asked him what it was like for him to be talking to me about these issues. With some reluctance, he told me that my evident excitement at his willingness to address his sexual conflicts had left him feeling that I was imposing a project on him, perhaps for reasons of my own. Talking about sex was supposed to be good for him, he said, but it was like working out at the gym, not necessarily something he'd choose to do for its own sake.

I immediately recognized the quality of enthusiasm my patient had attributed to me. I *had* been excited, partly because he was choosing to take on an important psychological challenge and partly because

I (not uniquely) find sex an engaging topic. But I suspect I was also enthusiastic because I felt that a conversation about sexuality would satisfy my impulse to bring the two of us closer together. The background for this assumption was my experience with my father, a sociologist who had researched and written extensively about sexual behavior. His openness and curiosity about sex had made it a subject around which we could easily connect. Probably, I had unconsciously assumed that around a similar conversation my patient and I could experience a similarly valued connection.

I chose not to disclose these details during the session, but used them to understand—and thus more readily acknowledge—my role in an enactment in which, as it turned out, while I was playing my (good) father, my patient was experiencing me as his (bad) mother.

When he was a teenager, his ordinarily remote mother had confided to him that his father was a sexual failure: If she wanted to be intimate, she'd have to chase him around the bedroom and even then he'd usually be unable to perform. From his mother as well as a previous girlfriend or two, my patient had gotten the uncomfortable message that providing sexually for a woman was the obligation of a man, if he were really a man. My rooting for Daniel's erotic exploration had made it easy for him to place me in their company, while at the same time he "knew" I wasn't really echoing their sentiments.

In discussing our interaction, Daniel was disturbed to notice once again the impact of his already familiar need to turn good things bad. He was struck by how automatically he could experience sex ("of all things") as an unwanted obligation and his therapist's (admittedly overenthusiastic) help as a burdensome imposition. We came to understand that his side of the enactment reflected, above all, his guilty need to match his mother's suffering—her "happiness strike"—with his own. "It's like I have to join my mother on the cross," he said. To which I replied by citing a lyric from Tom Waits: "Come down off the cross, we can use the wood." Along with the sober exploration that preceded it, my patient's uproarious and satisfied laughter at the Waits' line seemed to loosen the grip of our jointly created enactment.

Enactments That Are Unrecognized

Of course, not every enactment has the kind of happy ending I've just described. To begin with, we can be as embedded in enactments as the patient is, and as unable to harness the mentalizing capacity that might help us recognize the motives that are unconsciously driving our behavior. Or we may simply fail to be on the lookout for enactments. For these reasons and others, many enactments go unrecognized.

Sometimes the consequences here are relatively innocuous or even be-

nign. Not every shared experience in therapy is—or should be—explicitly scrutinized for its unconscious meaning. Moreover, some unrecognized enactments are, as I'll shortly explain, exactly what the patient requires.

Often, however, the consequences of remaining oblivious to an ongoing enactment can be very problematic. Such obliviousness may result in a therapeutic relationship that fails to make room for those aspects of the patient most desperately in need of recognition. For example, the therapist who remains unaware of his role in perpetuating an emotionally distant relationship may inadvertently ensure that the dismissing patient remains a relative stranger to his own feelings. Often such a lack of awareness is reinforced by the therapist's unwarranted belief that he is actually gearing the treatment to address the patient's defenses against feeling. In this connection, think of the enactment I described with my patient, the physicist.

More problematic still are those unrecognized enactments that corrode or explode an ongoing psychotherapy. Here I recall with regret my relationship with a male patient with whom I played out an enactment that repeated aspects of his history with his withdrawn but intermittently volatile father. Bending over backwards to be a different kind of attachment figure, I unconsciously repeated aspects of my own history by failing to confront the patient's provocations. Meanwhile, without being aware of it, I was becoming increasingly resentful. Finally, a session came in which the patient was exceptionally disrespectful to me—and I blew up. The patient was initially speechless, then outraged. Despite my efforts to repair the damage done, that session was our last.

Enactments as Repetition, Enactments as Repair

The forces that would have us stay the same and those that would have us change interweave in the work we do with enactments. As discussed in Chapter 10, enactments reflect a dynamic tension between the old and the new, security and risk, the "repeated relationship" and the "needed relationship" (Stern, 1994).

Patients and therapists alike are unconsciously gripped by the need to repeat habitual patterns of relating, feeling, and thinking. Our internal working models and the rules encoded in them amount, as I've suggested, to a kind of invisible straitjacket that leaves us at once confined and ignorant of our confinement. In an enactment of transference–countertransference, then, both partners play their roles without initially being aware of these ubiquitous constraints. This is the repetitive dimension of enactments.

On the other hand, most therapists and patients are also unconsciously (as well as consciously) motivated to experience new ways of being that are more inclusive and expansive than those they learned in their formative re-

lationships. Arrayed against the "repetition compulsion" (Freud, 1914/ 1924a) and the tendency of insecure working models to be self-perpetuating (Bowlby, 1969/1982; Main, 1995) are the mind's "self-righting" tendencies (Siegel, 1999), the competency motive (White, 1959), and the innate drive to develop (Weiss & Sampson, 1986), as well as the presence of biologically based behavioral systems that incline us to attach and explore (Bowlby, 1988). These motivations underlie what I would describe as the reparative dimension of enactments.

Sometimes an as-yet-unrecognized (and perhaps never-to-be-recognized) enactment reflects the direct impact of such "progressive" motivations. For example, the therapist who deliberately provides the attuned responsiveness conducive to secure attachment, and the patient who evidently makes good use of it, may be playing out complementary unconscious needs in an enactment that is primarily reparative. Such enactments are probably crucial in generating the background of safety and the experiences of heightened "fittedness" (Stern et al., 1998) that are essential in making therapeutic change possible.

More dramatic and emotionally charged than enactments like these, however, are those *repetitive* enactments that are recognized, explored, and thus transformed into *reparative* ones.

> For a number of years, I had seen in treatment a male patient—I'll call him Al—who nearly two decades earlier had molested his eight-year-old daughter. As an adult, the same daughter had on several occasions enlisted her father's participation in three-way sessions with her therapist. These difficult, but evidently productive meetings along with the changes occasioned by Al's personal therapy had contributed to partially resolving her trauma. Now Al's adult son, Clark, was requesting a similar discussion about the impact of his sister's trauma both upon his own experience of growing up and upon his current relationship with his father. When my patient proposed to his son that they might talk to each other either alone or in the presence of a therapist, his son chose the latter alternative, adding that he would prefer to meet with his father's therapist rather than his own.
>
> In the session immediately preceding the one with his son, Al began by saying that he was feeling apprehensive about the impending meeting. When he asked me if I might give him some guidelines to help ensure that the session would be helpful, I answered that I thought it would be useful first for him to say more about his feeling of apprehensiveness. Rather than do so, he told me that he needed to be clear about what he wanted to say to his son. Then in strikingly subdued and deliberate tones he began to speak, almost as though he were rehearsing the lines or perhaps as if his son Clark were already in the room with us, and making him uneasy. His words themselves did not lack for meaning, but Al's formality as he spoke seemed to vitiate

their emotional impact. He could almost have been talking about someone else as he described his crazy father, the pain of his own past, and the refuge he had found as a child in sexualizing his relationships.

As I listened, I became aware that I was having an unusually hard time empathizing with him. Having known him for several years, I typically found it relatively easy to feel emotionally in synch with him, to sense his emotional comings and goings, and to make sense of them. Now, however, the presence of his son in my mind—and probably in his own mind—seemed to have changed things. All of a sudden, it seemed to me that I had never before allowed myself to fully feel the gravity of what Al had done. It occurred to me that in order to feel I could be with him and be of help, I had needed to place myself at a safe emotional distance from the facts of his past. In so doing I was repeating aspects of my own past just as his emotional distance repeated aspects of his. Together, it appeared, we had enacted a collusion of defenses that—perhaps—we could now do without.

Here I recall interrupting him to say something like the following: "Al, I'm not sure if you're having an experience that's akin to mine. But I have to say that for me—and I'm guessing for you too—it's as if Clark is already here in the room with us. And for me, the sense that he is already a presence here makes infinitely and painfully more real the facts of what you've had to grapple with and what you've done. And all this has me seeing how much I've needed—and maybe how much *both* of us have needed—to make those facts feel less real in order to somehow make them feel bearable at all."

At this point, looking stricken and a little confused, Al averted his gaze. Then he said, "I don't want my father . . . I mean, I don't want . . . I mean, I don't want *Clark* to have to keep dodging the reality of what's gone on."

I said, "But I think your slip just now—first, it's your father, then it's you, then it's Clark—probably means you feel you *have* had to keep dodging the reality." Here he replied rather plaintively with a question: "Do you know what my father said when I asked him why he was always drinking? 'Go ask your mother.' " Parenthetically, when Al was a boy, this father had refused for several years to converse at all with his wife: Al, the oldest of seven children, had been enlisted as the go-between, who was required to carry his father's words to his mother, and vice versa.

I said, "You know, if I try to imagine what it might feel like to talk to my son about something that I felt so utterly, mortifyingly ashamed of . . . Jesus. . . ." And here I trailed off, at a loss for words to describe feelings that were difficult to bear, even in the imagining. Looking at Al, I saw his head tilt back, his face contorted in anguish. Then came a long silence that I ended, inquiring if he could say what was going on.

In a voice choked with feeling, he replied that he was recalling

that as a 14-year-old at school, he'd been asked by a friend if he was okay—and he had simply broken down, sobbing. And not just about his father, he told me, and the lies and silence, and the filthy house, and the grotesque family in which he was growing up. Or rather, it was that, but even more it was the dreadful crushing burden of shame and guilt about who *he* was that he had constantly to keep pushing away.

I responded by noting a terrible paradox: In order to somehow protect himself from the external sources of his shame, he had behaved sexually in ways that made his shame less a matter of what he had been forced to endure by others and more a matter of what he had forced others to endure. Al said then that his shame about what he had done was so unbearable he sometimes still just had to push it away. "You push it away," I said, "but you also carry it."

We went on to discuss what it might mean for him not to push his painful feelings away—and the possibility that they might then come to be experienced as a painful part of him, but only a part, rather than the shameful disavowed core of him. As the hour ended, there was a shared sense that we were standing together on new ground. The fact that I had finally been able to tolerate fully feeling the enormity of what he had done (I had already felt the enormity of what was done to him) allowed him both to bear more of his own excruciating shame and to feel that he could be known and accepted in spite of it.

As we were about to part, he asked me if I would give him a hug. "Of course," I said. I would only add here that for much of our relationship I would not have wanted to hug him, I assume because the feelings I was defending against made it impossible for me to fully embrace him, emotionally or otherwise. Now the hug between us felt entirely natural and appropriate: a bodily expression, I believe, of the shared recognition of the depth of emotional understanding and connection our session had newly made possible.

In clinical hours like this one, the therapist has an opportunity to transform a repetitive enactment into one that is reparative or needed. Often, as was the case in my relationship with Al, the path to this transformation begins with the therapist's recognition of his own participation in the enactment.

By witnessing the "trauma of transgression" (Kramer & Akhtar, 1991) through the eyes of one of its victims, rather than the eyes of the perpetrator, I was able to become aware of feelings about Al's behavior that I had unconsciously avoided. For me, such avoidance reflected a new version of an old need to keep at bay the emotional impact of the worst of my own experiences growing up. This defensive exclusion was part of my countertransference in relation to Al. In a similar way, Al had managed at times—but only at times—to soften the impact of his feelings about molesting his daughter by muting or avoiding them: These defenses were a self-protective

feature of his transferential mistrust in relation to me. The repetition here arose as it arises in nearly all enactments through the overlap—the fit, actually—between aspects of the therapist's countertransference and aspects of the patient's transference.

It is the fact of this predictable fit that makes the therapist's awareness of his own role in the enactment such a powerful resource. Recognizing the nature of our participation can enable the patient to become articulate about facets of experience he has previously been unable or unwilling to put into words.

Acting on Our Awareness of Enactments

As therapists, once we recognize our role in an enactment, we are usually liberated, at least to some extent, from its grip. Exactly how we should then proceed to make use of our awareness is not often a matter that can be prescribed on the basis of theory. Theory may well offer us some general clues, but what actually turns out to "work" will invariably depend on the particularities of a specific therapist in a relationship with a specific patient. The unique "interactive matrix" (Greenberg, 1995) made up of their intermingling subjectivities is the context within which the therapist's interventions with the patient acquire their meanings.

What does this patient need? And given our own psychological makeup, what are we capable of providing? Depending on our answer to these questions, as well as our feeling for the requirements of the moment, we will tend—either more or less reflectively—to respond with a deliberate disclosure about our experience, an empathic comment about the patient's experience, or an observation about the interaction. Alternatively, I suppose, a useful response might involve interpretation, humor, receptive silence, the setting of a limit, or, for that matter, any other technique that seems likely to serve the patient by loosening the hold of the enactment.

Processing Internal Experience, Sharing Internal Process

By encouraging an experimental and improvisational approach to therapeutic intervention (Renik, 1999a; Ringstrom, 2001), relational and intersubjective theories have opened up a wide range of "relational moves" (Lyons-Ruth et al., 2001; Stern et al., 1998). Specifically with regard to enactments, the key for us as therapists is to intervene in ways that demonstrate to the patient our newly acquired *freedom* to move—that is, our freedom to think, feel, and act now in ways we simply could not before we recognized our constrained (and constraining) participation in the enactment.

Such relational moves can be implicit and subtle, or they can be very direct. They can come easily or with considerable difficulty, depending on

the tenacity of the grip of both our own unconscious needs and those of the patient. And they can evoke responses from the patient suggesting either that the therapist's moves are useful and liberating, or that they are disruptive and unwelcome. What is potentially therapeutic about these relational moves—whatever their form—is their demonstration that the therapist has changed and is no longer straitjacketed by the enactment. As the therapist changes, the relationship usually changes, and so, at times, does the patient. Of course, this doesn't necessarily occur immediately or quickly. Working with our awareness of enactments is a process, not an event.

In the literature on enactments, a number of writers have suggested that in order to weaken the grip of repetition, so that something new can be learned and experienced, we would do well to alternate flexibly between two stances: one that is interpretive and one that is personally expressive. Hoffman (1992, 1994) discusses these alternating therapeutic stances in terms of the dialectic composed of authentic self-expression, on one hand, and disciplined theoretically informed understanding, on the other. Burke (1992) explores the same territory in sketching the "mutuality–asymmetry dilemma," while Mitchell (1995) describes the contemporary Kleinian and interpersonal approaches to interaction.

When in an interpretive stance, the therapist is cast as participant *observer*, while in the expressive stance the therapist is cast as observing *participant*. The emphasis in the first is on containing and internally processing our experience of the enactment well enough to be able to understand it and communicate that understanding to the patient. The emphasis in the second is on responding to the patient with an expressiveness and authenticity that is emotionally compelling enough to "break the spell" of the enactment.

Let me give you an example of each approach. Both involve the same unresolved patient—a woman I'll refer to as Ellen—who was traumatized by parents who were, by turns, neglectful and abusive. I have seen her in treatment for seven years. The clinical hour described below illustrates an interpretive response to enactment.

> In one session I became aware of a pattern of interaction that had occurred repeatedly in my relationship with Ellen. Around interruptions in the therapy, in particular, recognizing her dependency upon me would leave her feeling a nearly intolerable blend of fear, shame, and anger. Often she would react by telling me that she should be coming to see me less frequently. Sometimes she would pick a fight or threaten to quit therapy. In response, I would communicate both implicitly and explicitly not only my recognition of her difficult feelings and defenses against them, but also my conviction that her dependency, while real,

was not something shameful or out of the ordinary, but instead re-flected a healthily growing capacity to make use of what I had to offer her.

In considering my apparently attuned and appropriate—but by now, all too predictable—responses to the fear and anger Ellen felt about her dependency, I finally recognized my role in an enactment. I saw in my behavior my own wish to "save" her, that is, to lead her out of her wary self-protective solitude into the world of relationship. I suspected that in complementary fashion what she longed for, but knew she could not possibly live out, was a "real" relationship with me in which, figuratively, she would be walking with me out of her old world into a new one.

When I communicated this understanding to her, her immediate reaction was one of relief, I suspect because my words allowed her to feel less trapped in a pattern of response that had troubled, but also deeply confused her. She said she had never thought about the meaning of her dependency in this way, but that it helped her make sense of her feelings of anger and shame as well as fear whenever our therapy was interrupted. She also said this understanding enabled her to see that perhaps, out of her anger at not getting *everything* she wanted from me, she was actually stopping herself from getting *some* things from me that she could quite realistically expect to get. But, she told me, un-derstanding herself in this way was also disturbing. That turned out to be an understatement. In retrospect I was able to see that our conver-sation in this session marked a crossroads in the therapy.

The next session I'll present had occurred two months earlier. It illus-trates the use of personal expressiveness in attempting to "transcend" an enactment.

Ellen entered my office, appearing tense and glancing at me with what appeared to be a slightly suspicious look. Sitting down, she said in what I took to be a rather challenging tone that she hadn't felt like coming to therapy today. In fact, she'd thought she wouldn't come. As it happened, I was feeling more relaxed than usual with her that after-noon, for reasons I'll explain in a moment. So while I certainly had the familiarly resigned thought, "Here we go again," I also felt that we could likely have a productive conversation about her conflicted desire to meet with me. "Well," I said, probably with the trace of a smile, "I'm sure we'll be talking a lot about that when we get back." I was re-ferring to the fact that we were about to meditate, as we had regularly been doing for five or ten minutes at the beginning of each session. To my sincere but slightly facetious comment, she responded by rolling her eyes, whether with mock irritation or real annoyance, I couldn't tell. Then we meditated.

Before continuing, I should say that for several sessions immediately preceding this one, we'd been struggling to manage and make sense of her feelings of anger, but also mine. I had thought she had been getting in her own way by ignoring a number of risky medical issues. I had tried to understand her experience. I had set some limits to ensure that she would be safe. I had also become exasperated. For her part, Ellen had angrily experienced me as punitive and intrusive, but ultimately not unhelpful.

Shortly before the present session, I had recognized—with considerable relief—my probable role in a jointly created enactment. I saw that I was angry with Ellen in ways that reflected both my own conflicts about dependency and my childhood anger at my parents. Ellen was angry with me, I supposed, in ways that reflected not only her conflicts about dependency, but also her rage both at her intrusive, abusive father and at her neglectful, malingering, and help-rejecting mother. From her side, I was her father, while she was struggling not to be her mother. From my side, I was with my demanding, but ferociously self-sufficient mother, while struggling not to be my overtly tolerant, covertly resentful father. Obviously this analysis oversimplifies the exceedingly complex relationships that Ellen and I each had with the other and with ourselves. Nevertheless, my understanding here permitted me to experience the present session feeling lighter and clearer, as if for the first time in a while I now had room to move.

After we meditated, and our eyes were open again, Ellen and I gazed at each other. In our contact then I experienced a very striking—and moving—sense of the deep connection between the two of us. Privately I guessed that she felt the same. Her facial expression had softened, as if with a kind of acceptance. I had never before seen Ellen looking as calm and open as she did in those moments.

Then she shifted on the couch and began to talk in a somewhat perfunctory way, but at some length, about her reluctance to meet with me. She seemed to be continuing the rather contentious discussions of the preceding sessions, but with nothing remotely like the same intensity of feeling—as if, perhaps, the fact of my extricating myself from our enactment had implicitly been communicated to her and had already partially freed her from its grip. Clearly her words were not without meaning, but they didn't seem any longer to match what was going on in the room—certainly not for me. I think she sensed what I was sensing. At this moment, an interpretation seemed out of place. She asked me what I was thinking.

"I was thinking that at the same time that you're talking about your reluctance to be here and your anger—and those have certainly been a big part of our recent experience together—you also seem very capable of being present here today and you don't actually seem angry. I don't know, it just seems to me that there's a very strong and unusual

feeling here now of connection and acceptance between the two of us. Certainly that's what I'm experiencing. And I'm guessing that you may be, too."

"You're very perceptive." Then a long silence. "So what do you think it is?" she said.

"I think it's called love." The words were out of my mouth before giving them a thought. I was aware that I had spoken with a kind of lightness as if to somehow convey that I meant what I said, that it was an important thing, to be sure, but that it was also not so very out of the ordinary either—and certainly not so out of the ordinary that it couldn't be said.

Looking directly at me with tears in her eyes, she nodded her head.

I told her that I was still back with the look we had shared after meditating. "I just felt extraordinarily connected to you, as if we were both very present here together and very calm. You had a look on your face that I don't think I've ever seen before, you looked so utterly peaceful. Obviously I can't know, but I'm guessing that your experience then was similar to mine . . . I wonder, is that so?" Smiling and tearful at the same time, she agreed, saying it had felt to her like a special moment: very relaxed, very close, and very moving.

"But it seemed like you felt you had to turn away from the experience, as if you couldn't be comfortable staying with the feeling of connection and calm."

"I can't trust it."

"Of course you can't. Your parents certainly gave you no reason to. Very much the opposite. It must feel impossibly risky to stop waiting for the other shoe to drop. Much less to hope for what you're sure you're not going to get."

After another long silence, she said, "David, you've been profoundly important to me. It's gotten easier to hope now than it's ever been before. I don't have the same knee-jerk reactions, or assume that everything is what it appears to be. Even though my feelings might be very strong, I don't always have to believe them. Monday I wanted to hurt myself but I thought of you saying, "This will pass," and that was the only thing that stopped me from hurting myself. It's like you're always with me. I still sometimes feel like things are closing in, but I can regain perspective, I can recover much more quickly than before."

When the hour was nearly over, I found myself spontaneously telling her that she was beautiful. The fact seemed undeniable. She replied, "Beautiful on the inside, you mean."

"Actually, that's not what I meant. But I'm sure that's true, too." Just before the session ended, we hugged. Gazing at each other, we were both clearly moved. She touched me lightly on the cheek. Then she left.

By way of a postscript. Discussing this session when we met again, Ellen told me she was worried that I would think that she had crossed a boundary in touching my face. I replied that the thought had never occurred to me. These words apparently reassured her. When I raised the possibility that the touch might have worried her quite apart from my reaction to it, she demurred. As we explored what the session had meant to her, she said that she had left with a feeling of joy: Experiencing so powerfully the depth of my caring for her raised the possibility that there might be others who could also care deeply for her. Yet she had noticed how quickly she had to suppress this sense of possibility. All the same, she said, she could still refer to it in her mind when she chose to.

Juxtaposing these two sessions with Ellen helps to illustrate several key points regarding our work with enactments. I'll very briefly take up each in turn. Meanwhile keep in mind that in the final chapter of this book I revisit these sessions, to tell (some of) the rest of the story of my therapy with Ellen and consider further the extremely complex issues it raises.

Corrective Emotional Experience or Enactment?

Frequently it's both. Transcending an enactment can certainly make possible a corrective emotional experience. Yet that experience itself will often be seen, in retrospect, to have been part of a new enactment.

The session with Ellen that I just described, for example, seemed to have involved a transformative "moment of meeting" (Stern et al., 1998). Having recognized and temporarily extricated myself from our familiarly contentious enactment, I became aware of a very different dimension of my relationship with Ellen. In this dimension, our interconnectedness, commonality, and, yes, love for each other were in the foreground. From Ellen's side, experiencing my changed sense of our relationship allowed her own experience to change—as if, in my response to her as a lovable and beautiful being, she had glimpsed a new image of herself and a new sense of possibility.

While Ellen's experience with me in this session clearly appeared to have had a healing impact, it could also be understood in hindsight to have been part of an enactment. Here I played out my (rather grandiose) desire to rescue Ellen from her past, while she felt seduced by the false hopes I inadvertently encouraged—not only what she regarded as the foolish hope for a full-scale relationship with another man, but the impossible hope for more than a therapeutic relationship with me. In this enactment, she felt teased by my implicitly tempting her to imagine a different and brighter future than the one she believed was her lot. Understandably she was angry and ashamed when interruptions in the therapy made the limitations in our

relationship undeniable. Yet recognizing the enactment enabled both of us, for the moment, to transcend it and to perceive the real possibilities concealed behind the experience of deceptive promises.

The Old in the New, the New in the Old

The past and the present interweave in enactments. From one angle, the scenarios we enact with our patients are old wine in recycled bottles. For me, "saving" Ellen and seeing her for the moment in an altogether new light reflected familiar and temporarily reassuring experiences with my mother. For Ellen, my raising of certain-to-be-disappointed hopes echoed experiences with her father who could be seductive at one instant and sadistic in the next.

From another angle, enactments as repetitions are also the raw material from which new experiences can potentially arise, as can emotionally vivid insight into old ones. Often, the very fact that therapist and patient can now discuss the scenario they are enacting—almost certainly in a way that neither could in the original edition—transforms into a new experience what might otherwise feel only like a simple repetition.

And from still another angle, there is the paradox that new experience—arising, say, from the exploration of a repetitive enactment—can drive patient and therapist alike more deeply into the realm of the old. The session in which I extricated myself from a contentious enactment with Ellen and made possible a moment of meeting may be a case in point. Partially satisfying her suppressed desire for love and connection, our encounter gratified her. But it also encouraged her to take risks that were terrifying. In their light she was primed to turn defensively to the view that her therapist in the present like her father in the past was coaxing her onto dangerous ground.

Interpretation, Personal Expressiveness, and the Therapist's Ability to Change

Ideally the therapist has the flexibility and awareness to respond to enactments both expressively (as in the earlier session with Ellen) and interpretively (as in the one that came two months later). Such flexibility may be necessary to loosen the grip of repetitive enactments. The same flexibility makes possible a relationship in which the patient's encounters with the therapist are emotionally alive but also hospitable to reflection. Finally, flexibility enables us to function for our patients as models for identification in at least two ways.

To the extent that, in a relatively controlled fashion, we can "show some emotion" (Maroda, 1999), we provide patients with living proof that

feelings in a relationship can be safely felt and expressed. In this way, we model effective affect regulation. And to the extent that we can reflect aloud upon enactments, on our own participation as well as the patient's, we can model the capacity to mentalize.

When we recognize an enactment and make the implicit explicit by putting it into words, we communicate to the patient that behavior has a graspable psychological meaning—a context of feeling, thought, and desire within which it can be seen to make sense. Further, when we explore the enactment, we awaken or deepen the patient's awareness of unconscious mental models, enabling the patient to become more aware of the existence and impact of the representational world. In these ways, for therapist and patient alike, enactments provide a context within which to exercise the reflective function.

While the flexibility that allows us to intervene expressively and/or interpretively is doubtless desirable, it is also desirable that what we each choose to do in the patient's interest should be consistent with who we are as people. Given the predictable human responsiveness to nonverbal signals, it is not only what we actually do that will affect the patient but also our perceived feelings about what we do. If, for example, we choose to express our emotional reactions even though we're uncomfortable with such deliberate self-revelation, the patient will likely pick up on our discomfort and feel disconcerted at the lack of fit between our conduct and our unspoken attitude about that conduct.

But, of course, such lack of congruence is also the stuff of which enactments are made. As therapists, when we find ourselves behaving in ways that go against the characterological grain, we need to consider why. What are we enacting? And how does our experience of the interaction relate to the patient's? Yet it is in significant measure the therapist's capacity to change in particular ways—to go against the characterological grain, at times—that makes change possible for the patient. Recall here the research demonstrating that the attachment classification of young children can change if their caregivers change (Marvin, Cooper, Hoffman, & Powell, 2002).

Transference–countertransference enactments arise out of a dynamic system in which change in one partner's behavior inevitably affects the behavior of the other. Ideally, the therapist is something of an expert at "changing the system from within." In practice, this means being capable not only of recognizing the enactment in which we are embedded—itself often no mean feat—but also of changing the nature of our participation so as to be able to think, feel, and relate with greater freedom and awareness.

When a history of insecure attachment has imposed a lack of flexibility on an individual, the intersection of that individual's vulnerabilities with those of the therapist will result in a narrowing of options for the therapeu-

tic couple. That's when enactments occur. But the therapist who finds the wherewithal to think, feel, and relate more freely can open new options for the patient. Every time we change enough to extricate ourselves from the dual grip of our own limitations and the pressures of the enactment, we demonstrate that change is possible and thus facilitate, by degrees, the changes the patient herself both desires and fears.

CHAPTER 16

The Nonverbal Realm II
Working with the Body

> *. . . change ultimately requires connection to bodily experience that has been dissociated.*
> —WILMA BUCCI (2002, p. 788)

Psychoanalysis—the "talking cure"—and talk therapies, generally, have done an inadequate job of integrating into clinical work a focus on the body. The fact is that all of us experience ourselves and the world through our bodies. Filtered through our mental models, our initial impressions of events register by way of the five senses as they interact with the proprioceptive "internal sense" that informs us about goings on in the interior of our bodies—heart rate, respiration, muscular tension, visceral sensation, and so on. It is largely this internal sense that allows us to know how we feel. We feel our emotions in our bodies, and these feelings shape our reality. Thus, our lived experience as well as our memories of experience— emotional experience, in particular—are fundamentally rooted in the body.

The importance of including a focus on the body within an attachment-oriented framework should be clear: Emotions are an experience of the body (Siegel, 1999; Damasio, 1994, 1999), and attachment relationships are the context within which we learn to regulate emotions (Fonagy et al., 2002; Schore, 2003). It is this interactive psychobiological regulation that gradually enables us to "translate" bodily sensations into feel-

ings that can be recognized, named, contained, and interpreted (Krystal, 1988).

Originally the infant learns about the emotional meaning of bodily sensations through experiencing the attuned bodily behavior (touch, gaze, facial expressions, and tone of voice) of the sensitively responsive attachment figure. When our patients lack such early attuned responsiveness, especially when they have also experienced trauma, they are usually burdened by a compromised capacity to regulate emotion. To the degree that they experience their emotions only as somatic sensations or physical symptoms, their bodies keep the score rather than their minds (van der Kolk, 1996). In that world, feelings are facts because they are physical realities. As such, they can be overwhelming or they can be denied, but they cannot be reflected upon.

For many patients it is important—and for patients with unresolved trauma it is essential—for the therapist to include in treatment a focus on bodily experience. Translating the language of the body into the language of feelings helps foster the interactive regulation of emotion that enables the patient to experience the therapist as a new attachment figure and a secure base. Reciprocally, the patient's confidence in the therapist as a secure base can facilitate a deepening exploration of bodily experience and a growing sense that feelings can be tolerated. Over time such interactive emotion regulation helps the patient learn to decode her somatic sensations so that affects can begin to be used as signals to the self and to others. When, in this way, feelings can be recognized as communications about experience—as interpretable symbols rather than immutable facts—then the door is opened to mentalizing and to the insight, empathy, and internal freedom mentalizing can bring.

In addition to elevating the patient's capacity to regulate emotions, focusing on the body has the potential to facilitate the integration of experiences that the patient's original attachment relationships could not accommodate. Through bodily states (such as numbing or agitation) and bodily expressions (such as yawns or gestures) patients reveal feelings—and defenses against feelings—that they have been unable or unwilling to acknowledge.

Moreover, the body remembers as well as reveals (Rothschild, 2000; Hopenwasser, 1998). Dissociated memories are often stored somatically not only as sensations that can be relived in the present but also as bodily postures and incipient movements associated with patients' original experiences of trauma. For example, a depressed patient with chronic neck and shoulder pain initially came to recognize that he regularly held himself with his right shoulder raised and turned/pulled inward, as if in self-protective retreat from a blow. Later we saw his right hand becoming a fist—the fist, he said, "that wanted but had never dared to strike back"—as he connected

emotionally for the first time with the rage he felt toward his physically abusive father.

Thus, along with what our patients evoke in us and enact with us, what they express through their bodies can be a route to the integration of feelings and memories they have previously had to dissociate. In fact, it is largely through activating bodily and sensory experience in the session—and linking such experience to images and words that can be reflected upon—that we facilitate the integration that is the basis of therapeutic change (Bucci, 2002, 2003; Bromberg, 2003; Ogden et al., 2005). Forging links between our patients' bodily sensations, their feelings, and the meanings they ascribe to their feelings also contributes to the integration of subcortical and cortical regions of the brain. Such work can potentially enable patients to be present in an integrated way with both their bodies *and* their minds. This may be critical for unresolved patients, who lack the ability to reflect on somatic experience and thus live in a "mindless" rather than a mindful body. For avoidant patients who often seem lodged in a disembodied mind, work with the body may be crucial in reconnecting them to the affective and somatic experience from which they have been estranged.

MINDING THE BODY

For the body to become a therapeutic resource, mindfulness is required of the therapist (Linehan, 1993; Kurtz, 1990; Ogden, 2006). With a mindful stance we deliberately direct attention—our own and that of the patient— to the details of here-and-now experience, particularly *internal* experience. And we do so with an attitude of acceptance and intense curiosity about what we observe rather than a desire to change (or interpret) it. The therapist who suggests to the patient, "Stay with what you're sensing and get to know it better," is putting this attitude into practice. Such a stance allows us to make effective use of the body, rather than find that its sensations are either overwhelming or inaccessible. When bodily sensations *are* felt (or feared) to be too strong to bear, mindfulness can serve as an antidote to panic or dissociation. When these sensations have been habitually numbed or avoided, mindful attention to them can function as an antidote to feelings of unreality, devitalization, and disconnection.

We cultivate such mindfulness in our patients by intervening in ways that require them to be mindful—that is, to be consciously aware of their experience while they are experiencing it (Ogden & Minton, 2000). In drawing attention to the present moment, however, most therapists are more accustomed to focusing on their patients' emotions than on their bodies. Questions or comments about emotional experience ("What are you feeling right now?" or "You seem sad ") are likely more familiar a feature

of the therapeutic conversation than questions or comments about bodily experience ("What are you aware of in your body right now?" or "Your breathing seemed to change a moment ago"). Given the body's eloquence and the fact that somatic sensations often point to disowned or dissociated experience, this skew calls for correction.

Reading the Body

Observing the moment-by-moment changes in the body—our own as well as our patient's—is a way of accessing the nonverbal subtext of the therapeutic dialogue. Reading the body helps us to know our own feelings and those of the patient. It also helps us gauge the degree of connection between the therapeutic partners and the degree to which both are (or are not) connected to their own experience. Finally it can help us evaluate whether the patient's state of mind is such that fully expressing her anger, say, or her grief, is likely to be useful—or whether such abreaction may instead be overwhelming or retraumatizing.

An Affective Lexicon

From Darwin (1872/1998) to Ekman (2003), scientists have observed that each of the so-called "categorical" or "basic" emotions (happiness, sadness, fear, anger, disgust, shame) has a signature set of somatic expressions. These universal expressions register internally as visceral sensations and externally as muscular/skeletal responses that are visible (on the face and in posture) and audible (in the pitch, tone, and rhythm of the voice). In addition, each emotion tends to be expressed in particular kinds of behavior or impulses to act.

The following summary (see Rothschild, 2000; Ekman, 2003) may be helpful in translating body language into feelings that can be spoken about:

> *Happiness*: Breathing is deep; sighs; smiles; laughter; eyes bright.
> *Sadness*: Choked up feeling, lump in the throat; turned-down lips; wet, reddened eyes; slowed body movement; crying.
> *Fear*: Racing heart; mouth dry; rapid shallow breathing; trembling; eyes wide with lifted eyebrows; impulse to flee.
> *Anger*: Muscular tension, particularly in jaw and shoulders; pursed lips, clamped jaw (often thrust forward), lowered eyebrows drawn together, glaring eyes, upper eyelids raised; reddened neck; yelling; impulse to fight.
> *Disgust*: Nausea; nose wrinkled, raised upper lip; turning away.
> *Shame*: Rising heat in the face; blushing; averted gaze; impulse to hide.

Somatic Countertransference

> ... *much of what we pick up from our patients, we may first feel in our bodies and perhaps most immediately in our breathing.*
>
> —LEWIS ARON (1998, p. 28)

Observing our own bodily experience is no less important than observing the patient's. Because the brain's mirror neuron system ensures that we actually resonate autonomically with our patients, our somatic states may well represent unconscious responses to the patient's nonverbal communication. Our unconscious perception of a patient's fear, for example, may be relayed from the insula to the amygdala, priming us to feel afraid as our mirror neurons fire in sympathy with the fear we perceive in the patient (Iacoboni, 2005). In short, our bodily/emotional experience can simulate the bodily/emotional experience of the patient.

On the other hand, while countertransference (including somatic countertransference) is usually a two-way street, the flow of traffic can sometimes originate more from the therapist's side than the patient's. Therefore, we need to exercise caution, engage the prefrontal cortex, and sometimes initiate a dialogue with the patient in order to differentiate empathic resonance from the projection of our own feeling states onto the patient.

As therapists, awareness of our bodies has further significance. When we are comfortably "in our body" we can more easily be present and helpful. Patients don't have to read our mind, because they can read our body; knowing in this way that we are present, they can attend to their own experience, without having to worry too much about ours. On the other hand, *not* feeling settled in our own skin—as when we're uncomfortable, restless, drowsy, or too exclusively "in our head" —can signal a collapse of self-reflection, a lapsed ability to be fully present, and/or our disconnection from the patient. All of which will make it more difficult, in turn, for the patient to be present, to reflect, and to feel connected to us (Looker, 1998).

I referred earlier to the "mindful body"—by which I mean the body we can inhabit in the present moment with awareness and acceptance. And there is indeed a tie-up between the ability to be in the body, on one hand, and to be present, on the other. To be in the body is necessary if we are to be present. How can we be fully in the moment if we are not in our body? Eigen (1977/1993), attending specifically to the link between the "*breathing* body" and the capacity to be present, writes, "The self structured by an awareness of breathing . . . does not run after or get ahead of time, but, instead, seems simply to move with it" (p. 146). And Dimen (1998) says, "Mindfully inhabiting the breath is . . . also to inhabit the body, relatedness, desire, the unconscious" (p. 89), adding, "If you breathe, you feel" (p. 90).[1] The important point, for patients and therapists alike, is that

awareness of the breath—particularly, respiration that is deep and rela- tively slow—is a gateway to more mindful experience, including experience of the body. It can bring us back to the here and now.

The Window of Tolerance

Siegel (1999), Rothschild (2000), and Ogden and Minton (2000) argue that clinical interventions are generally effective, in the short run, to the extent that they help keep the patient's autonomic arousal within a tolerable range; in the long run, effective interventions can expand the "window of tolerance" so that increasing levels of arousal can be experienced without disrupting the patient's ability to think, feel, and act. As therapists, focusing attention on bodily sensations and the breath may be particularly impor- tant when the traumatic past and fearfully imagined future seem to flood the patient's experience of the present. Such flooding may be apparent to the therapist even when the patient is unwilling or unable to acknowledge it. The evidence is in bodily signs—respiration, skin color, heart rate—that reveal the hyperactivation of either or both branches of the patient's auto- nomic nervous system (ANS).

Signs of sympathetic nervous system (SNS) hyperactivation include in- creases in respiration and heart rate as well as dilated pupils and loss of skin color as blood rushes from the head to the limbs. In this state, the pa- tient may feel overwhelmed and disorganized. Parasympathetic nervous system (PNS) hyperactivation is reflected in a marked slowing of respira- tion and heart rate, constricted pupils, and a flushed face. In this state, the patient often feels numb and/or shut down.

Recall that the amygdala ("survival central") reacts to perceived threats by triggering neuroendocrine responses that prepare the body for fight, flight, or "freezing" (tonic immobility) when the first two options are closed off as is so often the case in trauma. We know the patient is feeling overwhelmed when we see signs of simultaneous hyperactivation of both branches of the ANS—the SNS that facilitates fight or flight, the PNS that promotes immobility. The patient, for example, whose breathing is rapid but whose face is flushed is probably feeling flooded by trauma-related emotion. This is probably the time to put on the brakes.

One approach here is to ask the patient to specifically attend to and describe her bodily sensations, rather than her feelings (Rothschild, 2000; Ogden & Minton, 2000). If this inward focus on the body proves too much, then the patient's attention can be directed outwardly to, say, her sensory impressions of the therapist's office. A third approach is to engage the patient in a breathing exercise that slows and regulates respiration (see Weil, 2004). All these approaches may help ground the patient in the imme- diacy of the present moment, loosening the grip of old, often trauma- related emotions. When successful, such interventions restore the patient's

level of autonomic arousal to the "window of tolerance" within which her "prefrontally mediated capacity for response flexibility" can potentially be reengaged (Siegel, 1999, p. 255).

Talking about the Body

Conversation about the body can be structured in several ways. We can observe the patient's body and comment directly on what we see. We can invite patients to notice and describe the sensations in their own body. And we can attempt to develop awareness of the connections between the patient's bodily sensations, feelings, and thoughts. But whatever shape the conversation about the body takes, it is sure to be quite fraught for some patients. Certainly it was for a woman whose attention I drew to the fact that her voice seemed to be coming from a place much closer to her throat than her belly. She responded that my observation made her quite uncomfortable, adding that she was well aware of her tone of voice and not the least bit unhappy with it. Suggestions about the body must be offered provisionally and respectfully, with awareness of their potential to leave the patient feeling exposed, self-conscious, or criticized.

In Chapter 8, I alluded to my work with "Eliot," a patient with a predominantly avoidant attachment style. During a recent session, as we were discussing his impulse to withdraw from his wife, Eliot yawned. And yawned again. I said, "You're yawning now. Maybe that's meaningful here. I wonder if you have a sense of what you might be feeling? Or perhaps not wanting to feel?"

Eliot spoke after a long pause: "I'm feeling tired."

"Hmm. Do you have any sense of what that tired feeling might be?"

Eliot was quiet, but looked a little angry. When I asked him what was going on, he said, "I didn't like it when you asked that question. It seemed manipulative, a kind of bait-and-switch. It felt like you had an agenda."

What gradually emerged was Eliot's sense that I had invited him to be vulnerable, by asking him about the yawning, and then had "mind-fucked" him: In response to his disclosing his experience, I had asked for something more and something different. He had revealed his feeling ("tired") and I had wanted him to interpret it—probably as dissociation. But it didn't seem like dissociation to him, he said, though he knew his yawning had previously had this significance.

I attempted to repair the rupture here by explaining that, partly on the basis of firsthand experience, it had been my sense that yawning and drowsiness often reflected the need not to be present. But not at all certain that this explanation applied universally, I had been genuinely curious about his own understanding of his yawns. I added that, to

me, "tired" was not so much a *feeling* as a physical sensation with a meaning we had yet to grasp. Finally I acknowledged the painful vulnerability associated with his letting me in on how he felt.

Here he seemed to relax, and told me about something he hadn't felt comfortable mentioning earlier—a poster affixed to a telephone pole that he'd noticed while approaching my office. From a distance, he'd imagined that the poster was one like a number he'd seen some months before in "Couch Hollow"—an area of San Francisco tenanted predominantly by therapists. Those placards had been like "Wanted" posters, apparently generated by a very aggrieved patient, publicly warning of the risks posed by the unethical therapist who had violated her boundaries. Eliot imagined that the poster near my office building was the work of a similarly aggrieved patient of mine. When he got within reading distance, he found that the poster was a plea for help in locating a lost dog.

Discussing his fantasy and his "irrational" sense of the danger of intrusion I posed, we were able to understand more about his anger and wariness in response to my query about his yawning, as well as their relationship to his need to withdraw from his wife. While averring that he still wasn't entirely reassured by my explanation for my behavior, he admitted that he no longer felt like yawning.

As therapists, we often have hunches about the meaning of the patient's bodily communication or experience. Generally I prefer to simply comment on what I think I see, letting the meaning emerge from the joint exploration the comment usually elicits. Not infrequently, however, it can be difficult to make the comment at all—as it was with a patient in one session who repeatedly brought his hand to his face, to scratch it or brush the hair from his eyes:

What struck me as he raised his hand to his face, again and again, was the single outstretched finger—the middle one—composing a gesture with which most of us are familiar. I had a hard time crediting the significance of this bodily communication, hence was reluctant to give it voice.

Then I remembered that in the previous session the patient had forgotten to pay me. Now as I found myself becoming a little annoyed, it occurred to me that perhaps what the patient was enacting with me, evoking in me, and embodying all conveyed an identical message. Emboldened by my silent interpretation, I shared my observation of his gesture.

The patient was incredulous—no less than I had been—until he recalled recently seeing a fellow student repeatedly push her glasses off the bridge of her nose with the same infamous finger. He had wondered how she could possibly be unaware of what she was doing. Unsurprisingly the two of us wound up discussing how it could be that others were often aware of his anger long before he was.

The context for our every comment about the patient's body is, of course, the therapeutic relationship. Ideally the therapist functions as a secure base whose presence makes safe exploration of the patient's bodily experience possible. Paradoxically, it is this very safety that establishes the conditions under which the unspoken dangers in the relationship can sometimes be given voice.

Struck one day by the posture of a patient with a history of trauma, I endeavored to put into words for him what I had observed in his body as he entered my office. When *telling* him my impression failed to adequately convey it, I asked if he would be open to my trying to *show* him what I'd seen. With his assent, I stood up and attempted with my own body—chest and chin thrust out—to mirror the way he held his:

Clearly unsettled by my miming of his posture, he said it looked angry and aggressive, adding that he was feeling uncomfortable here now—physically uncomfortable. I asked if he could describe the sensation. "It's like there's this tension all through here," he replied, moving his hand across his chest, shoulder to shoulder. "It feels like wanting to hit and hold back at the same time."

Here I saw his jaws clamping and his right hand repeatedly clenching. He arched his back, stretching, and shuddered briefly as if half shaken by, and half trying to shake off, the feeling. Then his seated body bent forward, his head dropped to his chest, and he rested his forearms on his thighs. In the same motion he brought his right hand (no longer a fist) to his left. Holding them tightly together and slowly rubbing them, he now appeared the very image of resignation. I asked if he were aware of what his body was doing.

He shook his head and said, "You know, I'm just very uncomfortable going there. It doesn't feel okay to have these kinds of feelings here. The physical stuff when I've gotten into it before, it seems like you've just gotten totally detached and clinical, like you were dissecting it."

I knew what he was referring to: During several earlier sessions, his body had erupted in what appeared to be virtually involuntary, seizure-like movements of enormous power that had (to my eye) an intimidating if not an angry cast about them. With a mixture of disquiet and relief at the opening he'd given us to address the "underside" of our experience of these episodes, I told him that I had probably felt scared by him, fearful that things might get out of control or even that he might attack me. I shared my guess that the detachment he'd sensed from me was the result of my inability to fully acknowledge this fear, either to myself or to him.

He responded that he was relieved to hear my admission now because he'd felt then that I wasn't being real with him. Later in the session, he told me (with considerable difficulty) that he had repeatedly had the fantasy of "beating the shit" out of me but hadn't been able to tell me about it before.

Tracking our patients' bodily sensations in an ongoing way is vital because they almost always change, unpredictably and meaningfully. When we enable our patients to stay with difficult sensations we allow them to learn that attending to bodily experience can transform as well as illuminate it. Thus, in fostering mindfulness of the body, we potentially promote both self-regulation and awareness of dissociated experience. In addition, following the body as its sensations shift sometimes opens the door to new experience:

> A patient whose early attachments left little room for healthy dependency was angry that his pregnant wife was so easily upset. He complained that—on the verge of leaving him and their one-year-old son for a two-week business trip—she was now burdening him with her worries about where she would stay, how she would get there, and the like. Helping him recognize the probable sources of his wife's anxiety (she was about to be separated from her husband, her infant son, and her obstetrician) evoked his concern about how difficult it was for him to empathize with her. When our efforts to understand the meaning of his angry obliviousness went nowhere, I suggested that he focus on the sensations in his body.
>
> He became aware of "butterflies" in his stomach that he read as fear. Encouraged to stay with the sensation in his belly, he said he felt it "welling up." There was a pressure behind his eyes: tears and sadness. He was quiet. Asking him then what he was aware of, I was surprised to hear that he was simply feeling his sadness. He said that an entirely different quality of emotion was opening up. He felt the desire to be close to his wife and had an image of her love "radiating" toward him.

Obviously not every exercise in bodily awareness is so fruitful. Avoidant patients like this one often simply draw a blank when invited to tune in to the body. Yet perseverance furthers, and even the awareness of no sensation in particular can illuminate a patient's alienation from the body as a potential wellspring of energy and information. Frequently it is helpful to suggest to patients that they notice what they are experiencing in their body while keeping in mind what they are presently feeling, thinking, or imagining.

Mobilizing the Body

It is a cornerstone of attachment theory that we are biologically preprogrammed to seek the "safe haven" of a stronger or wiser other when we are threatened with danger. If no such protective figure is available, then our active options narrow to fight or flight; when neither of these options can be acted on, the only remaining alternatives are freezing or immobility. Helpless passivity—the inhibition of active coping in the face of over-

whelming threat—is at the root of much trauma. Undoing such inhibition by mobilizing the body may be essential to reversing the impact of trauma, including the relational trauma triggered by a frightening—and immobilizing—attachment figure who can neither be safely approached nor escaped (Ogden et al., 2005).

Immobilizing trauma, as you may recall, can deactivate portions of the brain, stilling the will (dorsolateral prefrontal cortex), and silencing the voice (Broca's area) for as long as danger persists. Yet the temporary paralysis and "speechless terror" (van der Kolk, 1996) associated with trauma can leave a lasting legacy. Thus many of our patients suffer from a chronic compulsion to comply as well as an ongoing inability to set appropriate boundaries or initiate effective action on their own behalf—including the action of approaching others for support. While these patients have truly been victimized in the past, their habitual inhibition keeps them victims in the present (albeit frustrated and intermittently enraged ones). "Going limp" is a figure of speech that suggests how the inhibition borne of trauma continues to be expressed through the body. In attending to bodily sensations, however, patients often discover dissociated impulses to act self-protectively in ways that were previously too dangerous to risk (Ogden, 2006). Enabling them to take action on these thwarted impulses—including the action of speaking out—can help to break the habit of inhibition, as illustrated in the following vignette:

Feeling tyrannized by his boss, "Lowell"—a patient with a childhood history of physical abuse—made the decision to quit his job, yet was unable (as he suggestively put it) to "pull the trigger." For several sessions, we explored his fears of catastrophe should he express his wish to leave: His boss would become enraged. He wouldn't be allowed to quit. Or if he was, he would be blacklisted somehow and never work again. Alternatively he worried that his boss might be utterly devastated. Coming to grasp the irrational nature of these contradictory fears, Lowell eventually determined to act—only to find himself thrown into a panic of traumatic intensity. He felt like he was going crazy. Adding to Lowell's anxiety was his fear of my condemnation should he prove "too much of a wimp" to quit.

I conveyed my empathy for his distress and suggested that we take his actual decision off the table for the moment, to concentrate instead on helping him to get a grip on his panic and a better handle on its meaning. Guessing that a focus on his here-and-now bodily experience might both calm and illuminate, I asked Lowell if he would be willing to undertake something of an experiment here: Would he try paying attention to the sensations in his body? We agreed that if at any point he felt himself becoming more distressed, we would stop and reconsider our tack.

Initially in a tight, subdued voice, Lowell described a sensation of tension in his belly and said he felt depressed. I asked, Could he stay with the sensation in his body and get to know it better? He said he

felt like there was something inside him . . . a pressure . . . that it was rising, that the tension was moving up from his gut to his shoulders and his arms. Still speaking with a constricted voice, he said he felt like he wanted to push something away—to just get it away (this said with slightly more force).

"And if you just let your body do what it wants to do?" "It feels scary." "I wonder if you're worried you'll do something that's too much somehow, too big or too strong." "Maybe." And then his hands formed fists as he leaned into the couch for support while his legs kicked out and he repeated several times in strident concert with the movements of his body: "Get the fuck away from me!"

The power and fury of his words and gestures hung in the air like an echo slowly fading. I asked what was going on inside him, what was he aware of now. With the flicker of a smile he said, "I'm aware I'm not feeling depressed anymore." Processing this experience together made emotionally real the linkage between Lowell's panic at the prospect of "pulling the trigger" on his boss and the fear he had felt as a child about unleashing what would have been his virtually suicidal violence toward his vicious and terrifying father. Shortly thereafter he spoke to his boss, who became more accommodating. Yet Lowell continued to consider quitting.

In addition to actually physically disinhibiting adaptive defenses, it can be of use for the patient to *imagine* doing so. Contemporary neuroscience, in dissolving the presumed boundaries between perception and motor action, demonstrates that—as far as the brain is concerned—there is much less difference between lived and imagined experience than we have previously supposed. The implication here is that therapeutic change may be promoted through imagining new behavior as well as by actually behaving in ways that are new (Siegel, 2004). Therefore, we might do well to ask patients, for example, *What is it like if you visualize yourself as a child, effectively confronting your father's rage by fighting back or speaking up for yourself?* Or, *What do you experience now if you imagine successfully protecting yourself from your brother's abuse by telling your mother he was fondling you?* We open new possibilities for our patients when we can help them to behave—or imagine behaving—in hitherto unimaginable ways.

DESOMATIZATION AND THE UNRESOLVED PATIENT

Emotion is essentially psychosomatic.
—JOYCE MCDOUGALL (1989, p. 96)

"Desomatization" (Krystal, 1988) is a term that describes a key facet of the therapeutic process with patients who have been traumatized. These pa-

tients regularly experience their emotions as somatic sensations or physical symptoms rather than feelings. While human consciousness has been described as a "theater of the mind" (see Blackmore, 2004), unresolved patients often appear to live in a "theater of the body" from which dissociation and "psychosomatic explosions" can seem the only exit (McDougall, 1989). Desomatization—the reintroduction of the psyche into the somatic experience of these patients—potentially offers another way out.

Clearly the legacy of unresolved trauma and disorganized attachment is biological as well as psychological. Chronically high levels of stress-related autonomic arousal can produce physical symptoms (such as muscle tension, elevated blood pressure, difficulty breathing) and impair the functioning of the immune system. Unmodulated affects as risk factors for illness and disease often leave our traumatized patients feeling victimized by their bodies (Scaer, 2001). To be able to be as helpful as we can with these patients, it is essential to understand the vicious circle of emotional dysregulation and somatic distress in which they often find themselves trapped.

Traumatic stress and unregulated emotions directly affect the brain. They suppress activation of the hippocampus or even cause it to atrophy, leaving the amygdala to react to perceived dangers indiscriminately. Unchecked by the contextual framing, explicit memory, and control the hippocampus ordinarily makes possible, the amygdala of the traumatized patient operates on a hair trigger, promiscuously activating the autonomic nervous system in response to signs most of us would appraise as neutral—a car backfiring or, for that matter, the heart beating faster from excitement or exertion. The result of unresolved trauma can be a life lived as an ongoing emergency—the body taxed by real or imagined crises and the mind with no space to translate somatic states into feelings that can be shared, reflected upon, and modulated. With unresolved patients it is the therapist's job to provide the relational space that opens the mental space within which this translation—desomatization—can occur

The desomatizing process depends, first and foremost, on the therapist's ability to enable these patients to tolerate rather than dissociate from their bodily sensations. Dissociation is the patient's response to levels of arousal that threaten to exceed the window of tolerance. In the relative safety of the therapeutic relationship, we modulate such excessive arousal and help undo dissociation both by encouraging the patient to observe the body's sensations as they change and by translating the language of the patient's body into words. In so doing, we help the patient build a vocabulary that describes physical experience.

Such a vocabulary has two important functions for unresolved patients. In the face of their tendency to *equate* somatic reactions with emotional ones, the ability to differentiate bodily sensations from feelings can help liberate these patients from the tyranny of "somatic equivalence" in

which, for example, a racing heart *is* terror—rather than, perhaps, a conditioned autonomic reflex devoid of emotional meaning. In the face of their tendency to *decouple* somatic and emotional reactions (a racing heart is simply a cardiac symptom, never a marker of fear), the ability to *relate* their sensations to their feelings can help these patients to use internal experience as a basis for understanding themselves and communicating with others.

To illuminate the relationship of the body to the emotions, it may be particularly helpful to describe for patients their patterns of facial expression, posture, gesture as well as vocal prosody that seem recognizable as affects— that is, visible or audible signs of emotion. Once these bodily sensations and affects are made part of the therapeutic conversation, the goal is to link them to the patient's feelings (and defenses against feeling), as well as the contexts that evoke them.

Marla had a history of early loss, neglect, and trauma. In one session she seemed to be even more out of touch than usual, with no sense of feeling or thinking much of anything. When I asked her what she was presently aware of in her body, she said she noticed a sensation of tightness in her upper belly, just beneath the rib cage.

As we explored the sensation, she realized that the tension in her stomach muscles made it difficult for her to take a full breath. (In light of Dimen's [1998] "If you breathe, you feel" I found myself thinking that breathing less was a way for this patient to feel less.) She said the sensation of tightness was familiar and associated it with social interactions that made her anxious, particularly interactions in which she wanted something from the other person.

The work with her body was a way for us to begin to bring her dissociated emotions directly into our relationship—specifically, emotions that might provoke the dependent needs her formative experience had taught her to deny.

Desomatization involves not only recognizing and containing bodily sensations and affects, but also interpreting or making sense of them. At the most fundamental level, making sense of sensations and affects involves interpreting them as feelings (as Marla said, "if my stomach is tight and my breathing shallow, I'm probably feeling scared"). At another level, interpretation means linking bodily and affective experience in the present to its antecedents in the past. One patient, for instance, came to associate his testicular pain with childhood experiences of terror when feeling "tortured" psychologically by his mother.

Desomatization is an important dimension of psychotherapy with unresolved patients that results, in the best case, in a strengthened capacity not only for emotion regulation but also for reflective self-awareness. Enhancing these twin capacities can gradually enable these patients to cease

oscillating between experiences of being either trapped by their bodies or dissociated from them. It can also diminish their reliance on somatically focused responses (such as self-medication or self-mutilation) to difficulties that are essentially psychological. In sum, it can make it possible for our unresolved patients to process difficult experience with their minds as well as their bodies.

"Resomatization" and the Avoidant Patient

Recall the studies showing that dismissing adults can appear calm during discussion of their attachment history—while physiological measures reveal emotional distress that they sense only dimly, if at all (Dozier & Koback, 1992). Patients like these are frequently as disconnected from their somatic sensations as they are from their feelings—presumably as a result of their "deactivating" attachment strategy that demands the tuning out of *all* internal signals that might evoke awareness of their need for others. Living largely "in their heads" and occupying bodies that *do* rather than *feel*, such patients often appear low on life and affectively muted, limited in their capacity for excitement, particularly in the context of relationships. As Siegel (1999) suggests, they may have "an excess in overall parasympathetic tone" (p. 283). Usually lacking early experiences of being physically held and nurtured, they have no such nurturing or receptive relationship to their own bodies.

Part of the work with patients like these must be aimed at reclaiming the body that feels. This requires that the therapist attend to the body in ways the patient has not. By communicating our interest in the patient's somatic experience, we convey that what the body *feels* actually matters, both in its own right and as a signal about the patient's emotional experience. Rather than ignore the patient's body, we need to inquire about it and observe it, and when the body "speaks" without words we need to let the patient know what we hear. When we can help our avoidant patients become more grounded in their body we also help them become more present—in relation to their feelings, to other people, and to themselves. This is one more way in which, by generating a therapeutic relationship that is inclusive, we enable our patients to integrate experiences—in this case, bodily and emotional experiences—that they have previously been unable to claim as their own.

NOTE

1. See also Epstein (1995) and Aron (1998).

CHAPTER 17

Mentalizing and Mindfulness

The Double Helix
of Psychological Liberation

The contents of the mental stream are not as important as the consciousness that knows them.
—MARK EPSTEIN (2001, pp. 6–7)

Attachment theory research strongly suggests that our relatively abiding states of mind as well as our moment-to-moment subjective experience may be influenced as much—or more—by our *stance* toward the internal and external circumstances of our lives as they are by those circumstances themselves.

Relationships of secure attachment foster the capacity to adopt a reflective mentalizing stance that allows for flexible attention, openness to new information, and the ability to consider multiple perspectives on the same experience. Such a stance is essential if we are to understand each other and ourselves. In particular, it makes possible a *psychological* perspective that allows us to recognize (1) that there is an internal world that shapes behavior and (2) that this internal world is a representational one related, but by no means identical, to the external world it models. A reflective stance also promotes internal freedom—an awareness of the fluidity and pliancy of subjective experience as well as the possibility of exercising personal agency, that is, attempting deliberately to influence the nature of our experience.

In contrast, insecure attachment and/or unresolved trauma lead to rigid,

307

and sometimes brittle, attentional strategies that restrict our ability to update old internal models on the basis of new information and to consider experience from multiple perspectives, including—most important—the psychological perspective without which it is impossible to make sense of our own behavior or that of others. The stance here is one of embeddedness that leaves us so confined by our narrow view of the experience of the moment that any other view becomes emotionally irrelevant. Lodged in such a stance, we are unable to interpret our experience, but are instead simply defined by it.

Many of the patients who seek our help are chronically or intermittently embedded in their experience, with the result that they feel helpless on their own to affect the suffering, symptoms, or limitations that bring them to therapy. Such patients, when unable to grasp the difference between raw experience and their reactions to it, are liable to feel imprisoned by their emotions and beliefs as if these had all the unyielding literalness of facts. Unlike objective facts, of course, subjective experience—a fluid multimodal composite of bodily sensation, emotion, and thought—arises only as the uniquely personal representational world we each inhabit filters our perceptions of internal and external reality. Yet our patients often find themselves unable to access, or benefit from, an awareness of the impact of the representational world. As such, they wind up embedded in that world, living as if the map were the territory.

At worst, they are unable to think anything they don't already believe, unable to imagine feeling anything they don't presently feel, and unable to consider any perspective or course of action aside from the one to which they are currently committed. A stance of such embeddedness inevitably undermines affect regulation and response flexibility, as well as the sense of personal agency that might allow these patients to feel they could have a hand in shaping their own experience.

As therapists, we too will find ourselves embedded at times, with the result that our capacity to freely think, feel, and act will be severely abridged. Enactments of transference–countertransference are instances of *shared* embeddedness. When simply embedded in experience, we are gripped both by our own internal representational world *and* the world of external reality, including the behavior of other people. A mentalizing stance and/or a mindful one can potentially loosen the grip of the internal and external circumstances in which we find ourselves thus doubly embedded.

MENTALIZING AND MINDFULNESS
AS PROCESSES OF "DISEMBEDDING"

Recall the clinically crucial finding that an adult's capacity to think about thoughts—metacognition—and to interpret human behavior in terms of

underlying mental states—mentalizing—is a better predictor of attachment security and the ability to raise secure children than the remembered facts of that adult's own attachment history (Fonagy, Steele, & Steele, 1991). Evidently a well-developed ability to adopt a reflective stance can trump personal history, even when that history is quite horrendous.

A patient of mine was psychologically scarred by childhood neglect and abuse nearly grotesque in its severity. Yet, remarkably resilient, he was in no way disabled by his history of trauma. Key to his emotional survival was his recognition at age five or so that his mother was "crazy." This early mentalizing softened the impact of what might otherwise have been developmentally disastrous circumstances.

Throughout our lives, mentalizing has the potential to free us from embeddedness in the internal world and external reality by fostering awareness of the interpretive depth and representational nature of subjective experience in ourselves and others. My patient, for example, was able to offset his internal experience of shame and guilt by reading his mother's unstable mind. Rather than regard her as sane and himself as bad, he redescribed her as "crazy" and thus preserved the possibility of his own goodness.

The "representational redescription" (Karmiloff-Smith, 1992) and interpretation that mentalizing makes possible illuminate not only the implicit mental underpinnings of here-and-now lived experience but also its context in terms of the remembered past and the imagined future. Mentalizing facilitates the "mental time travel" (Wheeler, Stuss, & Tulving, 1997) that allows us, paradoxically, to more fully inhabit the present moment. When we lack the capacity to mentalize, our present experience may too often be lived in the shadow of the dispiriting past or the imagining of a catastrophic future.

By enabling us to consider such experience in light of underlying mental states and their history, mentalizing makes possible a disidentification from reflexive and self-defeating responses that have previously ensnared us. In this way, it contributes to a "deautomatization" (Deikman, 1982) of our habitual patterns of thinking, feeling, and doing. Because it opens a mental space—and often an interval of time—between our experience and our responses to experience, mentalizing is "disembedding"(Safran & Muran, 2000).

While the reflective stance that signals mentalizing figures prominently in attachment theory, mindfulness has gotten only glancing attention from attachment theorists. It too is a stance toward experience that facilitates disembedding and disidentification from problematic mental states. But unlike mentalizing which focuses attention on the psychological *depth* of experience—including its unconscious dimension and its history—a mindful stance loosens the grip of internal and external circumstances by concentrating attention, deliberately and nonjudgmentally, on the *breadth* of experience in the present moment.

In a mindful stance, rather than *thinking* about the meaning of experi-

ence (as we do when we intentionally mentalize), we simply *attend* to the panorama of the here and now, allowing ourselves to deliberately inhabit our immediate experience as fully as possible in order to apprehend it as directly as possible (Bobrow, 1997). This requires acceptance, surrender (Ghent, 1990), or what is sometimes called faith (Eigen, 1981/1999)—particularly when the experience we're attending to is distressing. But if we choose to turn toward it, rather than resisting it, we can become aware of the passing parade of thoughts, feelings, and bodily sensations that continuously shapes and reshapes our experience from one moment to the next.

Deliberately choosing where and how we direct our attention is key to a mindful stance—and the possibility of conscious choice here depends upon first *locating* our attention. Once we have done so, we can attend to experience in a way that strengthens the sense of the distinction between awareness and the objects of awareness. In the process, we also strengthen our identification with the *awareness of awareness* that can function as an internal secure base. As mindful attention reveals the kaleidoscopic, ever-changing nature of experience (*impermanence* in the Buddhist idiom), it usually renders such experience less solid—less monolithic, more elastic—and allows us to move through it more easily, thus facilitating the process of change.

At the same time, a mindful stance can also cause our experience of ourselves and others to feel *more* solid—more full-blooded, accessible, and experientially "real." Such transformation occurs when the past and future are subjectively sheared away from the experience of the present moment. Then the here and now may suddenly feel charged with a quality of liberating timelessness, rather than suffocating permanence.

In this atmosphere, there is a paradoxical sense both of the "lightness of being" and the urgency of responding to experience in a more compassionate, grounded, and present-centered way. This vitalizing double sense of freedom and urgency can break the trance of helplessness that arises at times as our internal world interacts with our external reality. Mindfulness fosters a kind of awakening that allows us to note and disidentify from our previously automatic and unconscious responses to experience. In this way, for patients and therapists alike, a mindful stance—like a mentalizing one—can be a powerful resource for disembedding and for change.

Mentalizing is, of course, a staple of psychotherapeutic practice. Responding to behavior in light of underlying mental states—making sense of experience in terms of the feelings, beliefs, and desires that give it meaning—this is what we do every day with our patients. Mindfulness, unquestionably of value in its own right, can also make us better "mentalizers" by enabling us, as therapists, to be more fully and calmly present. This quality of "open presence" (Epstein, 1995) facilitates a heightened receptiveness to that which is most emotionally salient in our patients and in ourselves. Through a wide, rather than a narrow, focus of attention, a mindful stance makes possible a di-

rect sort of knowing that is integrative and seems as much the product of the body as the mind. This integrated knowing can help us help our patients both to think about their feelings and to experience the feelings evoked by their thoughts. Thus mindfulness—by enhancing our own mentalizing—can help us strengthen our patients' capacity to mentalize.

DEVELOPING MENTALIZING AND MINDFULNESS IN A RELATIONAL CONTEXT

As Bowlby suggested, relationships of attachment are so powerfully influential as contexts for development because they are experienced as so necessary. As Ainsworth clarified, it is the quality of communication in the (initially nonverbal) developmental dialogue—its inclusiveness, flexibility, and effectiveness in regulating affects—that determines its potential to confer security or insecurity. And as Main demonstrated, our early interpersonal dialogues are internalized as working models and rules for deploying attention that shape, among other things, our stance toward experience.

In psychotherapy, as in childhood development, the stance toward experience, particularly experience that is emotionally charged, is shaped—and can be reshaped—in the matrix of attachment relationships. The therapist (or parent) capable of disembedding from experience can create a relationship within which the patient (or child) can learn to be similarly capable. For the patient and child alike, the key to the development both of security and mentalizing is the experience of a relationship in which the attachment figure has your mind in mind (Fonagy et al., 2002). Such an experience in psychotherapy depends upon the mentalizing stance of the empathically attuned therapist, which—like that of the sensitively responsive parent—has both implicit and explicit dimensions.

Implicit mentalizing involves the ongoing intuitive reading of nonverbal affective cues—a specialty of the right brain that allows us to respond to behavior in light of its psychological meaning. We mentalize implicitly, usually outside conscious awareness, when we reflexively "mirror" the patient's emotional state with a corresponding expression on our face or shift in our tone of voice. Automatically interpreting and responding to behavior in this way—that is, empathically—is vital for fostering a relationship in which the patient feels felt and understood.

Explicit mentalizing is a contrastingly *conscious* process that enlists the linguistic resources of the "left-brain interpreter" (Gazzaniga, Eliassen, Nisenson, Wessuger, & Baynes, 1996) to deliberately reflect upon the meaning of behavior and its psychological underpinnings, often making the implicit explicit (as when the therapist comments on the disavowed resent-

ment revealed in a patient's angry tone of voice). We mentalize explicitly, and invite the patient to do the same, whenever we put into words our efforts to understand the experience of the patient or, for that matter, our own experience of the therapeutic interaction.

It is, specifically, the therapist's mentalizing, implicitly and explicitly, in the context of an increasingly secure relationship of attachment that gradually strengthens the patient's ability to adopt a mentalizing stance. Similarly, the therapist who is capable of mindfulness can use the relationship to help foster the patient's own capacity to be mindful.

As suggested earlier, mindfulness can be "catching." In the presence of another who is calm and accepting, it is easier to find calmness and a modicum of self-acceptance in ourselves. When as therapists we can be mindful, we often find the patient meeting us on common ground. All this can occur implicitly. We can also *explicitly* invite patients' mindfulness—when, for example, we suggest to them that they stay with their experience of the present moment, or pose questions that they can't answer without focusing on here-and-now experience. Whenever we direct attention neither to what *has* happened nor to what is *going* to happen but, rather, to what *is* happening, we create opportunities for our patients to be mindful. And every time they are enabled to "inhabit" the present moment with awareness and acceptance they strengthen their capacity for mindfulness.

THE DOUBLE HELIX: A CLINICAL ILLUSTRATION

Teach us to care and not to care
Teach us to sit still.
                —T. S. ELIOT (1930/1991a)

The relationship between a mentalizing and a mindful stance in psychotherapy can be likened to a double helix: a pair of partially overlapping spirals that converge and diverge, again and again. Mentalizing and mindfulness are distinct, but complementary and interweaving, ways of knowing and responding to experience—and each potentiates the other: "Insight induces calming and calming induces insight" (Cooper, 1999, p. 74). Both a mentalizing stance and a mindful one can enhance the therapist's capacity to help the patient to regulate affects more effectively, to feel a sense of agency, and to integrate previously dissociated experience. And both can enhance awareness and internal freedom by allowing us—as therapists and patients alike—to recognize the ways in which the mind mediates our experience of the world.

The point, of course, is to diminish suffering and to be able to help our patients to feel more alive—more connected to themselves and others. The

suffering in which our patients are embedded takes many forms and has many causes. Much of it stems from the attempt to avoid suffering. The deactivating and hyperactivating strategies associated with insecure attachment, as well as the dissociation and "acting out" associated with unresolved trauma, can be seen as automatic, defensive measures to reduce both present suffering and the probability of suffering in the future. The therapist's mentalizing and mindfulness are ways of being with the patient's suffering—and ways of avoiding suffering—that can make room for, and potentially diminish, both.

But therapists, like their patients, are vulnerable to emotional pain and liable, at times, to find themselves embedded in their own habitual defenses against such pain. The result is that, as therapists, we regularly slip in and out of periods during which we are simply embedded—very much as our patients are—in self-protective patterns of thinking, feeling, and relating that play out as if by rote.

"Thank You for Another Year"

These words ended a Christmas note to me from Ellen, a patient obsessed with suicide whose therapy I began to discuss in Chapter 15. There (pp. 284–288) I summarized two sessions with Ellen: the first marked by an enactment *cum* corrective emotional experience, the second by an interpretation which crystallized around an image of myself taking Ellen by the hand to lead her out of her safe but barren isolation into a new world of relationship. These sessions set in motion a sequence of hours whose review is meant to illuminate the complex relationship between enactments—the embeddedness shared by patient and therapist—and the mentalizing and mindfulness that can help to loosen their grip.

The life-and-death stakes in my long relationship with Ellen, the sense of slow, but steady progress, and the partial "overlap" in our experience have combined to generate a powerful bond between us. After a number of years, she is profoundly, if not *entirely* securely, attached to me, while my affection for her now is considerable and my commitment unshakable. This, following a protracted siege—involving suicide threats and gestures, middle-of-the-night phone calls, police, medics, hospitalizations—and, later, the relative calm after the storm.

The issue we have struggled with, virtually from the inception of treatment, is dependency. Who will take care of whom? This is the question. Ellen has felt compelled throughout her life to take care of others. Very early on, this was the role assigned to her by parents who demanded that she care for her younger siblings as well as the two of them, at a time when by rights they ought to have been taking care of her. As an adult, having others depend on her has been a constant of her emotional job description.

In therapy, fighting her need to depend on me, she was like a drowning woman resisting rescue.

And yet she also longed unconsciously to be rescued—just as I, apparently, longed unconsciously to be able to rescue her. It was my image of myself as Ellen's knight in shining armor that first allowed me to glimpse my need to "save" her as well as her own hope of being thus saved. In the hour I described in Chapter 15 as a turning point in the therapy, I shared this image with her and my guess as to its meaning.

For several sessions thereafter, Ellen complained familiarly, and rather angrily, that she had allowed herself to become too dependent on me. She could make little use of my suggestion that her upset had directly followed our discussion of my wish to magically save her—and hers to be magically saved. She seemed to have no mental space in which to consider the meaning of her upset. She appeared instead to be utterly embedded in the claustrophobic world of psychic equivalence in which feelings are facts to be acted on, rather than mental states to be felt, but also understood. The only solution she could imagine was to see me less frequently: once weekly, rather than twice.

I found myself mildly frustrated that she wouldn't—or couldn't—think with me about what she was feeling. Yet suggesting to Ellen that her difficulty in doing so was tied to the very hopes we'd touched on in that disturbing hour was useful for me. When I proposed (without using the word) that her "mentalizing" was blocked partly by her "relentless hope" to receive from me what she had missed as a child (Stark, 2000), it helped deepen my empathy for her plight and took the edge off the urgency of my need to save her. What I had yet to grasp more fully were the roots of this need in my own psychology.

"No One at the Wheel"

In the first session of the four I'll sketch, Ellen says she knows that *I* feel something important has been occurring in therapy, but *she's* not so sure. She asks me to explain again what I've been thinking.

> I respond, "I'm sure you remember that hour in which I told you about my image of somehow 'saving' you by taking your hand and leading you into a better world. It's my guess that your hope for something like that makes it hard for you to want to work with me to understand what you struggle with. I think instead there's the hope that you could somehow be saved just by being with me and experiencing here what you didn't experience with your parents—all the love and care you needed to grow up feeling safe and strong."
>
> When she says she knows I have this idea, but doesn't know if it's

really true, I persist. "More than once, we've talked about how reluctant you are to stay with your feelings and try to get to know them, to put them into words with me in order to at least try and get a handle on them."

This idea is one she has no trouble relating to. "I'm not just reluctant—I've got a positive aversion to paying attention to what I'm feeling." Long silence. "So that part of what you're saying seems true." Another silence. "It just feels very challenging." Silence.

"And what's it like to feel challenged?"

"It makes me nervous. Like there's this thing I could do that I'm not doing. But why should I bother when I can't believe it would make any difference? It's too late for me. There's no reason to hope. I don't feel like I have a future. It seems like it would take so much work that the only point would be if I saw a future ahead of me. But I don't."

Hearing these words, I too have a sense of hopelessness, as though whatever I say will be insufficient to reach her. Recognizing once again how profoundly difficult, perhaps impossible, it is for Ellen to mobilize her own resources on her own behalf, I feel myself sinking—until, unbidden, a mental picture of Ellen sitting in the driver's seat of a car comes to mind.

An image or metaphor like this one is quite often the form taken by the therapist's mentalizing. Sometimes such an image becomes a vital part of the therapeutic conversation where it has the potential to contribute to the strengthening of the patient's own mentalizing capacity. How so? Images and metaphors—like mentalizing itself—involve symbols. That is, they stand for something else and, while meaningfully representing (we hope) some aspect of emotional reality, they can also be played with. When we work with such initially nonverbal symbols in therapy we are "playing with reality" (Fonagy & Target, 1996)—a pretty good description of what we do when we mentalize. I decide to share my image with Ellen.

"Just now as you were saying you couldn't see a future ahead, I had a mental picture of you sitting in the driver's seat of a car. And the car's not moving. You're in the driver's seat, but you're feeling reluctant, or maybe just unable, to really take the wheel. Using your words, it's like you've got a 'positive aversion' to looking through the windshield to see what might be in front of you and a positive aversion to looking into the rearview mirror to see what's behind you. And without being able to look ahead or behind, it's obviously going to feel very dangerous to drive. In fact, you're probably going to want someone else to take the wheel so that you might actually be able to get somewhere safely."

"I don't want to drive, you're right . . . I want somebody else to get me there." She says this in a particular tone and with a look that

seem to express, in turn, her angry entitlement to have someone else to do the driving and her shame at having given voice to such a desire.

Sensing her painful double feeling, I say, "I know. Of course, you want that. I think you must feel both that you deserve it and that it's a shameful and humiliating thing to want it."

"I'm too scared to look ahead. It's just so bleak. And it's just overwhelming to look backwards. I haven't done it in so long." Now in tears: "Things would just get too out-of-control. I was always driving before I fell apart. I was always in control. But since then I've just been kind of waiting and hoping for someone else to take over." She is clearly struggling with her feelings.

I say, "I don't want to take over. But I'd like to be sitting next to you in the car, a little as if you were just starting to drive again and I was there to help you keep your eyes on the road and look in the rearview mirror."

"But if I look, if I actually pay attention to what I'm feeling and thinking, it's just going to be too much. I know it is."

"I think you're afraid you're not going to be able to put on the brakes."

We talk at some length about some ways in which she might be able to put the brakes on: visualizing a safe place, attending to her breathing, meditating as we do at the beginning of each session. When the hour is nearly over, she tells me that she's always had dreams about cars. As a little girl, she dreamed of being in the back seat, terrified because there was no one at the wheel. Now, as an adult, she has dreams of being in the car alone, but unable to get herself into the driver's seat.

"Standing at a Crossroads"

Several sessions later while we're meditating, a thought—all too meaningfully obvious in hindsight—crosses my mind: *I need to spend less time at the wheel myself in order for Ellen to experience her own sense of agency.* I'm quiet, and in a way that is exceptional, Ellen speaks first. When she says she feels tired, I ask what it's like for her now to be tired here.

Slowly and quietly, she says, "It feels mixed. . . . It feels safe and it feels comfortable. I like being able to just be here. . . . But I also feel like I want to get somewhere today."

Hearing what may be the faint stirrings of agency, I'm silent. My attention is as much on my breathing and on the interior of my body as it is on her words. I feel calm, present, and much less pressured than usual to act. I'm aware of my belly rising and falling, with the inhalation and exhalation. I have the sense of apprehending her viscerally, and of making space for her.

Pausing between ideas, she says, "I'm tired because my thoughts are just racing . . . My mind is always just jumping from one thing to another . . . I'm constantly distracting myself with extraneous thoughts so I don't have to be with what's actually going on inside me."

"I'm with you. I know the experience of scampering around in my own mind when I'm upset. Like I'm searching for some secure place or understanding or conclusion or framing."

"But you can look at your thoughts. I'm just running from mine . . . always turning away from my experience."

You'd do better if you were able to turn toward it, is what I'm thinking. Then I direct my attention inward again, toward my own experience of my breathing body. I'm not trying to figure anything out just now. I feel calm and open.

After a very prolonged silence, Ellen says, "I feel somehow like I'm standing at a crossroads. . . . But I can't define it very well."

I break another lengthy silence, saying, "You seem to have the sense of struggling with a choice or a direction."

"David, I'm struggling with giving up the idea that I'm going to kill myself."

Deeply and audibly, I sigh.

"And it's so hard . . . It's so hard to let it go, because that's been my only security, that's been what I could count on. . . . The only thing I've ever wanted was to feel secure, and I can't seem to feel secure anywhere in my life. . . . But it's just getting harder and harder to believe that my kids, my grown-up kids, would ever be okay with my suicide."

Her deepening empathy here seems to be a marker of mentalizing and of disembedding from her "pretend" world in which she imagines that her children—easily accommodating her need for the solace of oblivion— "would really be better off without me."

"Tell me if this is right. I have the sense that you're putting yourself in their shoes more and more. You're imagining what your suicide would feel like to them. And when you do it's impossible to sustain the belief that it wouldn't have an enormous and very destructive impact."

"That's right. And I think about you, too. But I don't know what to do with what I feel. I can use what I've learned here to tell myself when I'm panicking that it will pass. But it's like I lack something, some part of my brain, or some ability to think about my experience, some insight."

"I don't think you lack the ability. I think you lack practice. And it's hard to want to practice when you're terrified that paying attention to your feelings is simply going to leave you overwhelmed."

"But I've also had the experience of being less overwhelmed when I leave here having talked about my feelings."

What emerges as this session draws to a close is some clarity that the crossroads at which Ellen finds herself represents the disturbing possibility not only of giving up the "security" of suicide, but also of choosing to live. And this choice raises the specter of getting herself behind the wheel, and summoning somehow the courage and initiative to turn toward her experience, rather than away from it.

"I Don't Want to Think"

Early in the session, Ellen tells me that she's feeling very anxious about a Christmas trip she is about to take to visit her sister in another state. What specifically is she anxious about? She feels that she needs to be strong and perfect; she needs to be able to take care of her sister. Quite terrified that she might appear to her sister in any way incapable of living up to this image, Ellen seems unable or unwilling to question her feelings or ideas: They simply are what they are.

I feel frustrated to be once again in this concrete world. Can't she see that there's something to think about here? Why is it that I alone seem to be responsible for helping her dig her way out of her self-created misery? Believing mistakenly that I'm containing these discomfiting responses—or perhaps I should say concealing them—I manage to draw her into a discussion in which it becomes apparent that her sister is, if anything, *less* in need than Ellen is of a strong, supportive other. Then, noticing that she seems to be retreating into herself, I ask Ellen what it's like for her to be talking with me about her conviction that she needs to take care of her sister.

"I feel like you're scolding me, or chiding me," she answers.

I sigh, knowing that, of course, she's right. In the effort to repair the disruption here I say, "I'm sure you're picking up on something real. I think I just get impatient at times, or frustrated. You're just having your feelings, but I've evidently got my own need for you to do something more with them. So naturally you wind up feeling the target of that need. But I have to say, the last thing I want is for you to feel that my efforts to help actually wind up hurting you."

Tearfully, she says, "I don't think you want to hurt me. But I don't think you understand. I am trying to talk myself out of what I'm feeling, but it just doesn't work. I keep having the feelings."

"Of course you do. Why wouldn't you? Do you think I've been suggesting that you talk yourself out of what you're feeing? What I'm talking about is something quite different. I'm talking about not being so willing to take what you feel as the last word on the subject. I'm talking about thinking about what you're feeling."

In tearful protest she replies, "David, I don't want to think. I don't want to take responsibility. I want someone else to think. I want someone else to take responsibility. I took so much responsibility as a kid, I just don't want to do it anymore."

Here I'm experiencing empathy for her obvious pain, but also some of the same frustration that had her feeling scolded only a few minutes before. While still struggling with my difficult feelings, I'm able to grasp that the depth of her longing to be taken care of must be heard and *felt* by me, so that she might subsequently be able to consider additional perspectives on that longing. To open up a space for mentalizing, Ellen needs first to feel that I recognize the "reality" of her desperate, unfulfilled desire to have now what she deserved before, but was never given.

"It wasn't fair that you had to be a parent when you were still a child. To me, your desire for someone to take responsibility for you, to take care of you in the vital ways your parents could not, or at any rate, did not—that desire is entirely understandable and legitimate."

Now I sense both a trace of relief in her and another, though fainter, protest as she responds: "I don't have any confidence about taking responsibility. I just can't do it. I want someone else to take the wheel, someone to take care of me, and think for me, but I know that'll never happen, no matter how much I want it to . . . no one else is really going to be there to do that . . . I realize I'm the only one, that I need to do it for myself . . . But I just don't want to."

"Again, your wish—your hoping against hope—is completely understandable. It makes emotional sense. And obviously I do want to take care of you, and I think you feel taken care of by me, much of the time. But I think you pay a price when I do too much of the thinking for you here, because then you wind up feeling less self-assured, less self-reliant, less in charge of yourself."

"I just have no confidence that I can think in the way you think I can. I just can't do it."

Were she to be saying this years ago, months ago, perhaps even weeks ago, I would be even less certain than I am about the usefulness of responding in the way I do: "I wonder if you can join me in remembering that we've had conversations like this before. Conversations where you tell me you just can't think. But then you'll come back later, the next time we meet or in a phone call, with lots of thoughts. And you're clearly thoughtful when you're writing in your journal. So sometimes at least, it may be less a matter of being unable to consider your experience in a thoughtful way and more a matter of being unwilling to—maybe especially when we're here together."

"But maybe there's nothing to consider," she says. Then rather plaintively: "Maybe I'm just a very simple person. I don't have a lot of complexity, like a lot of your other patients probably do. You already know everything there is to know about me. There's nothing more to know. So there's really nothing more to think about."

I'm feeling frustrated again here, but I'm also engaged, mentalizing, and hopeful that I can engage Ellen's own mentalizing process. I say, "Actually I think there's plenty to think about. You're struggling to re-solve whether you should keep holding out for someone to take care of

you or whether you should start trying with my help—to do the best you can for yourself. Isn't this another version of the crossroads you're at? If you're not going to kill yourself, then what are you going to do with your life?"

A few words later, the hour concludes on what seems at best an uncertain note. I wind up feeling unsettled and a little dispirited, realizing once more that I've been working too hard at making a case. It feels like a step backward.

Then, the morning before we are to meet next, I make the following note to myself, for which the backdrop is some reflection—mentalizing—about my own history:

> What a tangled web we weave. I need Ellen to get better in order to get myself off the hook, while she needs to accentuate her helplessness to get me to feel helpless, in order to get herself off the hook. At the same time, she's waiting for me to fix her, which hooks my vulnerability to feeling entirely responsible. And then I get angry because she's not allowing me to fix her. The point is there's an enactment here and my problematic part will be diluted if I can be more mindful and less driven by my need to make her better. It'll help if I can have more modest aims and allow things to be what they are. Which might mean letting her have the feelings she's having while communicating my ability to cope (and by implication, my confidence in her ability to cope) with whatever her experience might be. Don't be so hooked by her stuff and don't hook her so in mine.

"A Different Kind of Sadness"

I enter the last of the four sessions I'm summarizing with what feels like a newly deepened understanding of my participation in our co-created enactment. I feel less embedded in my experience and freer from the largely unconscious compulsion to repeat with Ellen aspects of my relationship with my mother. In this roomier, more flexible state of mind, I find it much easier to be present with acceptance—to be mindful—rather than gripped by my need to make something happen or to change her.

> When I open my eyes after we meditate, and see that hers are wet, I ask what she's feeling. Almost whispering, she answers, "I'm feeling sad . . . and I'm feeling anxious. . . ." She shifts on the couch, leaving me with the impression that she's trying to get away from herself. Then she shakes her head slightly as if to say "no" to what she's feeling.
>
> "Can you stay with those feelings for a bit?"
>
> "I've been having such a hard time these last few days, it seems like I can't not stay with them."

"And when you do, do you have a sense of what you're sad about? Or what's been making you feel anxious?"

"I know I'm scared about this trip to my sister's, which is back to where my mother's buried...I always worry before trips, I don't like to travel, especially when I'm traveling alone. . . ."

"I'm guessing part of the context for feeling scared is that we won't be meeting together for a while."

"I know." Then looking directly at me, she says in a quiet, steady voice, "I depend on you so much." After a pause she adds, "I've been telling myself it's only three sessions . . . but it seems like such a long time. I know I can call if I need to . . . but even so. . . ."

I'm feeling calm, quietly taking in her presence without experiencing the familiar internal pressure to quickly respond. Staying with her, I'm also turning my attention to my breathing and my body. I have the not unfamiliar sense that I'm "knowing" her through my belly: My "gut sense" is that, as I'm relinquishing the lead, she's taking it.

"The sad feeling . . . it feels like it's about the past." There's a long pause, as if she's just now hearing her own words and allowing herself to recognize their significance. Then she continues, "The trip to my sister's is just bringing it all back . . . all my feelings about the way things were, feelings about my mother and father . . . and how they never, ever protected me. . . ." She cries hard, then almost in a whisper says: "I want someone to protect me."

"Mmm . . . Yeah . . . Of course you do." While she's speaking, I'm seeing images in my mind's eye from the past she's described to me—images of trauma and neglect that she's previously related as if in a rather dissociated state, or as if she were seeing images of her own that would freak her out if she stayed with them much longer. Along the way I'm making empathic noises. I'm also nodding my head in sympathy with her sadness and, later, shaking it a little, as if sharing her quiet outrage. And then, rather suddenly, I flash that Ellen is feeling her feelings, rather than avoiding or seeming to be overwhelmed by them. More striking still, she's talking not about being depressed, as she usually does, but about feeling sad.

Tearfully, head down, she says, "I'll go to my mother's grave and I'll be expected to grieve, but all I'll really feel like doing is spitting on her grave and saying, Fuck you . . ." Between quiet sobs she says in a pleading tone, "I just wish to God I'd been able to come to peace with them before they died. . . ."

"It sounds like you're trying to do that now."

Through tears she looks at me as if she could read in my face whether what I'm saying about her is true. Then she drops her face into her hands, crying harder.

When she settles, I ask her if what she's feeling now is an old familiar sadness, or if it seems new.

"It feels like a different kind of sadness." After a long silence, she

goes on, "I'm also feeling scared . . . I think my sister's going to ask me for money. I can't really afford to help her. . . . But I can't not help her." We explore her fear and her compulsion to take care of others. Ellen tells me that her brother would respond to her sister very differently than she does: "He'd say, 'Just let her see if she can take care of herself!' But I just can't do that . . . I can't."

"God, it's just so pervasive, this question. Can you allow your sister to take more responsibility? Can I allow you to take more responsibility? Apparently we're both struggling with this question. I think we both grew up in families where we were expected to take care of other people's feelings. And if we didn't there was a high price to pay."

Here she tells me her dream from the previous night: She's in a public place and she's about to kill herself with a bomb. A doctor is there who talks to her in such a way that she changes her mind. Then very much to her dismay, the doctor leaves her with the bomb, rather than taking it with him or getting her to a place where she will be taken care of. With his departure, she is left on her own to somehow keep the bomb from exploding—for if it does, others will die along with her.

Discussing the dream, I suggest that it touches on exactly what we've just been talking about. First, the dream seems to express her terror that if she fails to take care of everyone, then not only will they be on their own, but there will be a violent catastrophe. "That's what happened in my family, " she says. Later I add that the dream may also communicate her worry that, in expecting more from her, I'm actually leaving her on her own. She admits that she does indeed have this worry—to which I respond with what I realize is an overlengthy effort at reassuring clarification.

And then, as I become aware of how much talking I've been doing, and how little space I've been making for her, I say, "I've just been getting clearer and clearer about how—while I know I've been helpful to you—I've also been getting in your way. It's like my own compulsion to take care of you has led me to do so much of the thinking here that it's made it hard for you to get behind the plow with me so as to share the work. It's just very hard to leave the past behind . . . for both of us, obviously . . . for me, all the ways in which I had to take care of my mother or else there was hell to pay. . . . And for you, I think, something similar, or worse. . . ." After a silence, and seeing a hard-to-read expression on her face, I say, "I wonder what it's like for you to hear me talking about some of my own experience growing up?"

"It's reassuring. It's like you've got way of understanding me based on what happened to you. It makes me feel less crazy and more safe."

Even at this moment, I'm aware of how hard it is for me to hand over the reins to her. "I'm thinking about our conversation and how deep these old patterns run. I just keep doing it." With a smile, I add, "Apparently I can barely shut up. It's just hard to stop."

Also with a smile, she says, "And it's hard for me to start."

"Meaning?"

"Hard to start taking responsibility for my own life. It's just automatic to take responsibility for other people. . . ." She sighs.

"What's it like for you right now?"

"I'm feeling better."

"Hmm. Do you know how that happened?"

"Talking and crying." Looking a little tearful, she tells me how difficult it is for her to let herself cry: She's so used to turning away from these feelings. She's scared that if she looks back and grieves for all the ways in which her life could have been different she'll sink back into her old depression. She associates crying with being depressed, she says, and she's terrified of becoming depressed again.

"I think your crying now is sadness, it's not depression. Depression is not feeling. Allowing yourself to feel sad may be a way for you to avoid getting so depressed again." When she objects that looking back always leads her to blame herself for everything, I suggest that blaming herself may be another way that she avoids grieving the loss of what she deserved to have gotten as a child, but never did.

As the hour ends, she tells me she has very mixed feelings about giving up her depression and her commitment to suicide. "It's what I've done. . . . It's been a way of life for me. . . . And it's frightening, the intensity of sadness and anger I'd feel if I let myself . . ."

"I know. But you actually are letting yourself begin to feel those feelings now."

Enactments and the Double Helix

Therapeutic change is mysterious. Yet sequences of sessions like those I've just sketched tend to reinforce my sense that change in the patient depends on—and may need, in many instances, to be preceded by—change in the therapist (Slavin & Kriegman, 1998). Casting a look backward, it seems clear that Ellen and I were locked into an enactment to which my psychology probably contributed as much as hers.

Early in our relationship, it was as if she had needed me to save her from drowning, so overwhelmed was she by the tidal intensity of her emotions and the (admittedly) crushing external circumstances of her life. Later in the therapy, because this need of hers for saving so dovetailed with a need of mine to save, I was slow to see that what had previously been Ellen's profound difficulty in "feeling and dealing" (Fosha, 2000) was now at least as much a matter of her profound disinclination.

My own mentalizing and mindfulness gradually allowed me both to recognize my role in our enactment and to change my behavior accordingly. The image of the double helix is apt here because the reflective and mindful

stances interweave to foster the therapist's disembedding which is often a precondition for the patient's.

Mentalizing led to my initial image of taking Ellen by the hand to lead her into a new world as well as my second image of Ellen, sitting in her car, but waiting for someone else to take the wheel. Translating these images into words helped me grasp, by degrees, the nature of the scenario we enacted together: a different, personal amalgam for each of us our own versions of Main's (1995) controlling–caregiving strategy as well as Stark's (2000) relentless hope and refusal to mourn that have been identified as core issues in the treatment of preoccupied patients (Eagle, 1999; Blatt & Blass, 1996).

Deliberately adopting a mindful stance—focusing not only on my patient but also on my breathing body—allowed me some freedom from my compulsion to help, in part through making possible an acceptance of the present *status quo*, rather than a resistance to, and a need to change, it. With the benefit of such acceptance, I believe I was gradually more capable of offering Ellen the experience of a calm, rather than an anxiously intervening, attachment figure. A marked increment in her ability both to feel and to think about her feelings—that is, to mentalize—seemed to follow this change in the relational context, not coincidentally, I presume,

In psychotherapy, mentalizing and mindfulness have the potential to contribute to the kind of developmental dialogue that has been demonstrated to foster secure attachment (Lyons-Ruth, 1999). Specifically, as two distinct and complementary forms of "knowing," both can enhance the inclusiveness of the dialogue and upgrade that dialogue to new levels of awareness. Of particular importance to keep in mind are the ways in which mentalizing and mindfulness can contribute to affect regulation, self-agency, and integration.

Affect Regulation and the Double Helix

Bucci (2003) uses the term "emotion schemas" rather than "working models" to underscore how internal representations are welded to affects. Indeed, we must effectively regulate—that is, recognize, tolerate, and modulate—our own affects in order to disembed from the emotion schemas we enact with our patients. Doing so makes us more capable of functioning for the patient as a secure base, of generating a relationship within which the patient's difficult affects can be effectively regulated.

Mentalizing strengthens affect regulation. The more I could recognize, name, and understand my anxious desire to take care of Ellen, the more I could contain it. The more I could recognize, name, and understand Ellen's desires to be taken care of by me and to take care of others, the more capable she was of doing the same. And working with these anxious desires made room for the "deeper" feelings that lay beneath them—anger and,

most important, sadness. Thinking aloud with Ellen about the underpinnings of my behavior with her modeled a reflective stance toward experience, as did my implicit as well as explicit mentalizing in relation to *her* behavior. I'm certain the latter helped her to feel felt, understood, and cared for. I believe it also allowed her to begin to regard her troubling feelings as mental states to be understood rather than facts to be acted on. As such, these feelings could more easily be borne.

Mindfulness, too, can allow us to bear more feeling, for the essence of the mindful stance is a wholeheartedly open and compassionate awareness of experience *as it is*, including painful experience. As such, it involves the practice of "turning toward" difficult feelings and thoughts—in our patients and in ourselves—with an attitude of "radical acceptance" (Brach, 2003; Linehan, 1993). Radical acceptance is pragmatic because so much of our suffering grows out of our efforts to avoid pain. As one patient put it, "*pain × resistance = suffering*" (Siegel, 2005, p. 182). Thus, "softening" or "breathing" into painful experience—rather than attempting to avoid or change it—can actually diminish suffering. But note that surrendering to troubling experience is entirely different from endorsing or clinging to it. Acceptance also means "letting go." The paradox here is that our radical acceptance of experiences that we tend reflexively to reject creates a context within which letting go of such experiences becomes possible. In addition, mindful awareness of painful feelings is an education in their transitory nature. The growing realization that these feelings both arise and fall away diminishes their power to intimidate. Finally, as I've mentioned, simply attending to the breath can itself foster calmness, particularly when such attention is associated with a state of mind that has become familiar through meditative practice. In part, this was the rationale for encouraging Ellen to meditate, both inside and outside my office.

Deliberately adopting a mindful stance as I related to her enabled me to sit with my own anxiety in relative calm rather than act on it. In this frame of mind, I was able to note my feelings with acceptance and interest. Containing them in this way enabled me to provide for Ellen a larger container for her own emotional experience: Focusing a kindly attention on her difficult emotions in the here and now made room for them. At the same time, helping her to contain these emotions by "putting on the brakes" in various ways enabled her to feel less threatened by them.

Agency and the Double Helix

Personal agency is a cousin of will, choice, freedom, and responsibility. Agents *make* things happen. In psychotherapy, we can facilitate the development of different sorts of agency. The mentalizing therapist fosters the patient's sense of herself as a *mental* agent—that is, someone who recog-

nizes that her own experience and that of others admits of interpretation, that subjective experience is not something that "just happens" but is instead something that can be shaped and reshaped by the understanding we bring to it. In parallel fashion, the mindful therapist fosters the patient's sense of herself as an *attentional* agent—that is, someone who is in charge of her attention and focus, and is able, as such, to exert influence upon her experience.

Whether in a mentalizing or a mindful stance—but not an embedded one—we can choose the uses to which we put our awareness. Ellen, in the sessions I reviewed, revealed an increasing ability to exercise agency in deploying her awareness. She told me that she was putting things together that had previously seemed isolated; she was choosing, in other words, to *reflect* on her experience rather than take it entirely at face value. She also told me that she was deliberately choosing to turn her attention toward her feelings, rather than distract herself from them. And when these feelings became overwhelming, she was learning that she could choose to turn away from them, by focusing on her breathing or on the safe place in her imagination. In these ways, she was exercising mental and attentional agency.

Ellen was beginning to discover that she could *choose* to mentalize and/or to be mindful. Both developments represented a departure from her habitual embedded stance in which choice and intention played only the most minor role. As an agent, she could potentially feel less helpless, though not without considerable risk. For Ellen, as we came to understand together, taking the wheel for herself was also to take on the challenges of mourning her lost childhood and relinquishing the safe familiarity of her depressive cocoon.

Integration and the Double Helix

As therapists, we exercise agency when we consciously choose to adopt a mentalizing or mindful stance in relation to our experience with the patient. Such conscious choices are particularly important when we notice that we are embedded either in an avoidant or anxiously preoccupied state of mind. For example, when I found myself compulsively intervening with Ellen in order to fend off my own anxiety, it was vital to be able to *reflect* on our interaction—or, alternatively, to simply *be* with my experience in a mindful way rather than act on it. So long as we remain embedded in enactments with our patients, we make little room for accessing and integrating dissociated feelings or undeveloped capacities like Ellen's grief or her experience of agency.

The therapist's deliberate mentalizing and mindfulness and the patient's are mutually supportive facets of a single integrative process. Yet it is often the therapist's mindfulness that sets this process in motion. Success-

fully dropping into a mindful stance and "landing" in the present moment can allow us to "know" (to sense, feel, or intuit) what is most essential in our interaction with the patient. This sort of knowing blends awareness and acceptance. Through a kind of holistic, integrated, body-based receptivity, it gets beneath the words to the emotional heart of the matter and thus permits access to dimensions of experience that neither patient nor therapist has previously been able to articulate. Once accessed, this implicit or dissociated experience can be made explicit and it can be explored—that is, it can be mentalized. Sequences of such mindful apprehension and reflective understanding are instrumental in furthering the process of integration.

For example, in a recent hour with a new patient—an unhappy captain of industry—I became aware of feeling unaccountably remote without being able to figure out why; here, in other words, my mentalizing proved a dead end. Choosing deliberately to cultivate a mindful stance at this point, I found myself capable of being present in a way that had seemed impossible moments before. Almost immediately I connected both with my own experience of feeling controlled and intimidated by the patient, as well as what seemed to be the patient's experience of deep and abiding vulnerability. In putting all this into words, I initiated a shared process of mentalizing that helped the patient to recognize the fear and hurt that lay behind what he admitted was a hair-trigger temper. He also realized that he had never had a parent to whom he could turn when he was scared or upset. Of necessity, he had learned to take care of himself with whatever resources he could muster, including the anger he used to intimidate others and to keep his own vulnerability at bay.

The kind of "broadband" receptivity that mindfulness makes possible may be an essential precursor to deliberate mentalizing. Such receptivity might be said to make room for the "dissociated present"—the feelings and bodily sensations that patients and their therapists unwittingly tune out. This here-and-now experience must be accessed before it can be explicitly mentalized—and the therapist's mindful stance is perfectly suited to foster such access.

Mindfulness diminishes discursive thinking about past and future. The focus of awareness in a mindful stance is "not ideas about the thing, but the thing itself" (Stevens, 1954/1990, p. 534). This kind of awareness can open channels of interpersonal, somatic, and emotional perception and communication that lie beyond, and can sometimes be blocked by, the therapist's attempts to understand experience by thinking about it. Moreover, mindfulness is largely defined by the quality of acceptance that it can foster. This kind of acceptance in the therapist—both self-acceptance and acceptance of the patient—itself contributes to the emergence and awareness of previously implicit or dissociated experience.

As therapists, our mindful attention to the present moment can bring

such experience more sharply into focus. Our mentalizing can then bring multiple perspectives to bear on that experience, giving it an in-depth context that permits its meaning(s) to be more effectively grasped. This context may relate here-and-now experience to the past and future. It may situate the present moment in relation to the history of the therapeutic relationship and to life outside that relationship. Or it may relate what is now in the foreground to facets of the patient's psychology with which he or she is presently out of touch. In short, our mentalizing—along with that of the patient—can allow the patient's lived experience with the therapist to be gradually integrated into a new, more adaptive, and more coherent narrative. At an explicit level, such a narrative makes sense of the patient's experience. It also "locks in" the integration of dissociated feelings, thoughts, and desires that largely occurs implicitly through the attuned and inclusive attachment relationship the therapist is, one hopes, providing for the patient.

FOSTERING MINDFULNESS

. . . and all is always Now.
—T. S. ELIOT (1943/1991b)

Psychotherapy is an intimate partnership that provides, among other things, the setting for a shared exercise in mindfulness in which (initially) the therapist and (subsequently also) the patient attempt to be fully present and aware, with acceptance. Conceiving of therapy in this way, as a kind of two-person meditation, highlights the desirability of attending to what is actually occurring in the present moment—not our ideas about the experience arising in the therapeutic interaction but the experience itself. In a mindful stance, such attention can yield a liberating awareness of the distinction between what happens *to* us and what happens *in* us. Buddhist psychology holds that this practice of "bare attention"—observing moment by moment our experience and our reactions to experience—is, in and of itself, healing (Epstein, 1995). As therapists, there are a variety of approaches we can take to cultivating such a healing process in our patients and in ourselves.

The Mindful Therapist

The therapist who engages in formal meditation is exercising the muscle that makes mindfulness possible, not only when sitting in silence, but also when interacting with others, including the patient. Such practice awakens our *awareness of awareness* and enables us to grasp what it means to actu-

ally be present. It also strengthens our ability to adopt a stance toward experience that is described in related terms by the Zen master Suzuki as *beginner's mind* and by Freud as *evenly hovering attention*:

> If your mind is empty it is always ready for anything; it is open to everything. In the beginner's mind, there are many possibilities; in the expert's mind, there are few. (Suzuki, 1970, p. 21)

> The technique . . . consists in making no effort to concentrate the attention on anything in particular, and in maintaining in regard to all that one hears, the same measure of calm, quiet attentiveness—of "evenly-hovering attention." . . . For as soon as attention is deliberately concentrated in a certain degree, one begins to select from the material before one. . . . This is just what must not be done, however; if one's expectations are followed in this selection there is the danger of never finding anything but what is already known, and if one follows one's inclinations anything which is perceived will most certainly be falsified. (Freud, 1912/1924a, p. 324)

Giving flexible, relatively impartial attention to *whatever* is there to be observed diminishes not only our tendency to be overly influenced by our preconceptions but also our vulnerability to imposing our expectations upon our patients. Bion (1967/1981) describes this kind of attention in the most striking terms when he writes,

> The psychoanalyst should aim at achieving a state of mind so that at every session he feels he has not seen the patient before. If he feels he has, he is treating the wrong patient. (p. 259)

When we notice that our evenly hovering, present-centered attention has been hijacked by strong feelings or rigid thinking, we might mentalize (to make sense of what has occurred) or we might attempt to return to the here and now just as we do in meditation—that is, through acknowledging what has occurred, then gently turning attention to our breathing, or any other sensory experience that allows us once again to locate our attention— our conscious awareness. Subjectively, this can feel like "waking up" from the trance of operating as if we were on automatic pilot. Psychoanalyst Marion Milner (1960/1987) suggests in this connection that therapists would often do well to maintain an inward focus on their own bodily experience.[1]

It may also be possible for us to reinhabit the present moment in psychotherapy by stopping (or slowing down) the action. Rather than being caught up in the effort to move the therapy or the patient from point A to point B, we can simply attend with heightened focus and curiosity to the details of what is actually occurring right here, right now. Stopping in order

to pay attention to the experience of the moment—dropping the attempt to "make something happen" or "facilitate change"—can allow us to *be*, rather than do (see Germer, 2005). It can also help us to locate our conscious awareness—that "still point" inside that may function as a secure base. Deliberately paying attention to just one thing at a time—a "core mindfulness skill" in dialectical behavior therapy—can have the same impact (Linehan, 1993). By shifting to a more mindful, present-centered stance, we often lead the patient to become either more present herself or more aware of her difficulty in doing so.

Finally, it may be possible to enter the present moment more fully by imagining while sitting with the patient that the two of us have just *50 minutes to live* (or however many remain in the session). This mental sleight-of-hand can often ground me in the here and now in a way that shifts my experience of the therapeutic encounter in a decidedly mindful direction. If I have been preoccupied or distant, overly emotional or overly intellectual, this thought experiment usually brings me back.

The Mindful Patient

What works to cultivate mindfulness in the therapist may also work for the patient: meditating (inside or outside the session), focusing on bodily experience, stopping the action, focusing on one thing at a time, or even imagining that there are now just minutes left to live. Implicitly, as I've mentioned, we can help to foster a mindful stance through the mindful quality of our own presence as we relate to the patient. Explicitly, we can encourage a mindful stance through a variety of "meditative moves" (Aronow, cited in Germer et al., 2005). Considering that mindfulness consists of three elements—*awareness* of *present experience* with *acceptance*—we can focus our interventions on one or more of these elements at any given moment.

First, there are interventions that draw the patient's attention to here-and-now experience: *What are you feeling or sensing in your body at this moment? What do you want for yourself right now? What are you hoping for from me right now? Or, I'm aware that you've got a smile on your face just now while you're talking about something that I'm guessing you don't find amusing at all.* Whether with a question or an observation, the aim here is to help the patient simply to become aware of whatever is occurring in the present moment.

Second, we can intervene with the aim of cultivating the patient's acceptance of present experience. Frequently, of course, our patients (like all of us, at times) are reluctant to fully feel what they feel. They stiffen up self-protectively to avoid pain, or they space out, or they cling to one emotion (say, anger) in order to stay away from another that is more threatening (say, shame). Quite often, they are unaware of this (entirely understand-

able) reluctance to accept their experience as it is. Making conscious this frequently unconscious resistance to experience is usually a precondition for "softening" it. Once it is recognized and acknowledged, we may suggest that the patient attempt to get to know the resistance, in order to grasp what it's made of: *What are you aware of feeling or sensing right now? Are you aware of what you might be* afraid *to feel?* Then it may well be useful to ask the patient if he'd be willing to try to "move toward" or "relax into" the experience he's been attempting to steer clear of. In this connection, Germer (2005) proposes a form of "motivational interviewing" aimed at establishing a context in which the patient's ability to accept his experience can be cultivated collaboratively:

> Is the patient willing to suspend feeling calmer—perhaps even initially feeling *worse*, while exploring his or her experience more intimately—to eventually feel better? Can the patient entertain the notion that an ingrained habit of tightening up to reduce discomfort is the root of his or her problem? Is the patient willing to explore whether the feelings pass more easily if allowed to be just as they are? (p. 114)

In much the same spirit, I've tried to communicate to patients my understanding of the paradox that resisting painful experience keeps it fixed in place, while embracing such experience allows it to change. Putting this understanding into words can give patients a useful framework for understanding the healing power of simply accepting their experience as it is.

In addition, we can attempt to help our patients grasp the distinction between the (internal or external) events they experience and their reactions to these events: *Have you noticed that it's only when you're feeling low that you think of your wife's working late as a rejection? Do you notice how differently you think about it when your mood is different?*

Finally, we can intervene in light of the insights to which mindfulness affords us experiential access, in particular, that our thoughts and feelings are fluid, ever-changing mental events rather than concrete unchanging "realities": *Can you stay with what you're feeling right now? What do you notice? Are you aware of any shifts in what you're feeling?* Subjective experience that is observed nonjudgmentally (no mean feat) will usually change: Distressing experience will typically become less distressing and pleasurable experience less pleasurable (Segal et al., 2002).

FOSTERING MENTALIZING

Much of our patients' suffering involves the failure to develop, or the derailing of, a mentalizing stance toward experience. Depression and un-

resolved trauma, as well as personality disorders in general, can all be understood as examples of *"the mind misperceiving and misrepresenting the status of its own contents and its own functions"* (Allen & Fonagy, 2002, p. 28). Depressed patients, for instance, experience their hopelessness and self-doubt not as interpretable mental states but simply as accurate reflections of reality. In contrast to this depressive equation of the internal and external worlds is their decoupling, as we see in patients with dissociative or narcissistic defenses. Swinging between these two nonmentalizing modes are patients with borderline personality disorder who appear terrified of looking into their own mind or the minds of others. To help all these patients, we need to be able to kindle or restore their capacity to mentalize.

Key here is our own mentalizing competence. When we can generate multiple perspectives on experience rather than being embedded in only one, when we can relate internal and external realities rather than equating or dissociating them, and when we can make sense of each other and ourselves in terms of underlying mental states, then we can help our patients begin to do the same.

Teaching "Mind Reading" through Reading the Patient's Mind

To read the patient's mind we must resonate with, reflect upon, and accurately mirror—with body or words—the patient's internal experience. In so doing, we allow the patient to see a reflection of her own mind in our mind. Our *implicit* mentalizing—that is, our largely nonverbal responsiveness to the patient's largely nonverbal cues—plays a crucial role in this intersubjective process. A mindful stance may well heighten this kind of automatic, intuitive responsiveness. Our *explicit* mentalizing recruits language to highlight or explain facets of implicit experience that seem puzzling, contradictory, and/or troubling. Such mentalizing "explicates the implicit" (Allen & Fonagy, 2002; Boston Change Process Study Group, 2002).

Yet too much explicit mind reading on the therapist's part can undermine the patient's developing ability to read her own mind and the minds of others. Fonagy cautions against an "expert stance" in which the therapist tells the patient what is going on ("I think you're feeling angry now.") He recommends instead an "inquisitive stance" of "not knowing" in which the therapist clarifies the patient's experience by asking questions, noting aspects of the here-and-now interaction, restating facts, and the like ("The way you're behaving now, it just strikes me that the only way this makes sense is that you're feeling angry. Could that be right?") Regarding interpretation he suggests that "what matters is not the destination but the journey": Rather than enlightening the patient with our insight, the primary aim of whatever interpreting we do should be to en-

courage the patient's own interpretive process (Fonagy, personal communication, 2006).

> For example, when Ellen repeatedly arrived late for her sessions, I found myself becoming increasingly annoyed. On one occasion, rather than take this annoyance (or for that matter, her lateness) entirely at face value, I was able to interpret it in a way that piqued her curiosity. Admitting that I could become irritated at her lateness—in spite of wishing not to—I wondered aloud whether it might feel safer for her to pick a fight and create distance, rather than feel close to me and risk my rejection, She looked thoughtful for a few moments, then said that today, walking in, she *had* wanted a fight, she wasn't sure why: "All I know is I *hate* being dependent on you. . . . Maybe if I get you angry, then I can be mad at you, and all that stuff about being taken care of would be just . . . gone." Later in the therapy, Ellen began to note her impulse to pick a fight. Apparently, it was often with some difficulty that she stopped herself from acting on the impulse, and instead acknowledged it to me, allowing the two of us to try and make sense of it together.

The Patient's Mentalizing and the Therapist's Interventions

Trying to intervene in ways that match our patients' needs often means expecting just a little more from them than they may presently believe they are capable of. Thus, at any given moment in the session, our efforts to engage (or reengage) their mentalizing potential will be enhanced to the degree that we can accurately assess their present mentalizing capability (which fluctuates) and the predominant mode of experience (psychic equivalence, pretend, or mentalizing) in which they seem currently to be lodged.

Gauging the patient's mentalizing capability on the fly is no easy matter. As discussed in Chapter 4, the Reflective-Functioning Scale developed by Fonagy et al. (1998) can be a help, as can Main's (1991) observation that metacognitive ability is evidenced in the awareness that appearance and reality can differ, that people can have differing views of the same reality, and that these views can change over time. Yet we often have only an impression, an intuitive sense, about the extent of the patient's ability to make use of our words when these go beyond what the patient is just now thinking or feeling. Will it be helpful or not to present an additional perspective on the patient's subjective experience? Because the answer to the question can shift, moment by moment, I frequently find myself rethinking my clinical judgments and adjusting the "depth" of my intervention virtually in midsentence.

Whether or not I have gotten it right is a matter to be determined empirically, in collaboration with the patient whose implicit or explicit re-

sponses are often quite telling. Or perhaps "collaboration" is not quite the word for the anger, heightened fear, or shutting down that we may evoke by overestimating what the patient is capable of hearing. Misattuned interpretations are regularly experienced as accusations or abandonment when the patient's capacity for reflection is momentarily, or routinely, more compromised than we have guessed. At the very least, our overreaching in this way is likely to leave the patient feeling inadequate.

As a rule, offering alternative perspectives or interpretations is most useful when the patient's metacognitive capacity is strong. When, by contrast, this capacity is inhibited or has yet to be kindled, other interventions are probably in order.

We can clarify the patient's subjective experience by helping, most importantly, to identify the feelings that underlie the patient's behavior and the context for these feelings. When such clarification is successful, it can diminish the distress and confusion that might otherwise provoke actions on the patient's part that are self-destructive. For the patient, this can be a powerful object lesson—a lived experience of the value of mentalizing. The impact of this sort of experience is likely to be still greater when the patient's difficult feelings arise in relationship to the therapist, with whose help they are clarified, understood, and assuaged.

Expressively empathizing with the patient's subjective experience can also be helpful, but only so long as our empathy is not confined to the patient's manifest feelings, but extends to emotions the patient may as yet be unable to feel or express. This caveat is especially significant when the feelings expressed (say, anger or hostility) cover other feelings (of dependence or vulnerability, say) whose expression seems more problematic, but is potentially more adaptive. Often our countertransference responses can help us to recognize the feelings from which the patient is protecting herself (Bateman & Fonagy, 2006).

At other times, our countertransference mainly reflects our trouble tolerating the patient's reluctance (or inability) to mentalize. When frustration with the patient's tightly held, one-dimensional perspective has generated an empathic impasse, it may be helpful to offer the patient a rounded account of our reaction to her difficulty in considering more than one view of her experience. Here I might say: "As we talk now I feel torn: On the one hand, I want you to know that I understand the importance of your perspective and the reality of the pain you're in. On the other hand, I also have an additional perspective, but I'm worried that if I try to convey it, you might feel that I'm not hearing you or that I'm not really with you. So I'm not sure how to proceed." With these words I'm modeling mentalizing as well as inviting the patient's collaboration. I'm suggesting the presence of alternative perspectives, even should these remain unspoken. In so doing, I often find that my ability to empathize with the patient is restored. Often

patients feel some relief as well, for they are now less alone and more capable of joining with me in what has become a shared dilemma. While patients may fear what the therapist has to say, they also know at some level that they very much *need* another perspective, because their own has been insufficient to undo their suffering.

Given that our primary aim here is to generate with the patient a reflective process rather than particular insights, it follows that we should address constraints on the patient's freedom to mentalize before attempting to make sense of any particular mental states. Such constraints are almost always undergirded by a sense of psychological necessity. It is usually important, therefore, that the therapist should investigate, silently or collaboratively, the emotional logic of the patient's apparently limited ability to mentalize (Seligman, 1999).

When we encounter a temporary freeze-up of the patient's reflective function, it is often helpful to consider what has recently occurred in our relationship with the patient. Looking back in this way, we may find that we have inadvertently provoked the patient's shame, touched on a vulnerable area, or stepped into an enactment of (ordinarily) dissociated experience. All these may be short-term disruptions, but they require immediate attention and repair to ensure that the limits on the patient's collaborative mentalizing will, in fact, be merely temporary.

Sometimes, of course, the capacity for mentalizing turns out to be limited in more abiding ways. Different patients may have trouble thinking and feeling in the same mental breath. Some are fearful of being overwhelmed, or of disintegrating, should they allow themselves to freely think and feel. Some have a psychological need to maintain dissociation and are threatened by the integration mentalizing tends to promote. Some patients are constrained by the prohibitions against knowing that often accompany trauma and violation. Other patients, to protect their tenuous sense of identity, must sustain the fantasy that there is but a single view of reality—and the therapist shares it (Seligman, 2000). Finally, there are patients like Ellen for whom embracing the option to think and feel for themselves means relinquishing their relentless hope and taking up the painful, if potentially liberating, tasks of mourning.

Beyond appraising the patient's reflective capacity—strong or weak, temporarily inhibited or chronically constrained—it can be very helpful to note the nature of the patient's "prereflective" stance toward experience. At any given moment, is the patient equating the mind and the world—or decoupling them? And in an ongoing way, does the patient tend to live in a subjective reality that is predominantly concrete and uninterpretable—or one in which wishes and thoughts mainly hold sway?

Patients in a psychic equivalence mode equate what they feel and believe with what is real and true. As therapists, our task with such patients is

akin to that of the parent who engages with the child while implicitly offering two views of the child's play: It is "real" and it is simultaneously "pretend." We need to support the patient's ability to preserve a sense of her own experience *and* we need to present alternative views that take the complexity of that experience into account.

Allowing the patient's view while maintaining our own can be particularly challenging when we are uncomfortable being seen in the way the patient sees us. And yet this is precisely what we must attempt to do. A patient with a history of disorganized attachment and/or trauma is usually incapable, at least initially, of seeing the therapist as a trustworthy other. If we are ever to be experienced as trustworthy, we must be able to accept the patient where she is, uncomfortable for us as this may be. By conceding the plausibility of the patient's singularly dark view while also keeping in mind—and sometimes communicating—alternative views, we help create a safer space within which the patient may begin to consider herself and others in more complex terms. Naturally, it doesn't hurt when conducting ourselves in this way serves to raise the patient's doubts about her worst expectations: "The contrast between the patient's perception of the therapist as she or he is imagined and as she or he is may help to place quotation marks around the transference experience" (Fonagy et al., 2002, p. 370).

Presenting complex interpretations does little to enhance the complexity of the patient's thinking. The patient's tendency to simply equate feelings and beliefs with facts is likelier to be dislodged by the therapist's consistent efforts to note, name, and explore the moment-by-moment shifts in the patient's emotional experience. It can be particularly helpful when we are able to identify in real time the internal or interpersonal circumstances that plunge the patient into states of overwhelming distress. Understanding these triggers can, in and of itself, provide a measure of relief. Over time, it can also further by degrees the patient's liberating awareness that her internal experience is not a direct reflection of reality but rather the idiosyncratic product of subjective responses to the realities she confronts.

In contrast to patients like these whose experience of reality tends to be oppressively "real," patients in the "pretend" mode are all too capable of setting oppressive realities aside. The former might be described as preoccupied or unresolved, and are often too overwhelmed by their experience to think about it. The latter could be called dismissing, and are often too cut off from their experience to have feelings about it—or else they are fearful of acknowledging their feelings. It is essential to recognize those patients who function in the pretend mode since they often give the impression that they are doing the work of therapy when they are not: They may appear to be "working," but are unlikely to be productive because their insights and their experience of the therapeutic relationship are ungrounded in emotional reality.

The first priority for the therapist here is to avoid colluding with the pretense that an emotionally absent patient is actually fully present. Instead we may need to note how hard it is for the patient to acknowledge the impact of unwelcome experience or, perhaps more broadly, to experience deep feelings at all. And, of course, we must follow the red thread of affect, drawing our patients' attention to signs of feeling that they may be reticent about or unaware of. Some patients find it exceptionally meaningful when we can illuminate their reflexive flight from feelings that they actually *have* become aware of. Our key interventions here—including, at times, explicitly disclosing aspects of our own emotional experience—are geared not only to make the patient's experience when with us more "real," but also to make bridges between facets of experience that the patient has needed to keep apart.

Whether embedded in the mode of psychic equivalence or of pretense, our patients are relating to their experience in a *dis*integrated way. According to Fonagy and his colleagues, it is by integrating these prereflective modes that the child learns to mentalize—to "play with reality" (Fonagy & Target, 1996) rather than feel overwhelmed by, or cut off from, it. We further such integration in psychotherapy through the kinds of interventions I've just described and through providing a secure relationship within which the patient can come to see herself in the mind—and feel herself in the heart—of the therapist as an integrated thinking, feeling, and desiring being.

MENTALIZING, MINDFULNESS, AND THE CONTRIBUTION OF THE THERAPIST

Our ability to intervene in these ways and to offer such a secure relationship depends to a significant degree on our own capacity for integration. And just as our patients have been influenced by what their attachment figures could and could not think, feel, and desire, it is the history of our own attachments in childhood and beyond that largely determines the range of subjective experience we are able to allow ourselves and others.

The new attachment relationship we experience in our personal psychotherapy or analysis frequently figures prominently in this history for clinicians—whose choice of vocation is often a product, in part, of the unconscious hope to heal early attachment wounds. And in the new attachment relationship we aim to provide for our patients, repeated experiences of disembedding through mindfulness as well as mentalizing can establish a competing center of organization in both the mind and brain. In this way, such experiences can potentially replace the patient's insecure working models with "earned secure" ones.

The patient's mentalizing is both a crucial skill in its own right and a means for "rewriting" the patient's autobiographical narrative—the story the patient uses to make sense of his or her life. As such, mentalizing facilitates the achievement of a self-authoring mind. Mindfulness is a similarly valuable skill. Rather than "retelling a life," however, mindfulness transforms the author.

Through fostering these skills, psychotherapy when it is effective yields a new experience of security that can benefit every patient. But in relation to patients who have (or will have) children, the contribution of the therapist may well go much further, for it has the potential to break the chain of disadvantage that tends to burden each successive generation with the insecurity and trauma of the generations that have come before.

NOTE

1. In Milner's (1960/1987) view, this meditative "concentration of the body" generates a context within which the experience of patient and therapist can be known in the most profound way. In describing the sort of attention that this "whole body awareness" requires, she writes:

> I noticed the astonishing changes in the quality of one's perceptions, both of oneself and the outside world, that the deliberate use of a wide rather than a narrow focus of attention brings. . . . [The] inner ground of being, as a real psycho-physical background to all one's conscious thoughts . . . can be directly experienced by a wide focus of attention directed inwards. . . . [This] kind of attention deliberately attends to sinking itself down into a total internal body awareness, not seeking at all for correct interpretations, in fact not looking for ideas at all—although interpretations may arise from this state spontaneously. (pp. 236–240)

References

Ainsworth, M. D. S. (1963). The development of infant–mother interaction among the Ganda. In B. M. Foss (Ed.), *Determinants of infant behavior* (Vol. 2, pp. 67–112). New York: Wiley.

Ainsworth, M. D. S. (1967). *Infancy in Uganda: Infant care and the growth of love.* Baltimore: Johns Hopkins University Press.

Ainsworth, M. D. S. (1969). Object relations, dependency and attachment: A theoretical review of the infant–mother relationship. *Child Development, 40,* 969–1025.

Ainsworth, M. D. S., & Eichberg, C. (1991). Effects on infant–mother attachment of mother's unresolved loss of an attachment figure, or other traumatic experience. In C. M. Parkes (Ed.), *Attachment across the life cycle* (pp. 160–185). New York: Routledge.

Ainsworth, M. D. S., Blehar, M. C., Waters, E., & Wall, S. (1978). *Patterns of attachment: A psychological study of the Strange Situation.* Hillsdale, NJ: Erlbaum.

Allen, J. P., & Fonagy, P. (2002). *The development of mentalizing and its role in psychopathology and psychotherapy* (Technical Report No. 02-0048). Topeka, KS: Menninger Clinic, Research Department.

Amini, F., Lewis, T., Lannon, R., Louie, A., Baumbacher, G., McGuiness, T., et al. (1996). Affect, attachment, memory: Contributions toward psychobiologic integration. *Psychiatry, 59,* 213–237.

Aron, L. (1991). The patient's experience of the analyst's subjectivity. *Psychoanalytic Dialogues, 1,* 29–51.

Aron, L. (1992). Interpretation as expression of the analyst's subjectivity. *Psychoanalytic Dialogues, 2,* 475–505.

Aron, L. (1996). *A meeting of minds: Mutuality in psychoanalysis.* Hillsdale, NJ: Analytic Press.

Aron, L. (1998). The clinical body and the reflexive mind. In L. Aron & F. S. Anderson (Eds.), *Relational perspectives on the body* (pp. 3–38). Hillsdale, NJ: Analytic Press.

Austin, J. H. (1999). *Zen and the brain:Toward an understanding of meditation and consciousness.* Cambridge, MA: MIT Press.

Baer, R. (2003). Mindfulness training as a clinical intervention: A conceptual and empirical review. *Clinical Psychology: Science and Practice, 10*(2), 125–142.

Baron-Cohen, S. (1999). Does the study of autism justify minimalist innate modularity? *Learning and Individual Differences, 10,* 179–191.

Basch, M. F. (1992). *Practicing psychotherapy: A casebook.* New York: Basic Books.

Bateman, A., & Fonagy, P. (2006). Mentalizing and borderline personality disorder. In J. G. Allen & P. Fonagy (Eds.), *Handbook of mentalization based treatment* (pp. 185–200). Hoboken, NJ: Wiley.

Bateson, G. (1979). *Mind and nature: A necessary unity.* New York: Ballantine Books.

Beebe, B. (2004). Symposium on intersubjectivity in infant research and its implications for adult treatment, Part II. *Psychoanalytic Dialogues, 14*(1), 1–52.

Beebe, B., Jaffe, J., Lachmann, F., Feldstein, S., Crown, C., & Jasnow, J. (2000). Systems models in development and psychoanalysis: The case of vocal rhythm coordination and attachment. *Infant Mental Health Journal, 20*(21), 99–122.

Beebe, B., Knoblauch, S., Rustin, J., & Sorter, D. (2003). Symposium on intersubjectivity in infant research and its implications for adult treatment, Part I. *Psychoanalytic Dialogues, 13*(6), 743–842.

Beebe, B., & Lachmann, F. (2002). *Infant research and adult treatment: Co-constructing interactions.* Hillsdale, NJ: Analytic Press.

Belsky, J., Fish, M., & Isabella, R. (1991). Continuity and discontinuity in infant negative and positive emotionality: Family antecedents and attachment consequences. *Developmental Psychology, 27,* 421–431.

Benjamin, J. (1999). Recognition and destruction: An outline of intersubjectivity. In S. Mitchell & L. Aron (Eds.), *Relational psychoanalysis: The emergence of a tradition.* Hillsdale, NJ: Analytic Press. (Original work published 1990)

Bion, W. R. (1959). Attacks on linking. *International Journal of Psycho-Analysis, 40,* 308–315.

Bion, W. R. (1962). *Learning from experience.* London: Heinemann.

Bion, W. R. (1965). *Transformations.* New York: Basic Books.

Bion, W. R. (1967). *Second thoughts.* Northvale, NJ: Jason Aronson.

Bion, W. R. (1970). *Attention and interpretation.* London: Karnac.

Bion, W. R. (1981). Notes on memory and desire. In R. Langs (Ed.), *Classics in psychoanalytic technique* (pp. 259–261). Northvale, NJ: Jason Aronson. (Original work published 1967)

Blackmore, S. (2004). *Consciousness: An introduction.* Oxford, UK: Oxford University Press.

Blatt, S. J., & Blass, R. B. (1996). Relatedness and self-definition: A dialectic model of personality development. In G. G. Noam & K. W. Fischer (Eds.), *Development and vulnerabilities in close relationships* (pp. 309–338). Hillsdale, NJ: Erlbaum.

Bobrow, J. (1997). Coming to life: The creative intercourse of psychoanalysis and Zen Buddhism. In C. Spezzano & G. Garguilo (Eds.), *Soul on the couch: Spirituality, religion and morality in contemporary psychoanalysis* (pp. 109–146). Hillsdale, NJ: Analytic Press.

Bollas, C. (1987). *The shadow of the object: Psychoanalysis of the unthought known.* New York: Columbia University Press.

Boston Change Process Study Group. (1998). Interventions that effect change in psychotherapy: A model based on infant research. *Infant Mental Health Journal, 19,* 277–353.

Boston Change Process Study Group. (2002). Explicating the implicit: The local level and the microprocess of change in the analytic situation. *International Journal of Psycho-Analysis, 83,* 1051–1062.

Boston Change Process Study Group. (2005). The "something more than interpretation" revisited: Sloppiness and co-creativity in the psychoanalytic encounter. *Journal of the American Psychoanalytic Association, 53*(3), 693–730.

Bowlby, J. (1944). Forty-four juvenile thieves: Their characters and home life. *International Journal of Psycho-Analysis, 25,* 19–52.

Bowlby, J. (1951). *Maternal care and mental health* (WHO Monograph Series No. 2). Geneva: World Health Organization.

Bowlby, J. (1982). *Attachment and loss: Vol. 1. Attachment.* London: Hogarth Press and the Institute of Psycho-Analysis. (Original work published 1969).

Bowlby, J. (1973). *Attachment and loss: Vol. 2. Separation: Anxiety and anger.* New York: Basic Books.

Bowlby, J. (1980). *Attachment and loss: Vol. 3. Loss, sadness and depression.* New York: Basic Books.

Bowlby, J. (1985). The role of childhood experience in cognitive disturbance. In M. J. Mahoney & A. Freeman (Eds.), *Cognition and psychotherapy* (pp. 181–200). New York: Plenum Press.

Bowlby, J. (1986). *John Bowlby discussing his life and work.* (Videotaped by Mary Main, Department of Psychology, University of Virginia at Charlottesville, VA).

Bowlby, J. (1988). *A secure base: Clinical applications of attachment theory.* London: Routledge.

Brach, T. (2003). *Radical acceptance: Embracing your life with the heart of a Buddha.* New York: Bantam/Dell.

Brennan, K. A., Clark, C. L., & Shaver, P. R. (1998). Self-report measurement of adult romantic attachment: An integrative overview. In J. A. Simpson & W. S. Rholes (Eds.), *Attachment theory and close relationships* (pp. 46–76). New York: Guilford Press.

Bretherton, I. (1985). Attachment theory: Retrospect and prospect. *Monographs of the Society for Research in Child Development, 50*(1–2), 3–35.

Bretherton, I. (1991) The roots and growing points of attachment theory. In C. M. Parkes (Ed.), *Attachment across the life cycle* (pp. 9–32). New York: Routledge.

Bretherton, I. (1995). The origins of attachment theory: John Bowlby and Mary Ainsworth. In S. Goldberg, R. Muir, & J. Kerr (Eds.), *Attachment theory: Social, developmental, and clinical perspectives* (pp. 45–84). Hillsdale, NJ: Analytic Press.

Bretherton, I., & Munholland, K. A. (1999). *Internal working models in attachment relationships: A construct revisited.* In J. Cassidy & P. R. Shaver, (Eds.), *Handbook of attachment: Theory, research, and clinical applications* (pp. 89–111). New York: Guilford Press.

Bromberg, P. M. (1998a). *Standing in the spaces: Essays on clinical process, trauma, and dissociation.* Hillsdale, NJ: Analytic Press.

Bromberg, P. M. (1998b). Staying the same while changing: Reflections on clinical judgment. *Psychoanalytic Dialogues, 8,* 225–236.

Bromberg, P. M. (2003). Something wicked this way comes: Trauma, dissociation, and conflict: The space where psychoanalysis, cognitive science, and neuroscience overlap. *Psychoanalytic Psychology, 20*(3), 558–574.

Brothers, L. (1997). *Friday's footprint: How society shapes the human mind.* New York: Oxford University Press.

Buber, M. (1970). *I and thou* (W. Kaufman, Trans.). New York: Charles Scribners Sons. (Original work published 1923)

Bucci, W. (2002). The referential process, consciousness, and the sense of self. *Psychoanalytic Inquiry, 22,* 766–793.

Bucci, W. (2003). Varieties of dissociative experiences: A multiple code account and a discussion of Bromberg's case of "William." *Psychoanalytic Psychology, 20*(3), 542–557.

Buck, R. (1994). The neuropsychology of communication: Spontaneous and symbolic aspects. *Journal of Pragmatics, 22,* 265–278.

Burke, W. (1992). Countertransference disclosure and the asymmetry/mutuality dilemma. *Psychoanalytic Dialogues, 2,* 241–271.

Carlson, V., Cicchetti, D., Barnett, D., & Braunwald, K. (1989). Disorganized/disoriented attachment relationships in maltreated infants. *Developmental Psychology, 25,* 525–531.

Cassidy, J. & Shaver, P. R. (Eds.). (1999). *Handbook of attachment: Theory, research, and clinical applications.* New York: Guilford Press.

Coates, S. W. (1998). Having a mind of one's own and holding the other in mind: Commentary on paper by Peter Fonagy and Mary Target. *Psychoanalytic Dialogues, 8,* 115–148.

Cooper, P. (1999). Buddhist meditation and countertransference: A case study. *American Journal of Psychoanalysis, 59*(1), 71–85.

Cozolino, L. J. (2002). *The neuroscience of psychotherapy: Building and rebuilding the human brain.* New York: Norton.

Craik, K. (1943). *The nature of explanation.* Cambridge, UK: Cambridge University Press.

Crowell, J. A., Treboux, D., & Waters, E. (2002). Stability of attachment representations: The transition to marriage. *Developmental Psychology, 38,* 467–479.

Damasio, A. R. (1994). *Descartes' error: Emotion, reason, and the human brain.* New York: Avon Books.

Damasio, A. R. (1999). *The feeling of what happens: Body and emotion in the making of consciousness.* New York: Harcourt.

Damasio, A. R. (2003). *Looking for Spinoza.* New York: Harcourt.

Darwin, C. (1998). *The expression of the emotions in man and animals* (3rd ed.). New York: Oxford University Press. (Original work published 1872)

Davidson, R. J., Kabat-Zinn, J., Schumacher, J., Rosenkranz, M., Muller, D., Santorelli, S. F., et al. (2003). Alterations in brain and immune function produced by mindfulness meditation. *Psychosomatic Medicine, 65*(4), 564–570.

Davies, J. M. (1998). Multiple perspectives on multiplicity. *Psychoanalytic Dialogues, 8*(2), 195–206.

Deikman, A. J. (1982). *The observing self.* Boston: Beacon Press.

Dennett, D. C. (1987). *The intentional stance.* Cambridge, MA: MIT Press.

Dimberg, U., Thunberg, M., & Elmehed, K. (2000). Unconscious facial reactions to emotional facial expressions. *The American Psychological Society, 11,* 86–89.

Dimen, M. (1998). Polyglot bodies: Thinking through the relational. In L. Aron & F. S. Anderson (Eds.), *Relational perspectives on the body* (pp. 65–96). Hillsdale, NJ: Analytic Press.

Dozier, M., & Kobak, R. (1992). Psychophysiology in attachment interviews: Converging evidence for deactivating strategies. *Child Development, 63,* 1473–1480.

Dozier, M., Chase Stoval, K., & Albus, K. E. (1999). Attachment and psychopathology in adulthood. In J. Cassidy & P. R. Shaver (Eds.), *Handbook of attachment: Theory, research, and clinical applications* (pp. 497–519). New York: Guilford Press.

Eagle, M. (1999, November 15). *Attachment research and theory and psychoanalysis.* Paper presented at the Psychoanalytic Association of New York.

Ehrenberg, D. (1992). *The intimate edge: Extending the reach of psychoanalytic interaction.* New York: Norton.

Eigen, M. (1993). Breathing and identity. In A. Phillips (Ed.), *The electrified tightrope* (pp. 43–48). Northvale, NJ: Jason Aronson. (Original work published 1977)

Eigen, M. (1999). The area of faith in Winnicott, Lacan, and Bion. In S. A. Mitchell & L. Aron (Eds.), *Relational psychoanalysis: The emergence of a tradition* (pp. 3–36). Hillsdale, NJ: Analytic Press. (Original work published 1981)

Ekman, P. (2003). *Emotions revealed: Recognizing faces and feelings to improve communication and emotional life.* New York: Times Books.

Ekman, P., Friesen, W., & Ancoli, S. (1980). Facial signs of emotional experience. *Journal of Personality and Social Psychology, 39,* 1125–1134.

Ekman, P., Levenson, R., & Friesen, W. (1983). Autonomic nervous system activity distinguishes among emotions. *Science, 221,* 1208–1210.

Ekman, P., Roper, G., & Hager, J. C. (1980). Deliberate facial movement. *Child Development, 51,* 886–891.

Elicker, J., Englund, M., & Sroufe, L. A. (1992). Predicting peer competence and peer relationships in childhood from early parent–child relationship. In R. Parke & G. Ladd (Eds.), *Family–peer relationships: Modes of linkage* (pp. 77–106). Hillsdale, NJ: Erlbaum.

Eliot, T. S. (1991a). Ash Wednesday. In *Collected poems, 1909–1962* (pp. 83–96). New York: Harcourt Brace. (Original work published 1930)

Eliot, T. S. (1991b). Four quartets. In *Collected poems, 1909–1962* (pp. 173–210). New York: Harcourt Brace. (Original work published 1943)

Engler, J. (2003). Being somebody and being nobody: A reexamination of the understanding of self in psychoanalysis and Buddhism. In J. D. Safran (Ed.), *Psychoanalysis and Buddhism: An unfolding dialogue* (pp. 35–100). Somerville, MA: Wisdom.

Epstein, M. (1995). *Thoughts without a thinker: Psychotherapy from a Buddhist perspective.* New York: Basic Books.

Epstein, M. (2001). *Going on being: Buddhism and the way of change.* London: Continuum.

Falkenstrom, F. (2003). A Buddhist contribution to the psychoanalytic psychology of self. *International Journal of Psychoanalysis, 84,* 1–18.

Fonagy, P. (1991). Thinking about thinking: Some clinical and theoretical considerations in the treatment of a borderline patient. *International Journal of Psychoanalysis, 72,* 639–656.

Fonagy, P. (2000). Attachment and borderline personality disorder. *Journal of the American Psychoanalytic Association, 48*(4), 1129–1147.

Fonagy, P. (2001). *Attachment theory and psychoanalysis.* New York: Other Press.

Fonagy, P., Gergeley, G., Jurist, E. J., & Target, M. l. (2002). *Affect regulation, mentalization, and the development of the self.* New York: Other Press.

Fonagy, P., Leigh, T., Steele, M., Steele, H., Kennedy, R., Mattoon, G., Target, M., & Gerber, A. (1996). The relation of attachment status, psychiatric classification, and response to psychotherapy. *Journal of Consulting and Clinical Psychology, 64,* 22–31.

Fonagy, P., Steele, H., & Steele, M. (1991a). Maternal representations of attachment during pregnancy predict the organization of infant–mother attachment at one year of age. *Child Development, 62,* 891–905.

Fonagy, P., Steele, M., Steele, H., Moran, G. S., & Higgitt, A. C. (1991b). The capacity for understanding mental states: The reflective self in parent and child and its significance for security of attachment. *Infant Mental Health Journal, 12,* 201–218.

Fonagy, P., Steele, M., Steele, H., Leigh, T., Kennedy, R., Mattoon, G., et al. (1995). Attachment, the reflective self, and borderline states: The predictive specificity of the Adult Attachment Interview and pathological emotional development. In S. Goldberg, R. Muir, & J. Kerr (Eds.), *Attachment theory: Social, developmental and clinical perspectives* (pp. 233–278). Hillsdale, NJ: Analytic Press.

Fonagy, P., & Target, M. (1996). Playing with reality: I. Theory of mind and the normal development of psychic reality. *International Journal of Psycho-Analysis, 77,* 217–233.

Fonagy, P., & Target, M. (2006). The mentalization focused approach to self pathology. *Journal of Personality Disorders, 20*(6), 544–576.

Fonagy, P., Target, M., Steele, H., & Steele, M. (1998). *Reflective-functioning manual, version 5.0, for application to adult attachment interviews.* London: University College London.

Forster, E. M. (1999). *Howards end.* New York: Modern Library Classics. (Original work published 1910)

Fosha, D. (2000). *The transforming power of affect: A model for accelerated change.* New York: Basic Books.

Fosha, D. (2003). Dyadic regulation and experiential work with emotion and relatedness in trauma and disorganized attachment. In M. F. Solomon & D. J. Siegel (Eds.), *Healing trauma: Attachment, mind, body, and brain* (pp. 221–281). New York: Norton.

Fox, N. A., & Card, J. A. (1999). Psychophysiological measures in the study of attachment. In J. Cassidy & P. R. Shaver (Eds.), *Handbook of attachment: Theory, research, and clinical applications* (pp. 226–245). New York: Guilford Press.

Freud, S. (1924a). Recommendations for physicians on the psycho-analytic method of treatment. In E. Jones (Ed.) & J. Riviere (Trans.), *Collected papers of Sigmund Freud* (Vol. 2, pp. 323–333). London: Hogarth Press and the Institute of Psychoanalysis. (Original work published 1912)

Freud, S. (1924b). Further recommendations in the technique of psychoanalysis: Recollection, repetition, and working-through. In E. Jones (Ed.) & J. Riviere (Trans.), *Collected papers of Sigmund Freud* (Vol. 2, pp. 366–376). London: Hogarth Press and the Institute of Psychoanalysis. (Original work published 1914)

Freud, S. (1958). Remembering, repeating, and working-through. In J. Strachey (Ed. & Trans.), *The Standard edition of the complete psychological works of Sigmund Freud* (Vol. 12, pp. 147–156). London: Hogarth Press and the Institute of Psychoanalysis. (Original work published 1914)

Freud, S. (1962). The ego and the id. In J. Strachey (Ed. & Trans.), *The standard edition of the complete psychological works of Sigmund Freud* (pp. 3–62). New York: W. W. Norton. (Original work published 1923)

Freud, S. (1966). Project for a scientific psychology. In J. Strachey (Ed. & Trans.), *The standard edition of the complete psychological works of Sigmund Freud* (Vol. 1, pp. 295–397). London: Hogarth Press. (Original work published 1895)

Friedman, L. (1988). *The anatomy of psychotherapy.* Hillsdale, NJ: Analytic Press.

Fulton, P. R. (2005). Mindfulness as clinical training. In C. K. Germer, R. D. Siegel, & P. R. Fulton (Eds.), *Mindfulness and psychotherapy* (pp. 55–72). New York: Guilford Press.

Gallese, V. (2001). "The shared manifold" hypothesis: From mirror neurons to empathy. *The Journal of Consciousness Studies, 8*(5–7), 33–50.

Gazzaniga, M. S., Eliassen, J. C., Nisenson, L., Wessuger, C. M., & Baynes, K. B. (1996). Collaboration between the hemispheres of a callosotomy patient—Emerging right hemisphere speech and the left brain interpreter. *Brain, 119,* 1255–1262.

George, C., Kaplan, N., & Main, M. (1984). *Adult Attachment Interview Protocol* (1st ed.). Unpublished manuscript, University of California at Berkeley.

George, C., Kaplan, N., & Main, M. (1985). *Adult Attachment Interview Protocol* (2nd ed.). Unpublished manuscript, University of California at Berkeley.

George, C., Kaplan, N., & Main, M. (1996). *Adult Attachment Interview Protocol* (3rd ed.). Unpublished manuscript, University of California at Berkeley.

Germer, C. K. (2005). Teaching mindfulness in therapy. In C. K. Germer, R. D. Siegel, & P.

R. Fulton (Eds.), *Mindfulness and psychotherapy* (pp. 113–129). New York: Guilford Press.

Germer, C. K., Siegel, R. D., & Fulton, P. R. (2005). *Mindfulness and psychotherapy.* New York: Guilford Press.

Gerson, S. (1996). Neutrality, resistance, and self-disclosure in an intersubjective psychoanalysis. *Psychoanalytic Dialogues, 6*(5), 623–647.

Ghent, E. (1999). Masochism, submission, surrender: Masochism as a perversion of surrender. In S. A. Mitchell & L. Aron (Eds.), *Relational psychoanalysis: The emergence of a tradition* (pp. 213–239). Hillsdale, NJ: Analytic Press. (Original work published 1990)

Gill, M. (1983). The interpersonal paradigm and the degree of the therapist's involvement. *Contemporary Psychoanalysis, 19*, 200–237.

Gill, M., & Hoffman, I. Z. (1982). *Analysis of transference* (Vol. II). New York: New York International Universities Press.

Ginot, E. (2001). The holding environment and intersubjectivity. *The Psychoanalytic Quarterly, 70*(2), 417–446.

Goldbart, S., & Wallin, D. (1996). *Mapping the terrain of the heart: Passion, tenderness, and the capacity to love.* Northvale, NJ: Jason Aronson.

Goldstein, J., & Kornfield, J. (1987). *Seeking the heart of wisdom: The path of insight meditation.* Boston: Shambhala.

Goleman, D. (1988). *The meditative mind: The varieties of meditative experience.* New York: Tarcher/Putnam Books.

Goleman, D. (1995). *Emotional intelligence.* New York: Bantam Books.

Goleman, D. (Ed.). (2003). *Destructive emotions: How can we overcome them: A scientific dialogue with the Dalai Lama.* New York: Bantam Books.

Gopnik, A., & Astington, J. W. (1988). Children's understanding of representational change and its relation to the understanding of false belief and the appearance-reality distinction. *Child Development, 59*, 26–37.

Gopnik, A., & Slaughter, V. (1991). Young children's understanding of changes in their mental states. *Child Development, 62*, 98–110.

Greenberg, J. (1995). Psychoanalytic technique and the interactive matrix. *Psychoanalytic Quarterly, 63*, 1–22.

Grossmann, K., & Grossmann, K. E. (1991). Newborn behavior, early parenting quality and later toddler–parent relationships in a group of German infants. In J. K. Nugent, B. M. Lester, & T. B. Brazelton (Eds.), *The cultural content of infancy* (Vol. 2, pp. 3–38). Norwood, NJ: Ablex.

Grossmann, K. E. (1995). The evolution and history of attachment research and theory. In S. Goldberg, R. Muir, & J. Kerr (Eds.), *Attachment theory: Social, developmental, and clinical perspectives* (pp. 85–121). Hillsdale, NJ: Analytic Press.

Grossmann, K. E., Grossmann, K., & Zimmermann, P. (1999). A wider view of attachment and exploration: Stability and change during the years of immaturity. In J. Cassidy & P. R. Shaver (Eds.), *Handbook of attachment:Theory, research, and clinical applications* (pp. 760–786). New York: Guilford Press.

Hariri, A. R., Bookheimer, S. Y., & Mazziotta, J. C. (2000). Modulating emotional responses: Effects of a neocortical network on the limbic system. *Neuroreport, 11*, 43–48.

Hariri, A. R., Mattay, V. S., Tessitore, A., Fera, F., & Weinberger, D. R. (2003). Neocortical modulation of the amygdala response to fearful stimuli. *Biological Psychiatry, 53*, 494–501.

Haviland, J. M., & Lelwica, M. (1987). The induced affect response: 10-week-old infants' responses to three emotion expressions. *Developmental Psychology, 23*(1), 97–104.

Hawkins, J. (2005). *On intelligence: How a new understanding of the brain will lead to the creation of truly intelligent machines.* New York: Owl Books/Holt.

Hesse, E. (1996). Discourse, memory and the adult attachment interview: A note with emphasis on the emerging Cannot Classify category. *Infant Mental Health Journal, 17,* 4–11.

Hesse, E. (1999). The adult attachment interview: Historical and current perspectives. In J. Cassidy & P. R. Shaver (Eds.), *Handbook of attachment: Theory, research, and clinical applications* (pp. 395–433). New York: Guilford Press.

Hesse, E., & Main, M. (2000). Disorganized infant, child, and adult attachment: Collapse in behavioral and attentional strategies. In *Journal of the American Psychoanalytic Association, 48*(4), 1097–1148.

Hobson, P. (2002). *The cradle of thought: Exploring the origins of thinking.* Oxford, UK: Oxford University Press.

Hoffman, I. (1983). The patient as interpreter of the analyst's experience. *Contemporary Psychoanalysis, 19,* 389–422.

Hoffman, I. (1992). Expressive participation and psychoanalytic discipline. *Contemporary Psychoanalysis, 28,* 1–15.

Hoffman, I. (1994). Dialectical thinking and therapeutic action in the psychoanalytic process. *Psychoanalytic Quarterly, 63,* 187–218.

Hoffman, I. (1996). The intimate and ironic authority of the psychoanalyst's presence. *Psychoanalytic Quarterly, 65,* 102–136.

Hoffman, I. (2001). *Ritual and spontaneity in the psychoanalytic process: A dialectical–constructivist view.* Hillsdale, NJ: Analytic Press.

Holmes, J. (1996). *Attachment, intimacy, autonomy.* Northvale, NJ: Jason Aronson.

Holmes, J. (2001). *The search for the secure base: Attachment theory and psychotherapy.* New York: Brunner-Routledge.

Hopenwasser, K. (1998). Listening to the body: Somatic representations of dissociated memory. In L. Aron & F. S. Anderson (Eds.), *Relational perspectives on the body* (pp. 215–236). Hillsdale, NJ: Analytic Press.

Iacoboni, M. (2005). Understanding others: Imitation, language, empathy. In S. Hurley & N. Chater (Eds.), *Perspectives on imitation: From neuroscience to social science: Vol I. Mechanisms of imitation and imitation in animals* (pp. 77–100). Cambridge, MA: MIT Press.

Jaffe, J., Beebe, B., Feldstein, S., Crown, C., & Jasnow, M. (2001). Rhythms of dialogue in early infancy. *Monographs of the Society for Research in Child Development, 66*(2, Serial No. 264), pp. 1–132.

James, W. (1884). What is an emotion? *Mind, 9,* 188–205.

James, W. (1950). *The principles of psychology.* Mineola, NY: Dover Publications. (Original work published 1890)

Kabat-Zinn, J. (1990). *Full catastrophe living: Using the wisdom of your body and mind to face stress, pain, and illness.* New York: Dell.

Kabat-Zinn, J. (2005). *Coming to our senses: Healing ourselves and the world through mindfulness.* New York: Hyperion.

Kahn, M. (1963). The concept of cumulative trauma. *The Psychoanalytic Study of the Child, 18,* 286–306.

Kaplan, N. (1987, May). *Internal representations of attachment in six-year-olds.* Paper presented at the biennial meetings of the Society for Research in Child Development, Baltimore.

Karen, R. (1994). *Becoming attached: First relationships and how they shape our capacity to love.* New York: Oxford University Press.

Karmiloff-Smith, A. (1992). *Beyond modularity: A developmental perspective on cognitive science.* Cambridge, MA: MIT Press.

Kegan, R. (2000). What "form" transforms? A constructive-developmental approach to transformative learning. In J. Mezirow (Ed.), *Learning as transformation: Critical perspectives on a theory in progress* (pp. 35–69). San Francisco: Jossey-Bass.

Kernberg, O. F. (1984). *Object relations theory and clinical psychoanalysis.* Northvale, NJ: Jason Aronson.

Kernberg, O. F. (1995). *Love relations: Normality and Pathology.* New Haven: Yale University Press.

Koback, R. (1999). The emotional dynamics of disruptions in attachment relationships: Implications for theory, research, and clinical intervention. In J. Cassidy & P. R. Shaver (Eds.), *Handbook of attachment: Theory, research, and clinical applications* (pp. 21–43). New York: Guilford Press.

Kornfield, J. (1993). *A path with heart.* New York: Bantam Books.

Kramer, S., & Akhtar, S. (Eds.). (1991). *The trauma of transgression: Psychotherapy of incest victims.* Northvale, NJ: Jason Aronson.

Krystal, H. (1988). *Integration and self-healing.* Hillsdale, NJ: Analytic Press.

Kurtz, Ron. (1990). *Body-centered psychotherapy: The Hakomi method.* Mendocino, CA: LifeRhythm.

Lakoff, G., & Johnson, M. (1999). *Philosophy in the flesh: The embodied mind and its challenge to western thought.* New York: HarperCollins.

Lazar, S. W. (2005). Mindfulness research. In C. K. Germer, R. D. Siegel, & P. R. Fulton (Eds.), *Mindfulness and psychotherapy* (pp. 220–239). New York: Guilford Press.

Lazar, S. W., Kerr, C. E., Wasserman, R. H., Gray, J. R., Greve, D. N., Treadway, M. T., et al. (2005). Meditation experience is associated with increased cortical thickness. *NeuroReport, 16*(17), 1893–1897.

Le Doux, J. (1996). *The emotional brain: The mysterious underpinnings of emotional life.* New York: Simon & Schuster.

Libet, B., Freeman, A., & Sutherland, K. (1999). *The volitional brain: Towards a neuroscience of free will.* Exeter, UK: Imprint Academic.

Lieberman, M. D. (in press). Social cognitive neuroscience: A review of core processes. *Annual Review of Psychology, 58.*

Linehan, M. (1993). *Cognitive-behavioral treatment of borderline personality disorder.* New York: Guilford Press.

Liotti, G. (1995). Disorganized/disoriented attachment in the psychotherapy of the dissociative disorders. In S. Goldberg, R. Muir, & J. Kerr (Eds.), *Attachment theory: Social, developmental and clinical perspectives* (pp. 343–367). Hillsdale, NJ: Analytic Press.

Liotti, G. (1999). Disorganization of attachment as a model for understanding dissociative psychopathology. In J. Solomon & C. George (Eds.), *Attachment disorganization* (pp. 291–317). New York: Guilford Press.

Looker, T. (1998). "Mama, why don't your feet touch the ground?": Staying with the body and the healing moment in psychoanalysis. In L. Aron & F. S. Anderson (Eds.), *Relational perspectives on the body* (pp. 237–262). Hillsdale, NJ: Analytic Press.

Lyons-Ruth, K. (1999). The two-person unconscious: Intersubjective dialogue, enactive relational representation, and the emergence of new forms of relational organization. *Psychoanalytic Inquiry, 19,* 576–617.

Lyons-Ruth, K., & Boston Change Process Study Group. (2001.) The emergence of new experiences: Relational improvisation, recognition process, and non-linear change in psychoanalytic psychotherapy. *Psychologist/Psychoanalyst, 21*(4), 13–17.

Lyons-Ruth, K. (1998). Implicit relational knowing: Its role in development and psycho-analytic treatment. *Infant Mental Health Journal, 19*(3), 282–289.

MacLean, P. (1990). *The triune brain in evolution.* New York: Plenum Press.

Mahler, M. S., Pine, F., & Bergman, A. (1975). *The psychological birth of the human infant: Symbiosis and individuation.* New York: Basic Books.

Main, M. (1981). Avoidance in the service of attachment: A working paper. In K. Immelman, G. Barlow, L. Petrinovitch, & M. Main (Eds.), *Behavioral development* (pp. 651–693). New York: Cambridge University Press.

Main, M. (1990). Cross-cultural studies of attachment organization: Recent studies, changing methodologies and the concept of conditioned strategies. *Human Development, 33,* 48–61.

Main, M. (1991). Metacognitive knowledge, metacognitive monitoring, and singular (coherent) vs. multiple (incoherent) model of attachment: Findings and directions for future research. In C. M. Parkes, J. Stevenson-Hinde, & P. Marris (Eds.), *Attachment across the life cycle* (pp. 127–159). London: Tavistock/Routledge.

Main, M. (1995). Attachment: Overview, with implications for clinical work. In S. Goldberg, R. Muir, & J. Kerr (Eds.), *Attachment theory: Social, developmental and clinical perspectives* (pp. 407–474). Hillsdale, NJ: Analytic Press.

Main, M. (1999). Epilogue. Attachment theory: Eighteen points with suggestions for future studies. In J. Cassidy & P. R. Shaver (Eds.), *Handbook of attachment: Theory, research, and clinical applications* (pp. 407–474). New York: Guilford Press.

Main, M. (2000). The organized categories of infant, child, and adult attachment: Flexible vs. inflexible attention under attachment-related stress. *Journal of the American Psychoanalytic Association, 48*(4), 1055–1096.

Main, M., & Goldwyn, R. (1994). *Adult attachment scoring and classification system.* Unpublished manuscript, University of California at Berkeley.

Main, M., Hesse, E., & Kaplan, N. (2005). Predictability of attachment behavior and representational processes. In K. E. Grossmann, K. Grossmann, & E. Waters (Eds.), *Attachment from infancy to adulthood: Lessons from longitudinal studies* (pp. 245–304). New York: Guilford Press.

Main, M., Kaplan, N., & Cassidy, J. (1985). Security in infancy, childhood, and adulthood: A move to the level of representation. *Monographs of the Society for Research in Child Development, 50*(1–2), 66–104.

Main, M., & Solomon, J. (1990). Procedures for identifying infants as disorganized/disoriented during the Ainsworth Strange Situation. In M. Greenberg, D. Cicchetti, & E. M. Cummings (Eds.), *Attachment during the preschool years: Theory, research and intervention* (pp. 121–160). Chicago: University of Chicago Press.

Main, M., & Weston, D. R. (1982). Avoidance of the attachment figure in infancy. In M. Parkes & J. Stevenson-Hinde (Eds.), *The place of attachment in human behavior* (pp. 31–59). New York: Basic Books.

Mandal, M. K., & Ambady, N. (2004). Laterality of facial expressions of emotion: Universal and culture-specific influences. *Behavioural Neurology, 15,* 23–34.

Maroda, K. (1999). *Seduction, surrender, and transformation.* Hillsdale, NJ: Analytic Press.

Martin, J. (1997). Mindfulness: A proposed common factor. *Journal of Psychotherapy Integration, 7*(4), 291–312.

Marvin, R. S., & Britner, P. A. (1999). Normative development: The ontogeny of attachment. In J. Cassidy & P. R. Shaver (Eds.), *Handbook of attachment: Theory, research, and clinical applications* (pp. 44–67). New York: Guilford Press.

Marvin, R., Cooper, G., Hoffman, K., & Powell, B. (2002). The Circle of Security project:

Attachment-based intervention with caregiver–pre-school child dyads. *Attachment and Human Development, 4*(1), 107–124.

McDougall, J. (1978). *Plea for a measure of abnormality.* New York: International Universities Press.

McDougall, J. (1989). *Theaters of the body.* New York: Norton.

Meltzoff, A. (1985). The roots of social and cognitive development: Models of man's original nature. In T. Field & N. Fox (Eds.), *Social perception in infants* (pp. 1–30). Norwood, NJ: Ablex.

Meltzoff, A. (1990). Foundations for developing a concept of self: The role of imitation in relating to others, and the value of social mirroring, social modeling, and self-practice in infancy. In D. Cicchetti & M. Beeghly (Eds.), *The self in transition: Infancy to childhood* (pp. 139–164). Chicago: University of Chicago Press.

Meltzoff, A., & Moore, M. (1998). Infant intersubjectivity: Broadening the dialogue to include imitation, identity and intention. In S. Braten (Ed.), *Intersubjective communication and emotion in early ontogeny* (pp. 47–88). Cambridge, UK: Cambridge University Press.

Merriam-Webster dictionary. (11th ed.). (2003). New York: Merriam-Webster.

Mikulincer, M., & Shaver, P. R. (2003). The attachment behavioral system in adulthood: Activation, psychodynamics, and interpersonal processes. In M. P. Zanna (Ed.), *Advances in experimental social psychology* (Vol. 35, pp. 53–152). New York: Academic Press.

Milner, M. (1987). The concentration of the body. In *The suppressed madness of sane men: Forty-four years of exploring psychoanalysis* (pp. 234–240). London: Tavistock and the Institute of Psychoanalysis. (Original work published 1960)

Mitchell, S. (1993). *Hope and dread in psychoanalysis.* New York: Basic Books.

Mitchell, S. (1995). Interaction in the interpersonal and Kleinian traditions. *Contemporary Psychoanalysis, 31,* 65–91.

Mitchell, S. (1997). *Influence and autonomy in psychoanalysis.* Hillsdale, NJ: Analytic Press.

Mitchell, S. (2000). *Relationality: From attachment to intersubjectivity.* Hillsdale, NJ: Analytic Press.

Morgan, W. D., Morgan, S. T. (2005). Cultivating attention and empathy. In C. K. Germer, R. D. Siegel, & P. R. Fulton (Eds.), *Mindfulness and psychotherapy* (pp. 73–90). New York: Guilford Press.

Nathanson, D. (1992). *Shame and pride: Affect, sex, and the birth of the self.* New York: Norton.

Natterson, J., & Friedman, R. (1995). *A primer of intersubjectivity.* Northvale, NJ: Jason Aronson.

Nyanaponika, T. (1972). *The power of mindfulness.* San Francisco: Unity Press.

Ochsner, K. N., & Gross, J. J. (2005). The cognitive control of emotion. *Trends in Cognitive Science, 9,* 242–249.

Ogden, P. (2006, March 5). *The role of the body in the treatment of trauma.* Paper presented at The Embodied Mind: Integration of the Body, Brain, and Mind in Clinical Practice conference, UCLA Extension and Lifespan Learning Institute, Los Angeles, CA.

Ogden, P., & Minton, K. (2000, October). Sensorimotor psychotherapy: One method for processing traumatic memory. *Traumatology, 6*(3).

Ogden, P., Pain, C., Minton, K., & Fisher, J. (2005). Including the body in mainstream psychotherapy for traumatized individuals. *Psychologist/Psychoanalyst, 25*(4), 19–24.

Ogden, T. (1994). *Subjects of analysis.* Northvale, NJ: Jason Aronson.

Ornstein, R. (1997). *The right mind: Making sense of the hemispheres.* New York: Harvest Books.

Patrick, M., Hobson, R. P., Castle, D., Howard, R., & Maughan, B. (1994). Personality disorder and the mental representation of early social experience. *Development and Psychopathology, 6,* 375–388.

Person, E. (1988). *Dreams of love and fateful encounters: The power of romantic passion.* New York: Norton.

Polan, H. J., & Hofer, M. A. (1999). Psychobiological origins of infant attachment and separation responses. In J. Cassidy & P. R. Shaver (Eds.), *Handbook of attachment: Theory, research, and clinical applications* (pp. 162–180). New York: Guilford Press.

Porges, S. W. (2006). The role of social engagement in attachment and bonding: A phylogenetic perspective. In C. S. Carter (Ed.), *Attachment and bonding: A new synthesis.* (pp. 33–55). Cambridge, MA: MIT Press.

Putnam, F. W. (1992). Discussion: Are alter personalities fragments or figments? *Psychoanalytic Inquiry, 12,* 95–111.

Racker, H. (1968). *Transference and countertransference.* New York: International Universities Press.

Rauch, S. L., Whalen, P. J., Shin, L. M., McInerney, S. C., Macklin, M. L., Lasko, N. B., et al. (2000). Exaggerated amygdala response to masked facial stimuli in posttraumatic stress disorder: A functional MRI study. *Biological Psychiatry, 47,* 769–776.

Renik, O. (1993). Countertransference enactment and the psychoanalytic process. In M. Horowitz, O. Kernberg, & E. Weinshel (Eds.), *Psychic structure and psychic change* (pp. 135–158). Madison, CT: International Universities Press.

Renik, O. (1995). The ideal of the anonymous analyst and the problem of self-disclosure. *Psychoanalytic Quarterly, 64,* 466–495.

Renik, O. (1996). The perils of neutrality. *Psychoanalytic Quarterly, 65,* 495–517.

Renik, O. (1999a). Analytic interaction: Conceptualizing technique in the light of the analyst's irreducible subjectivity. In S. Mitchell & L. Aron (Eds.), *Relational psychoanalysis: The emergence of a tradition* (pp. 408–422). Hillsdale, NJ: Analytic Press. (Original work published 1993)

Renik, O. (1999b). Playing one's cards face up in analysis. *Psychoanalytic Quarterly, 68,* 521–539.

Ringstrom, P. A. (2001). Cultivating the improvisational in psychoanalytic treatment. *Psychoanalytic Dialogues, 1*(5), 727–754.

Robertson, J., & Robertson, J. (1971). *Thomas, aged 2 years 4 months, in foster care for 10 days* [Film]. Young Children in Brief Separation Film Series. (Available from Penn State Audiovisual Services, University Park, PA)

Rothschild, B. (2000). *The body remembers.* New York: Norton.

Rubin, J. (1996). *Psychotherapy and Buddhism: Towards an integration.* New York: Plenum Press.

Safran, J. D. (Ed.). (2003). *Psychoanalysis and Buddhism: An unfolding dialogue.* Somerville, MA: Wisdom.

Safran, J. D., & Muran, J. C. (2000). *Negotiating the therapeutic alliance: A relational treatment guide.* New York: Guilford Press.

Sander, L. W. (1980). Investigation of the infant and its caregiving environment as a biological system. In S. Greenspan & G. Pollack (Eds.), *The course of life: Volume I. Infancy and early childhood* (pp. 177–201). Adelphi, MD: National Institute of Mental Health.

Sander, L. W. (2002). Thinking differently: Principles of process in living systems and the specificity of being known. *Psychoanalytic Dialogues, 12*(1), 11–42.

Sandler, J. (1981). Countertransference and role-responsiveness. In R. Langs (Ed.), *Classics in psychoanalytic technique* (pp. 273–278). New York: Jason Aronson. (Original work published 1976)

Sapolsky, R. (2004). *Why zebras don't get ulcers.* New York: Holt/Owl Books.

Scaer, R. S. (2001). *The body bears the burden: Trauma, dissociation and disease.* New York: Haworth Medical Press.

Schafer, R. (1983). *The analytic attitude.* New York: Basic Books.

Schafer, R. (1992). *Retelling a life: Narration and dialogue in psychoanalysis.* New York: Basic Books.

Schachner, D. A., Shauer, P. R., & Mikulincer, M. (2005). Patterns of nonverbal behavior and sensitivity in attachment relations. *Journal of Nonverbal Behavior, 29*(3), 141–169.

Schore, A. N. (1994). *Affect regulation and the origin of the self: The neurobiology of emotional development.* Hillsdale, NJ: Erlbaum.

Schore, A. (2002). Advances in neuropsychoanalysis, attachment theory, and trauma research: Implications for self psychology. *Psychoanalytic Inquiry, 22,* 433–484.

Schore, A. N. (2003). *Affect regulation and the repair of the self.* New York: Norton.

Schore, A. N. (2004, March 27). *Advances in regulation theory: The role of attachment and right brain development in the etiology and treatment of borderline personality disorder.* Paper presented at the Traumatic Attachments and Borderline Personality Disorders: Implications for Clinical Treatment conference, UCLA Extension and Lifespan Learning Institute, Los Angeles, CA.

Schore, A. N. (2005, March 12). *Changes in the mind, the brain, and the body in various psychotherapeutic contexts.* Paper presented at How Psychodynamic Psychotherapies Change the Mind and the Brain conference, UCLA Extension and Lifespan Learning Institute, Los Angeles, CA.

Schore, A. N. (2006, March 5). *Attachment trauma and the developing right brain: Origins of pathological dissociation.* Presented at The Embodied Mind: Integration of the Body, Brain, and Mind in Clinical Practice conference, UCLA Extension and Lifespan Learning Institute, Los Angeles, CA.

Segal, Z. V., Williams, J. M. G., & Teasdale, J. D. (2002). *Mindfulness-based cognitive therapy for depression: A new approach to preventing relapse.* New York: Guilford Press.

Seligman, S. (1999). Integrating Kleinian theory and intersubjective infant research: Observing projective identification. *Psychoanalytic Dialogues: A Journal of Relational Perspectives, 9*(2), 129–159.

Seligman, S. (2000). Clinical implications of attachment theory. *Journal of the American Psychoanalytic Association, 48*(4), 1189–1196.

Seligman, S. (2003). The developmental perspective in relational psychoanalysis. *Contemporary Psychoanalysis (in memoriam, Stephen A. Mitchell, Ph.D.), 39*(3), 477–508.

Shapiro, F., & Maxfield, L. (2003). EMDR and information processing in psychotherapy treatment: Personal development and global implications. In M. F. Solomon & D. J. Siegel (Eds.), *Healing trauma: Attachment, mind, body, and brain* (pp. 196–220). New York: Norton.

Shin, L. M., Orr, S. P., Carson, M. A., Rauch, S. L., Macklin, M. L., Lasko, N. B., et al. (2004). Regional cerebral blood flow in the amygdala and medial prefrontal cortex during traumatic imagery in male and female Vietnam veterans with PTSD. *Archives of General Psychiatry, 61,* 168–176.

Siegel, D. J. (1999). *The developing mind: How relationships and the brain interact to shape who we are.* New York: Guilford Press.

Siegel, D.J. (2001). Toward an interpersonal neurobiology of the developing mind: Attachment relationships, "mindsight," and neural integration. *Infant Mental Health Journal, 22,* 67–94.

Siegel, D. J. (2004, November 6). *Understanding emotion and empathy in relationships:*

Connection and empathy: Ground-breaking discoveries. Paper presented at R. Cassidy Seminars, San Francisco, CA.

Siegel, D. J. (2005, June 3). *The mindful brain.* Paper presented at the Emotion Meets Spirit conference, Deep Streams Institute, Watsonville, CA.

Siegel, D. J. (2006, March 4). *Awakening the mind to the wisdom of the body.* Paper presented at The Embodied Mind: Integration of the Body, Brain, and Mind in Clinical Practice conference, UCLA Extension and Lifespan Learning Institute, Los Angeles, CA.

Siegel, D. J. (2006). An interpersonal neurobiology approach to psychotherapy: How awareness, mirror neurons, and neural plasticity contribute to the development of well-being. *Psychiatric Annals, 36*(4), 248–258.

Siegel, D. J., Siegel, A. W., & Amiel, J. B. (2006). Mind, brain, and behavior. In D. Wedding & M. L. Stuber (Eds.), *Behavior and medicine* (4th ed., pp. 3–22). Cambridge, MA: Hogrefe & Huber.

Siegel, R. D. (2005). Psychophysiological disorders: Embracing pain. In C. K. Germer, R. D. Siegel, & P. R. Fulton (Eds.), *Mindfulness and psychotherapy* (pp. 173–196). New York: Guilford Press.

Slade, A. (1999). Attachment theory and research: Implications for the theory and practice of individual psychotherapy with adults. In J. Cassidy & P. R. Shaver (Eds.), *Handbook of attachment: Theory, research, and clinical applications* (pp. 575–594). New York: Guilford Press.

Slade, A. (2000). The development and organization of attachment: Implications for psychoanalysis. *Journal of the American Psychoanalytic Association, 48*(4), 1147–1174.

Slavin, M. O., & Kriegman, D. (1998). Why the analyst needs to change: Toward a theory of conflict, negotiation, and mutual influence in the therapeutic process. *Psychoanalytic Dialogues, 8,* 247–284.

Smith, H. F. (1993). Engagements in analysis and their use in self-analysis. In J. W. Barron (Ed.), *Self-Analysis* (pp. 88–109). Hillsdale, NJ: Analytic Press.

Solomon, J., & George, C. (1999). *Attachment disorganization.* New York: Guilford Press.

Solomon, M. F., & Siegel, D. J. (2003). *Healing trauma: Attachment, mind, body, and brain.* New York: Norton.

Spangler, G., & Grossmann, K. E. (1993). Biobehavioral organization in securely and insecurely attached infants. *Child Development, 64,* 1439–1450.

Spezzano, C. (1995). "Classical" versus "contemporary" theory: The differences that matter clinically. *Contemporary Psychoanalysis, 31,* 20–46.

Spezzano, C. (1998). Listening and interpreting: What analysts do to kill time between disclosures and enactments. *Psychoanalytic Dialogues, 8,* 237–246.

Sroufe, L. A. (1983). Infant–caregiver attachment and patterns of adaptation in preschool: The roots of maladaptation and competence. In M. Perlmutter (Ed.), *Minnesota Symposium in Child Psychology* (Vol. 16, pp. 41–83). Hillsdale, NJ: Erlbaum.

Sroufe, L. A. (1996). *Emotional development: The organization of emotional life in the early years.* Cambridge, UK: Cambridge University Press.

Sroufe, L. A., & Waters, E. (1977a). Attachment as an organizational construct. *Child Development, 48,* 1184–1199.

Sroufe, L. A., & Waters, E. (1977b). Heart rate as a convergent measure in clinical and developmental research. *Merrill-Palmer Quarterly, 23,* 3–28.

Stark, M. (2000). *Modes of therapeutic action.* Northvale, NJ: Jason Aronson.

Stern, D. N. (1985). *The interpersonal world of the infant: A view from psychoanalysis and developmental psychology.* New York: Basic Books.

Stern, D. N. (2002, March 11). *The change process in psychoanalysis.* Presented at the San Francisco Psychoanalytic Institute, San Francisco.

Stern, D. N. (2004). *The present moment in psychotherapy and everyday life*. New York: Norton.

Stern, D. N., Sander, L. W., Nahum, J. P., Harrison, A. M., Lyons-Ruth, K., Morgan, A. C., et al. (1998). Non-interpretive mechanisms in psychoanalytic psychotherapy: The "something more" than interpretation. *International Journal of Psychoanalysis, 79*, 903–921.

Stern, S. (1994). Needed relationships and repeated relationships: An integrated relational perspective. *Psychoanalytic Dialogues, 4*, 317–346.

Stern, S. (2002). The self as a relational structure: A dialogue with multiple-self theory. *Psychoanalytic Dialogue, 12*, 693–714.

Stevens, W. (1990). Not ideas about the thing but the thing itself. In *The collected poems of Wallace Stevens* (p. 534). New York: Vintage. (Original work published 1954)

Stolorow, R., & Atwood, G. (1997). Deconstructing the myth of the neutral analyst: An alternative from intersubjective systems theory. *Psychoanalytic Quarterly, 66*, 431–449.

Stolorow, R., Brandschaft, B., & Atwood, G. (1987). *Psychoanalytic treatment: An intersubjective perspective*. Northvale NJ: Jason Aronson.

Sullivan, H. S. (1953). *The interpersonal theory of psychiatry*. New York: Norton.

Sullivan, H. S. (1964). *The illusion of personal identity: The fusion of psychiatry and social science*. New York: Norton.

Suzuki, S. (1970). *Zen mind, beginner's mind*. New York: Weatherhill.

Teilhard de Chardin, P. (1959). *The Phenomenon of man*. New York: Harper and Row.

Trevarthen, C. (1979). Communication and cooperation in early infancy: A description of primary intersubjectivity. In M. Bullowa (Ed.), *Before speech: The beginnings of human communication* (pp. 321–347). London: Cambridge University Press.

Trevarthen, C. (1998). The concept and foundations of infant intersubjectivity. In S. Braten (Ed.), *Intersubjective communication and emotion in early ontogeny* (pp. 15–46). Cambridge, UK: Cambridge University Press.

Tronick, E. (1989). Emotions and emotional communication in infants. *American Psychologist, 44*, 112–119.

Tronick, E. (1998). Dyadically expanded states of consciousness and the process of therapeutic change. *Infant Mental Health Journal, 19*(3), 290–299.

van der Kolk, B. A. (1996). The body keeps the score: Approaches to the psychobiology of post-traumatic stress disorder. In B. A. van der Kolk, A. C. McFarlane, & L. Weisaeth (Eds.), *Traumatic stress: The effects of overwhelming experience on mind, body, and society* (pp. 214–241). New York: Guilford Press.

van der Kolk, B. (2006). Clinical implications of neuroscience research in PTSD. *Annals of the New York Academy of Sciences, 1071*, 277–293.

van der Kolk, B. A., McFarlane, A. C., & Weisaeth, L. (Eds.). (1996). *Traumatic stress: The effects of overwhelming experience on mind, body, and society*. New York: Guilford Press.

van IJzendoorn, M. H. (1995). Adult attachment representations, parental responsiveness, and infant attachment: A meta-analysis on the predictive validity of the Adult Attachment Interview. *Psychological Bulletin, 117*, 387–403.

van IJzendorn, M. H., Schuengel, C., & Bakermans-Kranenburg, M. J. (1999). Disorganized attachment in early childhood: Meta-analysis of precursors, concomitants, and sequelae. *Development and Psychopathology, 11*, 225–249.

Varela, F. J., Thompson, E., & Rosch, E. (1992). *The embodied mind: Cognitive science and human experience*. Cambridge, MA: MIT Press.

Wallin, D. (1997). Clinical controversies: The analyst's right to privacy. *Psychologist/Psychoanalyst, 17*(1), 9–10.

Walsh, R., & Shapiro, S. L. (2006). The meeting of meditative disciplines and western psychology: A mutually enriching dialogue. *American Psychologist, 61*(3), 227–239.

Weil, A. (2004). *Natural health, natural medicine: The complete guide to wellness and self-care for optimum health* (rev. ed.). Boston: Houghton Mifflin.

Weinfield, N. S., Sroufe, L. A., Egeland, B., & Carlson, E. A. (1999). The nature of individual differences in infant–caregiver attachment. In J. Cassidy & P. R. Shaver (Eds.), *Handbook of attachment: Theory, research, and clinical applications* (pp. 68–88). New York: Guilford Press.

Weiss, J., & Sampson, H. (1986). *The psychoanalytic process: Theory, clinical observation, and empirical research.* New York: Guilford Press.

Wheeler, M. A., Stuss, D. T., & Tulving, E. (1997). Toward a theory of episodic memory: The frontal lobes and autonoetic consciousness. *Psychological Bulletin, 121,* 331–354.

White, R. W. (1959). Motivation reconsidered: The concept of competence. *Psychological Review, 66*(5), 297–331.

Winer, R. (1994). *Close encounters: A relational view of the therapeutic process.* Northvale, NJ: Jason Aronson.

Winnicott, D. W. (1965). The theory of the parent–infant relationship. In D. W. Winnicott (Ed.), *The maturational processes and the facilitating environment* (pp. 37–55). London: Hogarth Press.

Winnicott, D. W. (1971a). Mirror role of mother and family in child development. In Winnicott, D. W., *Playing and reality* (pp. 111–118). London: Tavistock. (Original work published 1967)

Wrye, H. K., & Welles, J. K. (1994). *The narration of desire: Erotic transferences and countertransferences.* Hillsdale, NJ & London: Analytic Press.

Index